The Complete Herbal Handbook
for Farm and Stable

The Complete
Herbal Handbook
for Farm and Stable

Juliette de Baïracli Levy

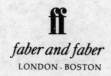

faber and faber
LONDON · BOSTON

First published in 1952
by Faber and Faber Limited
3 Queen Square London WC1N 3AU
Second edition 1963
Third edition 1973
Revised and first published as a Faber Paperback in 1984
Reprinted in 1988, 1990
Fourth edition 1991

Photoset by Parker Typesetting Service Leicester
Printed in Great Britain by
Clays Ltd, St Ives plc

A CIP record for this book is available from the British Library.

ISBN 0-571-16116-2

4 6 8 10 9 7 5 3

To PROFESSOR EDMOND BORDEAUX SZEKELY who shares my belief in the power of herbs and who has encouraged my work almost from its commencement and to THE PRINCE OF VENOSA, ITALY (Alberico Boncompagni Ludovisi) who took my veterinary herbal work, when it was yet young, to use on his famed dairy cattle (and pointer dogs) with much success, and who continues to praise herbs

IMPORTANT NOTE FOR READERS IN
GREAT BRITAIN

Since this book was written, the natural habitat of many wild plants has disappeared and some herbs have become rare in the wild because of building developments, intensive farming, and other pressures on land use.

In an effort to prevent these rare plants from extinction, the Wildlife and Countryside Act 1981 and its Variation of Schedule Order 1988 make it an offence for any unauthorized person to pick, uproot, destroy or offer for sale almost a hundred wild plants in Great Britain.

It is also an offence for an unauthorized person to *uproot any wild plant*, whether or not it is on the protected list.

The author strongly advises readers to grow their own herbs or obtain dried herbs from health food shops.

The Wildlife and Countryside Act 1981 and the Wildlife and Countryside Act (Variation of Schedule) Order 1988 can be obtained through HMSO bookshops. Alternatively, a list of the fully protected plant species can be obtained from the Department of the Environment, Tollgate House, Houlton Street, Bristol, BS2 9DJ.

Readers in countries other than Great Britain should check local regulations before gathering flowers in the wild.

Contents

Foreword

Such ailments as the now prevalent ones of scrapie in sheep and 'mad cow' in cattle are not going to find a place in this *Herbal Handbook for Farm and Stable*, despite the fact that many thousands of cattle in the UK have now been diagnosed as suffering from Bovine Spongiform Encephalopathy (BSE). My book teaches *natural* care of animals and totally shuns their exploitation (wherein they are treated as machines, instead of as living, sensitive and loving creatures).

This book wholly condemns the force-feeding of unnatural foods to any creatures. If a diet is unnatural, disease will keep company with those subjected to it: that is a fixed law. I state force-feeding because, when animals through hunger are driven to eat foods entirely unnatural to their species, such as giving meat offal to cows and sheep, that, to me, is force-feeding.

The Bible tells of God's instructions to Noah, that the preferred and natural foods of every creature were to be taken into the Ark for their nourishment. And to this day, animals fed on natural foods do not develop those horrible (almost satanic) ailments being reported in journals, on radio and television.

The usual, simple diseases, of the mucous membranes, digestive system and kidneys, are all easily curable by simple and safe herbal treatments, which never need cruel experiments on laboratory animals to prove their efficiency, experiments which are a detestation to me for I have the welfare of animals ever in my mind.

As I write this, when visiting England, television is showing *cats* suspected of having a similar disease to BSE in cattle. I do hope this fear proves to be unfounded. In any case, it is terrible that human acceptance and connivance in forcing the unnatural on our domestic animals bring much misery, pain and fear, all of which could be avoided.

Introduction

A book on herbal medicine for farm and stable could become a vast undertaking, the diseases of farm animals being manifold owing to man's mismanagement and ignorance of the simple and unchanging laws of nature; and, above all, his over-commercialization of the earth and the creatures that he has domesticated. Shelley rightly stated that man's dominance over the animals was one of disease and pain, for the animals. The ailments dealt with in this book are mostly unknown among the wild animal species from which the domestic breeds are derived; this providing a good example of the error of over-domestication of animals, with its consequent artificial rearing methods and medical treatments.

This herbal has been written for international use. But, as it is published in England, all British and other farmers who read this book, and who will find many references to their colleagues of other countries and also to gypsy herbalists, can be confident that particular care has been taken to give only common herbal remedies that can be found wild, or readily cultivated, or easily bought. Great care has also been taken to secure accurate naming and to use popular names of wide currency.

I am not going to compile a lengthy volume of herbal medicine, for I consider that such is unnecessary; I am content to confine my book to the common animal ailments. Professor Edmond Bordeaux Szekely, the great Hungarian doctor, has taught me that in human medicine it is erroneous to be concerned with, and to treat, merely local symptoms of disease; the whole body must be given a basic treatment. Local symptoms are but an indication of disorder of the whole body (apart from external injuries), for when one part of the body indicates sickness, then the entire organism is likewise sick. He teaches a basic treatment for all disease, which is the internal cleansing of the body by fasting and laxative treatment, and then the rebuilding of healthy blood and tissue by careful diet and natural foods. This theory is equally applicable to animals, and is indeed instinctive to them, for the wild animal with inherent intelligence fasts itself until restored to health, partaking only of water and the medicinal herbs which it seeks instinctively for cure of the malady from which it is suffering. In the wild, animal sickness is generally one of injury or wounding.

There must be reason for the present-day disuse of herbs and the popularity of chemical and vaccine therapy. Personally I think that apart from the prevalent lack of time, or laziness, which makes the modern farmer loath to busy himself with preparation of his own medicines, the cause is modern commercialism and the power of advertisement. The present-day farmer has been educated to consider disease as inevitable and the only scientific cure as being in the artificial remedies of the modern veterinary surgeon who, through over-rigid orthodox training and himself under the influence of advertisement, is too often a mere vendor of the products of the vast and powerful chemical and serum manufacturers. For the vested interests in modern medicine are stupendous. Businessmen who have never owned an animal fatten like breeding toads upon the ailments of farm stock which need not know sickness at all if they had daily access to the herbs of the fields. The true farmer should cultivate his own medicines in his own fields, and he should not consider himself as being a farmer if he has to resort to outside help for keeping his animals in health, and healing them when in sickness. Science is providing the ruination of true farming; the only thing that I, and countless others, have noted as flourishing alongside science, is disease! – disease of the earth, disease of crops and disease of the animal and people who feed on the diseased produce. I have made a study of the wild deer, and I have never yet met with one hind unable to rear her calf owing to mastitis of the udder, nor have I seen deer with skin disease or diseased feet. That is but one example of animal health, but everywhere in the woods one observes the wild animals rearing their young in health and freedom from sickness, whereas close by, the domestic animals frequently fail to breed at all, or lose their young at an early age through disease.

In his book, *Pleasant Valley*, the talented author Louis Bromfield well describes the true farmer: 'A good farmer in our times has to know more about things than a man in any other profession. He has to be a biologist, a veterinary, a mechanic, a botanist, a horticulturist and many other things. He has to have an open mind, eager and ready to absorb new knowledge, new ideas and new ideals.' Yet how many modern farmers are botanists? Few indeed.

The great doctor Paracelsus von Hohenheim forsook the medical universities of the world and lived with the gypsy and peasant herbalists in many parts of Europe in order to learn the *true* medicine. It is from such people that I have obtained much instruction in herbal medicine and the rearing of animals. From the gypsies and peasants of Mexico, France, Spain, Portugal, Greece, Israel, Turkey, Algeria, Tunisia, French and Spanish Morocco – and England. In all these countries I have sought gypsy and peasant herbal treatments. Grateful I am to my herbal teachers; they taught me far more than I ever learnt during nearly four years of scientific study at two universities. It was in thankfulness that I turned away from the places where vivisection is practised (the crying of animals in the vivisection laboratories!) and went instead, like Paracelsus, to the green fields and the woods for my medical education.

All the treatments prescribed in this book on herbal medicine are truly herbal, and all are harmless, for, as the result of careful observation, I have the strongest objection to the using of violent chemicals for the so-called cure or relief of any form of disease: chemicals, such as the sulphonamide group, which are habitually more dangerous to the delicate tissues of the animal body than are the diseases for which they are frequently prescribed as cure.

Professor Szekely had declared emphatically, that the curing of the ailments of his patients is often a simple task in comparison with the freeing of their bodies from the accumulations of chemical drugs lodged in their tissues – the drugs derived from orthodox medical chemo-therapy, and from the poisons sprayed upon fruits and vegetables by the modern farmer, or placed in tinned and bottled foods as preservatives. Many of his patients are Americans; and in present-day America the chemist seems to be running amok, spraying and poisoning everything edible.

In herbal medicine, too, we have violent-acting substances, usually derived from the poisonous groups of plants. I have excluded them altogether, influenced perhaps by the wild animals which instinctively avoid the poisonous herbs. Also nature has provided always a gentle herb to do the work in place of the ones of violent action. Furthermore, I wanted to be able to state with absolute certainty that this is a book of safe treatments; and having excluded the poisonous herbs, I can declare so in truth. There is not one treatment in this herbal which could cause any farmer to declare that through using the prescribed herbs he lost an animal. The herbs advised are all benevolent and beneficial.

Many of the herbal treatments are my own discoveries successfully used in my veterinary work in various countries; others are purely gypsy remedies taught me by my Romany friends; others are proved treatments taken from old botany books of many lands, of which I have made a study. They have been fully tested by myself or by other experienced herbalists, and only the fully proved treatments have been included. I found much interesting lore on animal husbandry in a very ancient book that I discovered in an Exmoor, Somerset, farmhouse, and subsequently put this into practice; the book is without mention of any author and is called merely *Rural Life*. It is still in use on that farm, in Porlock, which is known for its high standard of health and the fine animals reared there – especially Exmoor sheep.

The agricultural expert of whom I am such a sincere admirer, the late Sir Albert Howard, was greatly interested in the study of gypsy herbal medicine. He urged me to learn all that was possible in that unexplored field, feeling that such medicine could prove of great benefit to the farming world. He upheld his belief in herbs by advising farmers to write to me for help in curing their disease outbreaks. Invariably success was obtained, no matter how difficult the disease, because natural medicine is truthful and consistent. Nature changes not. Nature's remedies are not abandoned annually, and new ones lauded, as with chemicals; invariably they are perennial. One success which especially pleased Sir Albert Howard was my cure of over one thousand pedigree Swaledale sheep condemned as incurable by modern medicine, following the great snow of 1947. Later the Albert Howard journal *Soil and Health* published my paper, giving all details of the sheep treatment and farmers' testimony.

Sir Albert Howard, so far-sighted and knowledgeable above the agriculturists and scientists of his time, knew well that herbs grow upon the earth for good reason and are an important part of Nature's chart of wholeness. He believed, as I believe, that man's neglect of the medicinal plants is one of the basic causes of human and animal disease. After his death, his wife, Lady Louise Howard, wrote me: 'My husband told me that he thinks you have a unique knowledge on the raising and care of animals.'

To Sir Albert Howard and Professor Edmond Bordeaux Szekely, two great men who have encouraged me in my herbal medicinal work, I record my thanks, and to my many gypsy friends in far parts of the world, including the gypsy doctor, Paul Fenet of Provence.

Finally, is there any need for a herb book such as this? Is there not already a vast assemblage of learned books on animal husbandry? I believe that there is true need, for in spite of highly developed scientific medical treatments, a very large proportion of the domestic animals in the world today are wiped out by disease each year. Through ill-health, old-established and valuable strains are lost for ever, and likewise the peasant, because he has turned from the cures of his forefathers, loses his few animals which, often enough, are his main livelihood, and essential to the existence of his smallholding. I became well aware of this in Mexico when doing veterinary work with the peasants' cattle there. Those peasants could not afford to lose their sick beasts, which gave to them their daily food and the fertility of their fields. It was after my experience in Mexico that I resolved to write my herbal for cattle and horses, and began seriously to collect all possible herbal information. When I was staying at Ensenada, Mexico, the explorer, Gaston Fleury, introduced me to the great farmer, Thomas Robertson, a farming adviser to the President of Mexico. Thomas Robertson was immediately interested in my herbal work. While at Ensenada I was able to demonstrate to him the healing of the gangrenous wing of a wild pigeon which hunters had shot and left dying in the woods. I was told that the bird was beyond cure: but herbal medicine, as is general, enabled me to restore the bird to good health.

Thomas Robertson is author of a book on the subject of a pioneer agricultural colony in Western Mexico: *A South-Western Utopia*. He himself was reared in the colony and grew up with the Mexicans, and at an early age learnt of the famed and ancient herbal lore of Mexico. Only because my work was herbal did he speak so surely of its success and acceptance in Mexico. For the peasants there continued to show much suspicion and dislike towards orthodox chemical medicine. The peasants are intelligent because they want to know the exact nature of the substances that are being put into their animals. They accepted eagerly all the medicines that I prescribed because they were herbal. And we had no failures. This brings me to quote from a statement written by another well-known farmer who is opposed to unnatural medicine, G. P. Golden, of Leicestershire, famed for his pedigree Shorthorn cattle and Kerry Hill sheep: 'The prevalence of mastitis, or inflammation of the udder, and so many other diseases, is evidence of the low disease-resistant powers of cows today. The use of vaccines – by which the blood of cattle is interfered with from birth – for a progressively increasing number of diseases, is gradually undermining the health of stock. In the mistaken idea of stopping one disease the way is being paved for the inroads of other troubles. The general health of cattle today is unquestionably lower than twenty-five years ago. . . . There is not a shadow of doubt that the continual injection into the animals of all manner of poisonous materials for T.B. testing, abortion, mastitis, blackleg, etc., is gradually undermining the powers of disease resistance.' (The history of T.B. testing material is not impressive, and is of a kind typical of so many lauded benefits of the scientist, rooted in the amoral practice of vivisection. This precious T.B. testing substance has once been proffered to the public as a cure for tuberculosis, discredited, and then brought forth newly as a reliable test for cattle. I have known many false results given by this testing material. —J. de B.L.) 'Unnatural methods of feeding and rearing and the maintenance of stock under intensive conditions, combined with three or four times milking, have added their share to unwise veterinary practice. These false ideas have grown and are being maintained by propaganda put forth by vested and business interests and by the hosts of officials whose interests are bound up with it. Proofs for their claims are not in evidence. On the contrary, all the main facts which condemn this false system are excluded from the public.' True words indeed.

I feel that the most helpful contribution that this book can make to animal husbandry is in the fact that it dismisses the Pasteur-inspired beliefs that disease is inevitable, and gives assurance that the healthy, that is, the naturally reared animals, will not take any form of disease at all. This fact, I, and many other followers of natural rearing, including Sir Albert Howard and Lady Eve Balfour, have well demonstrated. One of the most effective examples of disease resistance by healthy stock was provided by Sir Albert Howard's cattle in India. They 'rubbed noses' with neighbouring stock suffering from foot-and-mouth disease and never took the malady at all. The book also does offer simple and effective herbal treatments when disease does occur, together with the promise that the treatment will produce a lasting cure not merely suppressing symptoms as in the case of orthodox chemical therapy.

My attitude to herbal medicine is almost worshipful, I have witnessed such remarkable cures resulting from the careful application of herbs. I have written this book to share my knowledge with others and above all to conserve the medical teachings of the gypsies and the invaluable work of the old-time herbalists. The passing of the 1949 Veterinary Act might well have ensured the end of all herbal medicine in England, both gypsy and peasant. It was necessary to write this book in order to help keep alive the ancient and valuable art of the herbalist in veterinary medicine.

But as time went by the Veterinary Act began to lose some of its threat. Qualified vets came forward and taught herbal and homeopathic treatments as a replacement for the traditional modern drugs therapy. Then the BBC, in its 'Science in Action' programmes, gave many talks in favour of herbs and other types of healing as opposed to the orthodox, now all classed together as 'alternative medicine', which would number millions among its followers if a census were to be taken. Personally, I meet them everywhere; they used to come to visit me when that was possible. Nowadays I have no address at which it would be convenient to welcome visitors.

I believe that this is the first veterinary herbal for farm animals and horses to appear in the English language, as the art of the ancient farrier and of the gypsy has been preserved by the spoken word only. And the old farming books have not been purely herbal, but have included chemical medicine with the plant treatments. I have not included the farm cat in my book, as its care and the treatment of its ailments are very similar to the dog, except that the cat, having a yet smaller stomach capacity than the small one of the dog, needs more frequent and lighter meals; three meals a day are advised.

I have given much thought to the inclusion of pigs in this book, but I have decided against it. Quite apart from religious beliefs inherent through my Turkish ancestry, where the pig is strictly prohibited as food for man, being considered as unclean and a potent source of disease to the human race, I know very surely that the animal will not easily respond to disease treatment by herbal methods. It is ill advised to proffer natural remedies for animals being reared habitually on an entirely unnatural diet, cooked foods being fatal to whole health, and breeding disease faster even than sour earth. The modern basic diet of the pig is boiled household swill from the refuse bins. It is prevented from feeding naturally by confinement and by the ringing of the nose. The animal is made by man internally filthy, and no herbal treatments are going to expel worms readily from intestines which are clogged with the mucus deposits resulting from unnatural diet, nor will herbs easily penetrate tissues clogged with fat and toxins from the same causes.

I have had no failures with herbs; be the patient a pigeon with a gangrenous wing or a Turkish camel suffering from scour. I have prescribed all treatments with confidence. However, if pig farmers, having witnessed the successful results of herbs upon other animals, are made desirous of applying such medicine to pigs, I can but advise them to follow fairly closely the prescriptions given for goats: they will be correct enough for pig dosage. And when pigs are allowed to live a natural life, free range exercise and rooting for their food, there is then no reason why herbal medicine should not keep them in excellent health or restore them when sick. The wild boars that I met with on the hills and in the lonely valleys of many parts of Galilee, Israel, are all memorable for their rugged strength and proud bearing.

Finally, I should like to state my thanks to E. P. Lewin for encouragement and help with this book, also to Lawrence D. Hills, who read my book in manuscript and gave much beneficial and constructive advice for its improvement. And thanks also to two deeply mourned friends, the late Ella Hatt who shaped this first of my Faber books, and the many other books which followed after, and to Kathleen F. Barker for valuable suggestions for improving the horse section. Also my thanks to Barbara Ellis, whose work on the revisions for this new edition deserves the highest praise.

1

Gathering and Preparing
Medicinal Herbs

The best method of giving herbs to the farm animals is by planting them in the pasture lands and alongside the hedgerows where the animals graze. Farmers who wish to have their farms entirely free from animal disease should plant medicinal herbs as surely as they plant corn, kale, cabbage and other foods.

Many of the big seed firms are now supplying herbal leys to meet popular demand; and it is hoped that in time the common ley of grasses devoid of all herbs will no longer be tolerated by farmers desirous of keeping healthy farm stock. Hunters of Chester are one pioneer firm in this respect. They are followers of Robert Elliott's 'Clifton Park' system of grass growing.

Then that excellent farming and gardening association, The Soil Association, of 86 Colston Street, Bristol BS1 5BB gives information on suppliers of herbal ley seeds, to members.

L. D. Hills, author of many books on organic gardening and farming states

> Apart from mixing deep-rooting herbs into temporary and permanent ley mixtures, direct sowing in the hedgerows to establish medicinal plants that are not available in the district, is both cheap and easy. Scattering with a fiddle drill, or by hand of the following herbs, seeds of which can be bought by the ounce or pound, at the rate of 2 to 3 ozs. per

chain (66 ft.) in March is well repaid. A 'hedge ley' is little trouble to establish; choose a sunny bank, or ditch side; no soil preparation is needed, and once established the herbs will seed themselves – those which do not do this easily are cheap to replace. This is recommended especially to farmers who consider herbal veterinary treatment out of date and worthless: their own beasts will convince them that there is a great deal in natural medicine.

Herbs for a hedge ley are recommended if these are not already found on the farm. A good supplier of these is Hunters of Chester Ltd, The Old Estate Office, Oulton Park, Tarporley, Cheshire CW6 9BL. They will send a list on receipt of a stamped addressed envelope. Many seeds can also be raised in the open in the farm garden, and spring sowing is advisable. Most good seedsmen also sell these medicinal herbs in small packets at reasonable prices.

Seedsmen Thompson & Morgan of Ipswich stock aniseed, balm, borage, dill, fennel (British perennial, not the Italian annual), horehound, hyssop, marjoram, tansy, vervain and wormwood, apart from ones you can buy from herb gardens. Plants of big-leaved Russian comfrey, also an excellent herb, are readily obtainable. Chicory and garlic seed are easy to get, and even fenugreek, which is not a native of Britain. The English garlic, 'ramsons', will readily root itself in shady places if transplanted from the woods where it grows wild throughout Europe. Other species of garlic are distributed world-wide and I have found it and used it in my herbal work in many parts of the world with the exception of desert places.

A gypsy horse-trader, Jack Vincent, said wisely, when discussing horse medicine with me, that he never had to 'medicine' his animals, because they took their own cures from the hedgerows where he grazed them daily, in different parts of the countryside. And his son, Jim Vincent, also highly know-ledgeable concerning horses, spoke to me in scorn of the general pastureland grazed by the present-day dairy herds, when we were walking over some typical closely grazed fields, almost without any herbs in their entire acreage, planted apparently with only one type of quick-growing grass. He said simply that he would never be able to induce any horse of his to stay in such places; that his horses were used to the good foods of nature and would leap out of any fields where they could not get hedgerow herbs and an abun-dance of 'weeds' and also hedge croppings. He and his father and brothers are all able to work their horses heavily on little more than such grazing; an impossible thing to achieve for the average horse kept on the modern herb-deficient grassland.

There is much truth in Edgar Saxon's description of the true herbalists, printed in *Health and Life* journal. 'Those who have an inborn intuitive insight into wild plants and their properties, an insight impossible to produce by academical training.'

The college room is the wrong place to study herbal medi-cine, the fields and the woods are the true universities, for there the wild animals can be observed and likewise can be discovered the wild herbs that they seek and consume. The gypsy people are part of the fields and woods. The gypsies always declare concerning their own horses (not those which pass through their hands for sale) that they get their own food and medicinal herbs from the wayside places and the hedgerows where they tether them, and they are able to work their animals heavily, hauling long distances the loaded, weighty, family caravans, on little more than wild field pro-duce. They especially value the hedgerows; and yet, more and more farmers in England and elsewhere, for reasons of commercial economy, are destroying these important growths, wherein are massed the vital herbs, all rich sources of natural vitamins, minerals and roughage, uprooting them for more yards of acreage for grain sowing, more ease for the big machines with which during the present day they cultivate (and bruise and trample) the earth over which they have dominance. Machines are one of the chief deprivers of the earth of the animal manure which is so essential to the keeping of the fields in good heart. Horse manure supplies additional soil fertility elements which cows cannot supply; although it must be admitted that the grazing of horses depletes the land more than cows or sheep. A most successful organic farmer whom I know, never trims his hedges other than the little required to keep them stock-proof, he encourages rampant growth, and allows kine and horses to do all the required trimming. He knows also that his hedgerows provide shelter for the birds which feed upon the insect pests, and which are essential to keep the natural balance of insect life in his fields, for it is only when the balance is disturbed that the insects deserve the name of pests. Furthermore, the hedgerows retain essential moisture in the fields, and the rotting leaves and the annual herbs which grow in their shelter make important compost material and aid the propagation of earthworms.

For me, the art of herbal medicine is always pleasurable; it is a happy thing to be able to go out into the fields and gather the herbs required for restoring to health the various animals that I am asked to treat. It gives one a sense of achievement to be able to take the herb-collecting basket, and from the fields obtain the exact herbs required, knowing where to find them, and further, when the required plants are in season, which plants of the many known to herbalists for specific cures are the best for the individual case under treatment. The gypsies are instinctive herbalists; the layman can acquire some of their skill by mingling with them and also with peasants and

4

foresters who possess herbal knowledge, and by walking the fields and woods and studying wild plants and their medicinal properties. Not only is such study fascinating, but it is of great importance to any serious follower of natural farming. It does seem to me most extraordinary and very foolish, that stock-keepers should go to such trouble to grow fodder for their animals and yet neglect entirely to grow crops for treatment of their common ailments. I am convinced that the time will come when all farmers will cultivate medicinal herbs for their animals just as surely as today they cultivate their crops.

Once a farmer has known the satisfaction of restoring to whole health his own sick animals, then he can go farther afield and cure the animals of his fellow farmers, and thus spread the teachings of natural medicine. For nothing is more impressive than example, and the very effective disease cures achieved by herbal medicine are most excellent proof of the power of nature. I suggest that those would-be students of herbal medicine who are without any knowledge of wild plants, and it is sadly true of the majority of farmers today, obtain a good illustrated handbook on the subject – the classic Bentham and Hooker is especially recommended – or borrow such a book from one of the postal libraries specialising in agricultural subjects. Because of the importance of farmers' being able to recognize the commonly used herbs of food and medicine. I arranged for almost a hundred illustrations to be added to my *Herbal Handbook*, which is primarily for humans but also useful for animals. I should also mention the several journals such as the 'Landsmen Library'. The Soil Association, founded by the organic farming pioneer, Lady Eve Balfour, issues an excellent and informative journal called *Mother Earth*, to members of the Association. It has its headquarters at 86 Colston Street, Bristol BS1 5BB, and is an international association with world membership and very long experience of organic farming and animal husbandry; indeed serious 'nature' farmers should not fail to associate with them. Also Lady Louise Howard publishes an informative bulletin on natural farming to followers of the great agricultural work of Sir Albert Howard.

My publishers, Faber and Faber, have for many years been issuing a long and successful list of books on natural farming and gardening methods. For the interest in natural farming grows daily. Farmers are coming to accept less calmly the disease which is a general companion of inorganic farming and unnatural animal husbandry.

In Europe, medicinal herbs grow wild in abundance, and in England especially, where I commenced my herbal education, herbs are of a quality often unsurpassed in other countries and can provide an important export trade when the world returns to herbal medicine once more. Cultivation and drying of the herbs could well become a foremost trade.

Every farmer and farmer's wife, and the children also, should be educated in the collection, storage and preparation of herbs. **A warning must here be given: as we live now in a chemical dominated, poisoned world, care must be taken when gathering herbs to ensure they have not been poison-sprayed.** Spraying by aircraft is specially dangerous, being very far-carrying, contaminating far more than the area they have contracted to spray. There should be heavy fines enforced for such careless contamination.

Collection of Herbs

The best way of utilizing herbs for the making of medicines is their collection in fresh undried form direct from the countryside or the herb garden. It is for this reason that leaves and plant stalks figure so largely in herbal medicine. But in some herbs the highest healing properties are contained in flower or seed, and collection (and subsequent storage) of such plant parts then becomes necessary during the usually brief flowering or seeding period, followed by careful preservation. Roots, except those of a bulbous nature, can usually be freshly gathered. However, as the majority of herbs are not evergreen, some foliage collection and preservation, even if only in limited quantity, is necessary to ensure that the herbalist is never without his supply of herbs during the late autumn and the winter months.

For herbal collection the following rules should be followed. A general law is that all plant parts should be gathered during those months when the species is at its fullest state of growth – usually during the spring and summer months. Early morning after the dispersal of morning dew, is the best period of the day. Herbs, if gathered when wetted by dew or rain, will turn mouldy.

The following rules are applicable to the different parts of the plants used:

Roots The best period to gather roots for preservation is before the sap rises in the spring, although they may also be collected after the shedding of the leaves in the autumn.

Leaves Leaves should be collected in the early opening stages of their unfolding. Leaf buds in the early opening stages possess concentrated powers. Yellowed (faded) leaves lack medicinal properties and should not be used. Snip off all stems and discard.

Flowers Flowers should be gathered in their early unfolding, before being much visited by bees and other insects. Flower buds are also invaluable for fresh use: they are difficult to dry. Faded flowers – as with faded leaves – should not be used. Snip off any thick stalks; they are not needed and prolong the drying time.

Seeds Seeds should be left to sun-ripen on the plant, and

then be collected before wind-dispersal, which does not usually occur before the fading of the plant leaves, yellowing leaves being a common indication of ripened seeds.

Barks As with roots, should be gathered in the early spring or autumn. Less damage to the tree then results, and also the medicinal properties of barks are at their highest.

Preservation of Herbs

The preserving of herbs for successful storage is dependent upon the following general rules. All parts of the plant should be gathered only when in good health – all mildewed, blighted or faded parts must be discarded. The plant parts should be entirely dry when collected, i.e. free from dew, rain or frost moisture.

Leaves and Flowers These should be hung in bunches in a cool, dry place where there is an ample current of air, or spread on tables or shelves and turned frequently. Drying between sheets of newspaper (not pressing) is also a useful method; or spreading on closely laid canes or wire netting placed on dry ground and covered with large squares of muslin held in place with stones; or in large shallow baskets. Place sheets of brown paper in the baskets before putting in the herbs, so that small insects can be seen more easily and removed. The leaves and flowers should be protected from bright sunlight during drying, to prevent fading and loss of medicinal properties. When the herbs are fully dried they can be stored in cotton bags or strong paper bags, or broken into small pieces and stored in jars or tins. The tall jars of dark glass and fitted with glass stoppers, as seen in old-fashioned pharmacy shops, are the best containers for herbs, which should then be finely broken to conserve space but not packed too tightly. Personally, as I am a traveller and cannot carry jars around, I always use cotton sugar bags, the necks tied tightly to prevent entry of insects.

A Note on Drying   This is important. Heat from a fire should be used with caution for quick drying destroys the medicinal powers of the herbs as surely as the drying of cereals artificially in a modern drying plant kills the true vitality of the grain. The natural drying of cereals or herbs should be a slow, mellowing process. It takes months for the moisture to evaporate naturally from corn in the stack, and weeks to evaporate from herbs in the drying shed. In a prolonged rainy season, when natural drying becomes impossible, then a gently heated oven can be used, the door always to be kept slightly ajar. As already stated, bright sunlight should be avoided in drying. Only in cold climates the weak sunlight of early morning and late noon can be used.

Seeds or Fruits   Treat as with leaves and flowers. Spread to dry on shelves or between newspaper in a cool airy drying place. A longer period is required than with leaves and flowers. Weather and other natural factors permitting, seeds and fruits of course can be sun-dried and similarly stored, directly off the plant or tree. Larger fruits can be smoke-cured or freshly sliced and dried off slowly in a gentle oven.

Roots and Barks   These require long and careful drying after removal of all dirt and other accumulations. They can be stored in boxes of wood or in cotton bags or in sacks.

(Guard against spoliation by vermin, who love to seek out and eat healthful medicinal herbs. Rodents, moths, beetles, mites and many other insects are spoilers of stored herbs. Mice, small moths and weevils are especially tiresome.)

9

Preparation of Herbs

Herbs when carefully dried will retain their medicinal properties for two years. They should then be discarded and sprinkled around favourite plants to make a healthy mulch. The preparation of herbal medicines from plants – leaves, flowers and seeds – is a simple process. In the case of leaves and flowers, these should be shredded finely with scissors before use. The shredded herbs should then be placed in an enamel pan, with the required amount of cold water, and heated over a slow fire until near boiling-point is reached. Do not near boil for more than one or two minutes, which is sufficient to break the cellulose of the plant cells. Cover tightly to prevent the vital oils present in most herbs from being lost in the escaping steam. Then remove from the heat and allow to steep (brew) in the water for at least three hours. Six hours is the best time period and can be achieved by overnight steeping.

I repeat that, throughout the time of preparation, while being heated over the flame and while brewing, the herbal liquid must be kept covered completely, so that no steam is allowed to escape; so many of the medicinal herbs have volatile aromatic properties which are lost in any escaping vapours. The prepared brew should then be stored in a jar covered with a paper lid: to cover with a fully airtight lid will often cause speedy fermentation which is not desirable. The herbal medicine is then ready for use as required. This is called the *standard brew*. For more exact quantities of individual herbs the second chapter (Materia Medica Botanica) should be studied.

It is necessary to say that on account of the vital properties of herb brews, the keeping properties do not extend usually beyond two to three days – less in hot weather. Fresh daily brews are preferable. In hot climates unless under refrigeration, twelve hours may be the maximum keeping period.

Bubbles seen in the brew or a 'winey' taste indicate fermentation. For external use fermentation does not matter: for internal use fermentation is harmful.

Seeds   Seeds require soaking for twenty-four hours or more, until the seed cover cracks preparatory to germination. They should then be brewed in the same way as leaves and flowers.

Roots   Careful washing to remove all soil and other foreign matter is the primary preparation. They should then be sliced finely and simmered at nearly boiling-point for one or more hours, keeping them covered. Then remove from the flame, brew for any period from three to six hours, and put in jars. The shredded roots can be left in the brewed liquid with advantage, for they will be found to sink to the base of the jar, and will not aggravate fermentation. Root medicines will generally remain fresh for longer periods than leaves or flowers; four days is the maximum. But fresh brews are always best.

Barks   Prepare as for herbs; grating finely with a vegetable grater before use.

Tinctures of Herbs

Tinctures are made by taking approximately two ounces of the powdered herb, placing in a large jar or pot, and adding one quart of alcohol; cheap surgical spirit or vinegar can be used, both possessing preservative properties. This should be allowed to stand for two weeks: the tincture is then ready. Tinctures should be stored in a dark place. The jars used must have tight-fitting lids, such as are used for fruit bottling. This is especially important if surgical spirit is used owing to its very high evaporative properties.

Essences of Herbs

Essences are made by dissolving one to two ounces of the essential oil extracted from the herb in one quart of alcohol; surgical spirit or vinegar can be used. Store in a dark place.

Both tinctures and essences are for external use, and the general dosage directions which follow do not apply.

Long-keeping Bottled Herbal Medicines

I believe in the use of all herbal medicines raw or freshly brewed. But for those who wish to preserve herbs the following is a 300-year-old recipe printed in the journal *Health from Herbs*.

Prepare your infusion and decoctions, etc. in the usual way. Before they are cold strain them through muslin; it is advisable to strain through a coarser metal sieve first.

The vessel to hold the preparation should have as small a neck as possible. It should not be more than an inch or one and a quarter inches across.

Pour in the liquid until it runs just over the top, to get rid of the froth. When the liquid is free from bubbles, pour off some which will leave the liquid about half an inch down the bottle neck.

Now melt some lard or white wax and gently pour on top of the contents. This will float at the top and effectively seal off the contents from the air. Now get a piece of parchment – mutton or beef skin will do even better – pull it over the top and tie down with string. Never use a cork for this purpose.

When the lard or wax is set, move to a dark, cold cupboard or cellar. It should keep indefinitely.

In Spain peasants preserve bottled, cooked, herbs, vegetables or roots, by pouring an inch-depth layer of olive oil on to the top layer of the jar contents when cooked and cooled. The oil floats on top and seals off all air.

General Dosage for all Herbs One heaped handful of herb, leaf, flower, seed, root or bark, brewed in one pint of water (preferably spring or well water). *Note.* A man's hand is the general measure. General dosage for the animals is: sheep and goats one pint of brew daily, given in cupful doses morning and night; cattle and horses a quart of herbal brew given daily, in pint doses morning and night. Many animals will drink the herbs freely, as a sort of herb tea, especially when sweetened with honey or molasses, *or most of the herbs can be fed fresh gathered and raw*, in handfuls, or finely cut and mixed with a mash of bran and molasses, for all animals. (See Chapter 2). All drenches should be given by means of the special drenching horns designed by the firms of instrument makers for the different animal species. Exact dosage is never very necessary in herbal medicine, and can be altered to suit the individual case. For instance when the animals crop their own medicinal herbs from the hedgerows or fields they cannot follow exact measurements. Also the quantity of medicine will naturally vary with the breed of animal and even with the degree of severity of the ailment being treated. More frequent dosage is required in special cases, for example, vomiting, dysentery, hysteria, pain relief, etc. When making brews for cattle and horses large gallon quantities can be prepared. But remember that herbal brews ferment rapidly and will not keep longer than two to three days, less in hot weather.

When honey is stated as an addition to the herbal brews it must be *pure* honey. And all molasses advised in the book should be cane molasses. Pure honey from the local bee-keeper is best. Common, cheap honey is frequently both pasteurized and adulterated with glucose – obtained by pouring sulphuric acid on starch. It thus becomes harmful instead of beneficial.

For external use there is the same twice daily usage of the herbs. Period of dosage is dependent upon the individual case. Nature is not generally quick-acting in her ways; herbal medicine never produces sudden suppression of mere symptoms as with chemical drugs, which generally passes for a 'cure'. Nevertheless, herbs can often cure – not suppress – in weeks, ailments which chemical treatments have been unable to remedy in months or years: again, all is dependent upon the individual case. But as a general guide it should be stated that the animal is usually required to take the prescribed herbs for several weeks, and for longer periods in deep-seated ailments. The same with external applications.

Pills Pills can be made on the farm. The required herbs need to be very finely cut, or the dried ones to be powdered. The herbs are then rolled into small balls of the required quantity, using as a binding agent a mixture of thick honey and wheaten flower or, instead of the flour, powdered slippery (red) elm bark. Slippery elm bark holds the herbs more firmly than does the wheat flour. It is present in quantity in the N.R. gruel, which I use when making my own pills. I stress, honey must be in thick form.

An important remark on the giving of pills to all animals: it is better to insert as many fingers as possible into the mouth, in a wedge, because fingers together are less likely to get nipped than a mere one or two within the mouth.

Injections Nil. I never give medicines (or nourishment) by injections. In my more than forty years of veterinary work, I have never owned a syringe. The body, human and animal, is wonderfully made and it is a deep and grave shock to the entire body for any substance to be injected suddenly into the bloodstream or limb tissues. The mouth, with its wonderful

14

selective powers to accept or reject all put into it, is the right channel for medicines, and the throat and stomach also co-operate, delicately, skilfully and protectively.

Poultices   The art of poultice-making is becoming lost to the present-day generations, and yet it is one of the most important methods of applying herbs to the body. The following is a basic recipe for all poultices in the method of preparation. It describes the making of a really good poultice. *Note.* When swabs or bandaging are mentioned, only cotton or linen should be used. No synthetic fabrics or wool.

Linseed Poultice   Take a bowl, warm it by gently rinsing with water just off the boil, then pour into it half a pint of boiling water. Using one hand, sprinkle slowly into the water a quarter of a pound of linseed. With the other hand, using a strong spoon, stir in the meal until a smooth dough is made, stirring quickly and strongly to prevent lumpiness. When the dough is fully mixed stir into it half an ounce of olive oil.

The meal should then be spread speedily on to a square of warm linen, the ends folded over, and the poultice applied to the area requiring treatment. Or the meal can be spooned into tightly sewn linen bags.

Never apply a poultice overhot, so as to scald the skin.

Herbal Poultice Bandages   These can be made by sprinkling powdered slippery elm bark (obtainable from herbalists) into a small bowlful of boiling herbal brew until a thin paste is formed. The brew is made from the chosen herb for the ailment being treated. The finely cut herb used to make the brew should be left in the water and included in the paste. This is then spread, warm, on a linen or cotton bandage and applied over the wound or area to be treated. Or N.R. gruel, which contains slippery elm and other healing herbs can be used for this. Or a green pulp can be made of the chosen herbs, finely cut, and the slippery elm or N.R. gruel, well worked in to form a firm paste. Also there is the gypsy method of placing fresh gathered leaves over wounds and binding in place with cotton bandages or lengths of old sheeting. Use big leaves of mallow, vine, cabbage, geranium, nasturtium, castor oil, shrubs, etc. Wash the leaves in cold water. Then place over them a long piece of cotton wool well soaked in cold water. Bind firmly in place with cotton cloths. Replace the leaves with fresh ones, at least four times daily. Leave unbandaged overnight. It is remarkable how the leaves heat up, drawing the fever from wounds, and also discolour from the impurities being drawn out from the wounds. This is *my favoured method of treating all types of wounds*, sores and gatherings. A main merit is that removal of the leafy dressings is painless and they do not tear off scabs, as is general with orthodox bandaging and plastering, which can set back the healing process with each dressing. This method is also recommended for all human wounds: compresses of fresh, medicinal leaves, placed directly on them.

Herbal Juices   Herbal juices are very beneficial in sickness and during convalescence, especially chlorophyll-rich nettle, alfalfa, and spinach juices, also the restorative juices of roots, such as beet and carrot, and of fruits, such as apple and grape. Freshly pressed juice from unsprayed grapes is a true life-restorer for all sick animals unable to accept any food, the grape juice being spoon or (plastics) cup fed, as a medicine, three times daily. The plastics cup, although rightly condemned for storage of juices, being an unhealthy material, is pliant, and thus can be pressed into convenient shape when giving medicines from it.

Fresh, raw juices from leaves, roots, fruits and berries can be made by convenient use of a juicing or blending machine, electric or hand pressing. More primitively, juices can be made by grating the herbs finely and then pressing them through a fine-mesh sieve, using the base of a heavy bottle for pressing, or squeezing them through butter muslin or cheesecloth. The residue from all these processes can of course be fed to some well animal as it contains valuable fibre and natural roughage and minerals.

Prepared Herbal Products

Prepared herbal products of good quality are becoming increasingly difficult to obtain. The problem is that destructive modernity has moved into herbs now that there is a worldwide demand for them, and it is likely to remain.

Formerly, herbal supplies were in the hands of true, caring herbalists, devoted gatherers who carefully air-dried the herbs in their own skilled way.

Presently, because herbs are now big-sellers, they are cultivated by the acre by quick-growing methods and are dried by electricity, instead of the former, gentle way.

This quick drying by artificial heat turns the herbs an unnatural bright colour and renders them very brittle. The delicate essential oils, which are the main medicinal part of herbs, are damaged and often totally lost.

Note: To prevent evaporation loss, herbal pills need to be given a sugar coating to seal in their contents (I am not an anti-sugar fanatic: a limited amount of sugar is harmless, and I prefer use of sugar to loss of essential oils of prepared herbs.) Herbal pills made at home for immediate use do not need coating.

Frequently I have purchased herbs by post and, on opening the packets, have thrown the herb out into my garden because for medicinal purposes they were useless, without proper colour and scent. Among such throwouts was an expensive purchase of French lavender. France was once famed for its lavender: the growers will have to return to natural drying if they want to keep their good name.

Therefore, one must be very careful as to what quality of herbs are going into commercial products. This also concerns my own formulae because in the past some former suppliers have broken faith and used sub-standard herbs and added chemicals to my recommended recipes.

When there is difficulty in obtaining high-grade herbal products by post, learn to make home remedies. One does not want one's animals to be deprived of important herbal helps because some people are exploiting them for commercial gain. One gives time to preparing daily food for one's family so some time can be given to preparing food for the animals. It does not take long to mix up some dried, powdered herbs and bind them into pills with flour and thick honey.

My basic advice for home-made remedies is not to use the very potent herbs, even though I recommend them in my books: they are for the experienced.

Substitute milder herbs instead.

Rue and wormwood are both very potent herbs – leave them out (though I love them both). Rue can be replaced by vervain or marjoram, and wormwood by the milder southernwood (of the same family). For *external* use, rue and wormwood are both appropriate, no precise prescribing being needed.

A home mixture for deterring skin pests can easily be made, and in lotion or soaked in hot oil, to treat sores and wounds; any of the wounds and skin treatment herbs mentioned in this book, all in equal amounts. Such herbs would include southernwood or wormwood, sage, rosemary, vervain, marjoram, nasturtium (especially the seeds), all types of mints; if being used in dry powder form, for bulk add powdered barks of eucalyptus and any type of pine-tree.

FURTHER NOTES (NON-HERBAL)

Honey (See also Chapter 9)

Honey is a great basic medicine as well as food, for all living creatures from man to every species of bird. The Arabian horsemen feed honey to their fabulous horses to give strength and stamina – and fertility. Hydromel, honey and water, and oxymel, vinegar and honey, were the basic medicines for most treatments of the great and immortal Greek doctor. Hippocrates, known as the 'Father of All Medicine'. Honey is a mildly laxative, body cleansing, soothing, restorative tonic. It is the first of the heart tonics (seconded by rosemary herb), and most animals eat it willingly. That vegetarian animal of great strength, the bear, is associated with honey. Honey is commonly adulterated for commercial reasons. Choose pure honey carefully. In the Canary Islands I found that the islanders generally kept a jar of honey handy for treatment of wounds, burns and scalds. A wise custom, for honey is antiseptic and soothing.

Honey Drinks

Two honey drinks, suitable for all animals and which most animals will take readily. Will give energy, soothe internal inflammations of throat and stomach, etc. Will reduce coughing. (Sage brew can be used instead of plain water.)

Barley-honey   Barley ½ lb., water one gallon. Boil slowly until reduced to ¾ gallon: when tepid add ½ lb. honey.

Blanche Water   Wet four handfuls of bran with hot water (boiling) and work it with the hands till it becomes clammy: then add one quart cold water. Strain, warm, and stir in ½ lb. honey.

Lemon Treatment

In order to prevent repetition in this book, it should be stated that whenever lemon juice is advised it is the pure juice from fresh lemons, not synthetic, tinned or bottled juice in any form.

Salt

All the herbivorous animals require a salt lick for health, unless they are living in a coastal area over which strong salt winds blow, depositing sea-brine on vegetation. Or give sea salt with bran. The requirement is a half teaspoon salt per average-size animal, or one teaspoon large-size animals (cow, etc.), several times weekly.

A Herbal Birthaid Brew

A life-saver in difficult births. It is bitter tasting, but always impresses me the desire that animals show to take it in quantity. The dosage given is for a medium-size dog. Increase the amount for larger animals.

A dessertspoon each of the following leaves, all finely cut: ivy (the inclusion of ivy is very important), southernwood (also important), sage, mint, raspberry, and six spice cloves. Mix well, then place in a pan with four cupfuls of cold water. Lid well. Heat slowly, remove from heat before boiling. Steep for several hours, unless it is urgent, when give without steeping. Strain, add a dessertspoon of honey. Give half a cup every hour.

Water

Do not use plastics or aluminium containers for drinking water troughs or for herbal brews. If stone troughs are not available, then use enamel or tin buckets. Put a large, heavy, smooth pebble or small rock into the bucket to prevent it from being knocked over readily. It will also help to keep the water cool. A sprig of rosemary placed under the pebble will also freshen the water. Water sealed in bottles – plastic containers are especially bad – soon becomes lifeless and loses much of its health properties: water needs air. When water is stored it should be sealed over with a piece of cloth, tied to keep it in position. Remember that pure water is the life force of every creature. Without good water there cannot be good health.

2

Materia Medica Botanica

I consider this chapter to be one of the most important in my veterinary herbal. It is a sorry thing that the majority of the world's farmers have so little knowledge of the medicinal herbs which grow upon their farmlands, and which are instinctively sought by the stock which graze those lands and which further are essential for the whole health of the animals and for the cure of all disease. Thus I have compiled a chapter giving brief descriptions of the chief medicinal and nutritive herbs, their medicinal properties and their preparation and dosage.

I think that this chapter alone justifies the writing of this herbal book; and I hope that many farmers will avail themselves of this knowledge now that after years of travel across the world it has been carefully collected and made available. This is the first chapter of its kind to be found in veterinary writings. I owe much of its contents to my gypsy herbalist friends and teachers. In order to keep this book of reasonable length and price, I have had to limit the number of herbs and medicinal trees, although many more herbs and trees have been added to this edition. However, in my *Illustrated Herbal Handbook for Everyone*, a very large section on herbs is available and all therein can be applied to animals. Like this farm and stable herbal, the *Illustrated Herbal Handbook* has also recently gone into another new edition and is now fully illustrated by a great botanical artist, Heather Wood. This book is likely to be available in most libraries for reference. It is published in America by Pantheon Books Inc. under the title of *Common Herbs for Natural Health*. It is now in an inexpensive paperback new edition.

Also I am always puzzled by the modern farmers' trusting attitude to orthodox veterinary medicine, a trust not shared by the true peasant. Farmers habitually permit the modern vet to inject into or feed to animals, substances about which they know nothing, and often enough of which the vet himself knows very little. The farmers' livestock is often the result of generations of careful planning and rearing, the worth of which cannot be estimated in mere money. Farmers should insist upon knowing the full nature of all drugs, vaccines and so forth, given to their animals; for it should be known that such potent and unusual substances often enough destroy permanently the former delicate natural balance of the animal organism. Professor Edmond Bordeaux Szekely rules that it is far more difficult to cure people of the after effects of unnatural medicines that they have taken, than to cure the disease for which the medicines were used. Recently I met on the Greek island of Crete, Roberto Alvarez, a young American medical student who came from a family of herbalists; he told me about an Afghan doctor working in a U.S. Military Hospital in West Germany. Whereas all the other doctors of the hospital were prescribing the latest drugs, the Afghan gave only simple drugless remedies, and explained his medical policy in words which I consider historic: the body and soul of both human and animal are made so completely and wonderfully that they are capable of providing their own medicines, and therefore it is an insult to the Creator to force on the body unnatural substances of any kind.

It is now necessary to add that scientists are beginning to interfere with the good reputation of many of the world's herbs. Using intensive dosage of herbs (probably badly grown or even chemically sprayed, for they believe in and advocate that unnatural type of plant culture!) on their test cases of laboratory animals (which animals are always unhealthy to begin with because no caged creature can ever be normal, mentally or physically) they are claiming that herbs cause internal tumours and other things. We herbalists, however, have tested herbs that are properly grown on animals and people leading normal lives, and proved herbal safety over the centuries. And there is God's emphatic promise in Genesis: 'Behold! I have given thee every herb bearing seed which is upon the face of all the earth' (Gen. 1:29).

Borage, comfrey, sassafrass, sage, among the greatest of all the herbs, have been condemned by scientists. The very name of sage, *Salvia*, comes from the Latin, to save, salvation, saviour. What more can one say!

Herbs can never destroy the normal balance of the body, for they are a natural part of animal bodies, and are a part of the blood, nerves and tissues of all herbivorous creatures. I have omitted the poisonous herbs from this book, although many of them possess excellent medicinal properties.

Furthermore, I have not included all of the herbal treatments learned on my travels, as I have utilized only those herbs which are general to the flora of the world, and not local to any particular country.

Most of the true peasant farmers of the world are herbalists. When treating animals in such countries as Mexico, Spain, Turkey and North Africa, I never met with any hostility from the farmers, although it was very unusual for a woman to be treating sick animals. I gained their co-operation because I was able to indicate to them the herbs growing in their own fields and prescribe their simple preparation and use. If I had been wishing to vaccinate their animals with unknown fluids, or proffering pills of unknown content, doubtless they would have declined my help. As it was, they co-operated willingly with me and together we achieved very excellent results. The only herbal pills that I gave to the farmers were purely made of several antiseptic herbs, or pills of grasses and meadow herbs. Before giving any such pills, I fully explained their contents and the herbal properties. I also swallowed many myself to prove their harmlessness, and the farmers tasted of them likewise! How few modern veterinary surgeons can explain fully the sera and drugs that they prescribe, and how few would themselves partake freely of such substances which too frequently are highly dangerous!

The Latin name of each herb has been given so that with the aid of a good illustrated botany book, readers can identify all herbs included in this chapter.

The dosage given is for sheep or goats. The dosage should be doubled or trebled for cows and horses, according to size.

The making of the standard brew, which is the basic method for all of the herbal brews, is fully described in Chapter 1. Honey or cane molasses can be added with advantage to all of the herbal brews without exception, as the natural sweetening agents energize the system and aid the work of the herbs. When the inclusion of honey or molasses is very necessary it has been given along with the individual herbs described in this chapter. Honey or molasses should be stirred into the brew when it is of tepid heat, not when hot. Heat spoils the sensitive powers, especially of honey.

Although the traditional herbal brews are often advised as drenches, etc., all parts – leaves, flowers, fruits, barks, roots – can be fed RAW, if the case will eat of such.

Finally, I should state that the herbs which I have given in the following five chapters of treatments for the various animal ailments, are not necessarily always the best or the only one. They happen to be my own selections mainly, and the ones which I have used most. All herbalists have their favoured herbs. I can declare that all the herbs described in this chapter have been fully tested by the world's herbalists: all are good, all are safe. If readers will make full use of them they can banish disease from farm and stable, though I must add, that a pre-condition for total health is also provision of sufficient daily exercise, because if animals do not move they surely rot. Exercise is as important as the daily intake of food.

Note   The herbs now described are arranged in alphabetical order of British popular names. There is not space to give local variations, but by looking up the Latin name in any botany book, further common names will be found. As Latin names are international, a book on wild flowers in *any* language will give local popular herbs wherever they may live. On pages 440 to 446 is a more compact list of herbs, giving both popular and botanical names, and useful for herb gatherers.

Further Note   When specific dosage is given, it is for an average-size animal, such as a goat. Decrease or increase dose for other animals depending upon their size. Dogs cannot take much vegetable matter and require far less (this is fully explained in my canine herbal, *The Complete Herbal Handbook for the Dog and Cat*, Faber and Faber Ltd., England, and Arco Publishing Inc., USA).

ADDER'S TONGUE (*Ophioglossum vulgatum*. Filices. Fern)   This is a fern-plant of fields and waste places. One broad leaf which grows with the stalk several inches from the ground. Distinguished by its dark, smooth, oval leaves, and flowering part resembling a small green tongue, being a thin, hard spike, and is the chief distinguishing feature of this plant, giving it its name. In France it is called la langue de serpent.

Use   A supreme wound herb. General preparation is infusing the leaf and spike in warm olive oil, brewing gently, not boiling. A fine balsam of a brilliant green colour is thus produced. French gypsies make adder's tongue ointment. Equal parts of olive oil, white wax (especially bees-wax) and fat (preferably nut fat as sold in vegetarian or health food shops. The herbivorous animals in general instinctively dislike the fat of other dead animals being used upon their bodies.) Melt over a slow fire until fully dissolved, making approximately one pint of melted fat, then put into it as much finely chopped adder's tongue as it will absorb, stirring well for about ten minutes. Run into jars and keep uncovered until well set. Apply to all wounds, sores, bruises, ulcers – the whole plant is used.

AGRIMONY (*Agrimonia eupatoria*. Roseaceae) This is a plant of hedgerow and field. Distinguished by its bramble-like thornless leaves. It bears spokes of small yellow flowers of rose form. The fresh flowers, have a scent of apricots. Sheep and goats will eat it, but horses and cows leave it alone. It is classed as a magic herb. The flower spines yield an attractive yellow dye.

Use Its chief property is a remedy for jaundice, from which it derives it botanical name – *Eupatoria*. It should be given to fasting animals as a drench, or finely cut and mixed with bran. It is also a valuable astringent to stem bleeding; and is a remedy for sore throats. Sprains are aided by a lotion made by boiling one handful of chopped agrimony in one quart of brew made from wheaten bran. Boil for thirty minutes then brew for two hours, finally stirring in two tablespoons of beer. Excellent for tired or strained limbs of horses, when well massaged into the flesh. The whole plant is used.

Dose Internal dose for jaundice: a half-handful of herb brewed in 1½ pints of water. After brewing for two hours, mix in half a pint of skimmed milk. Sweeten with molasses. Divide into two draughts and give morning and night, fasting.

ALDER (*Alnus glutinosa*. Betulaceae)   This is a tree of moist places and river banks. Distinguished by its short, stout form, shiny, oval leaves and green catkin flowers. The leaves and bark are cooling and astringent. The leaves pulped and bound over swellings reduce them and allay irritation.

Use   Treatment of blood ailments, rheumatic complaints, swellings. Lay the green leaves on swellings, bind in position. This treatment will also reduce breast swellings and inflammation.

Dose   One handful daily, fed in bran using leaves or bark.

ALFALFA (*Medicago sativa*. Leguminosae)   Known also as Lucerne. Found by waysides and in cultivation as a prolific and highly esteemed fodder crop, distinguished by its small grey-green foliage, and pale purple (sometimes whitish) pea-form flowers. Flowering time is early spring into late summer. In temperate climates will yield three or more harvests. Rich in nitrates and vitamins. Is a very tonic food and a kidney cleanser. Excellent for all animals and poultry. Increases speed of horses and greyhounds.

Use   Fodder, tonic, nervine.

Dose   Unlimited.

ALMOND (*Prunus dulcis*. Rosaceae)   A well-known tree wild and cultivated. Distinguished by its early blossoming, masses of pale pink rose-form flowers, and its green fruits wherein are the true almond nuts which are freed when the green pods split. The nut kernels and extracted oil are the parts used.

Use Nutrient, soothing, skin remedy, mild laxative for new-born animals; treatment of sores, lung ailments and cough.

Dose As a nutrient for young, sickly, animals, the kernels are finely grated and mixed into milk, one teaspoon of grated almond given twice daily. For very sick animals the almonds should be blanched, that is, their skins removed from the kernels by dipping in hot water. Or the extracted oil can be given, a quarter teaspoon in a tablespoon of tepid milk is a dose for a goat kid.

Externally. Apply a light smear of almond oil to wounds and sore places which refuse to heal on young animals and others. It is an excellent remedy for sore eyelids and for cracked noses and lips in canine distemper cases and for sore teats in milking animals. Almond oil is expensive, but is less costly than popular chemical salves etc.

ALOES (*Aloe communis*. Liliaceae) Not British. This is a plant of dry, sandy places and hillsides. Distinguished by its fleshy, cactus-like appearance. The leaves are very tall and spiney-toothed and the white or yellow flowers are borne in tall spikes. The aloes are native to warm climates. They are one of the most famed plants of Arabian medicine, used internally and externally. The juice is expressed (usually from the leaves) and sun-dried. It is the solid juice that is procurable from herbalists in Europe. From it exclusively is made the most famous of the old-time farrier's horse purge and conditioner – Aloes balls. Owing to its use in equine medicine the juice of aloes was once very popular in Europe. It is still obtainable from herbalists, and is used also in human medicine. The leaves and stems are used. It is claimed to be the only plant which survived from the Garden of Eden.

Use Treatment of constipation, indigestion, worms, urinary ailments, mastitis, and skin ailments. Externally: as a lotion for cure of corneal ulcers and keratitis. The pulp, applied as a salve for wounds, sores, bruises and tumours. In the Canary Islands it is effectively used as a mastitis treatment. The leaves are stripped of their outer skin and applied raw, as a pulp, massaging the udder with the pulp, cold, three times daily.

Dose Seven grains of powdered juice taken in one cupful of tepid milk-water, equal parts. Give fasting, morning and night. Aloes balls are made from six to eight drams of juice (1 dram of an ounce apothecaries' weight). The amount needed should be tested on individual animals for assessing good laxative effect.

ANEMONE (*Anemone nemorosa*. Ranunculaceae) A common woodland flower, known also as wind-flower. Distinguished by its two- or three-fringed leaves and a single, starry flower of white or rose from each rootstock. The French gypsies use the leafage to put 'the speed of the wind' into their horses.

Use Tonic. Head purge. Eye remedy. The whole plant is fed finely chopped to promote digestion. It is very potent, and therefore one plant daily, given in the cereals feed, is sufficient. As a head purge, the leaves, well bruised by pounding with a stone, are made into thin rolls, using a little fat, and pushed up the nostrils and kept there for several minutes, treating only one nostril at a time. This will aid cleansing of the sinus passages. The leaves can be made into an ointment (see adder's tongue) and if well rubbed into the eyelids, will strengthen the eyes and cure inflammations.

Dose One whole plant given each morning. Externally: as an ointment.

ANGELICA (*Angelica archangelica*. Umbelliferae) A beautiful and very powerful garden plant. Also found wild in woodlands. Distinguished by its large grey-green pleated leaves and umbels of creamy-gold flowers of intense and pungent sweetness. The scent of angelica flowers is unique and makes the plant very useful in farm gardens because, in addition to the medicinal properties of this plant, the flowers attract pollinating insects of all kinds, from bees to moths, and help produce heavy crops. Angelica certainly was a blessing for my bees and for my apple trees and bush fruits. The stems (which are peculiar, being hollow with prominent ridges) are a fertility aid, the seeds are a digestive tonic, and the roots (given raw, as shavings) remove stones and hard matter of the bladder and bowels.

Use A general tonic and fertility aid. Removal of internal obstructions. It is called the ginseng of Europe.

Dose A handful of stems, seeds and root shavings, daily, early morning.

ANISE (*Pimpinella anise*. Umbelliferae) This is a plant of hedgerows or moist places. Distinguished by its tall form, sometimes forming a small shrub. Feathery leaves, umbels of creamy flowers. The whole plant is strongly aromatic. The seeds and extracted oil are used. The seeds can be purchased from herbalists and grocers. Dogs like anise so much that it was once used as a bait by dog thieves.

Use As a carminative it is unsurpassed. An important remedy for all digestive ailments including colic. Especially good for young animals.

Dose Average dose is one heaped handful of seeds daily.

ARNICA (*Arnica montana*. Compositae) A plant of hillsides, stony plains and rocky places. Distinguished by its pale yellow, daisy-form flowers and pungent smell; its stem is slightly hairy. The whole plant is used but especially the flower heads. It is for external use only: this is important. It is one of the most famous remedies known to the herbalist for treatment of bruises, joint stiffness, wounds, swellings, paralysis. Arnica flowers are commonly sold in Spanish pharmacy shops for such use, and likewise arnica tincture. The tincture is considered a specific for chapped lips and for inflamed nasal passages.

Dose A handful of the flowers (or whole plant) brewed in two cups of water – not to be strained – and then massaged externally into the affected parts.

ARTICHOKE (*Cynara scolymus*. Compositae) A well-known vegetable with tall, serrated, fan-form, grey-green leaves. The fruits are borne at the ends of long stems and are eaten in their globe-shaped bud form before they open into purple thistle-type flowers. The ray flowerets will curdle goat and sheep milk strongly enough to make excellent hard cheeses. In Spain an aperitif, Cynara, is made from the artichoke. This Cynara is a bitter tonic and is also used for animals. Artichoke contains *cyanose*, which aids digestion. Rich in vitamin A and in iron.

Use Raw, finely sliced, remove inner, hairy core. A powerful digestive tonic and kidney, bladder and diabetes remedy; also an anaemia cure.

Dose Two or three of the globe heads daily; also feed several handfuls of the leaves and cut-up stems.

ASH (*Fraxinus excelsior*. Oleaceae) This is a woodland tree, distinguished by its many-fingered leaves and peculiar seed fruits known as 'keys'. It is altogether a wonderful tree and a favourite of mine. It is an acclaimed tree of magic powers and should never be felled, always allow to die a natural death. A shepherd's crook is made of ash-wood and is said to protect flocks and herds. A thrust with an ash-staff will overthrow an attacking wolf or snake. Before the discovery of quinine the bitter astringent bark from ash boughs was used as a febrifuge. The leaves are mildly laxative, also tonic. Farm stock should be encouraged to eat them. The strong waterproof wood makes the best churns and farming implements.

Use   Treatment of rheumatism, bowel torpor and fevers.

Dose   Let the animals feed off the leaves. Cut down some branches for the goats. In rheumatic cases feed several handfuls daily, chopped in a bran mash. The keys are used to remove internal wind, ten keys being brewed in half a pint of water and milk, equal parts: or fed raw. Gypsies use all parts of the tree as a remedy for adder bites.

ASPARAGUS (*Asparagus officinalis*. Liliaceae)   This is a plant of dry banks. The appearance of asparagus is familiar to all as a vegetable, distinguished by its thick, scaly shoots, and fine, ferny leaves. It grows wild in sandy places in England and Scotland, but it is rare. It is abundant wild in the Middle East where it is much sought by horses and cattle. Popularly cultivated in gardens throughout Europe. In medicine the small shoots, known as *sprue* commercially, can be used. The shoots contain a peculiar crystalline principle, *Asparagin*. The whole plant, including the root, exerts a most powerful influence upon the entire urinary system. It is apt to diminish milk yield.

Use   A remedy for all derangements and obstructions of the kidneys and bladder. Also beneficial in treatment of jaundice. It is aperient too.

Dose   A handful of the raw shoots twice daily.

Use The root is the strongest part medicinally. In Greece, asparagus fronds are used to close up mice and rat holes because they are very prickly.

AVENS (*Geum urbanum*. Rosaceae) This is a plant of the fields. Distinguished by its rough, rose-form leaves and round, yellow rose-like flowers and peculiar hooked seeds. A very safe and useful herb. The gypsies call avens 'the kind herb'. This plant should be sown in all cattle fields. It is a powerful heart tonic, strengthener of the stomach and intestines, cure for dysentery, and cleanser of the liver and spleen. The whole plant is used.

Use Treatment of heart ailments, digestive ailments and weakness, vomiting and jaundice.

Dose One ounce of finely sliced root boiled for ten minutes in a pint of cold water, and then brewed for two hours. Taken in quarter-pint doses, morning and night.

BALM (*Melissa officinalis*. Labiatae) This is a woodland plant, distinguished by its hairy, serrated foliage and whorls of creamy, hooded flowers. Very attractive to bees – the plant's name is derived from bee. Rubbed inside and outside of new beehives, it persuades bees to settle. It possesses tannin. This plant possesses strong tonic properties, especially good for the brain area. The Arabs say that it gives intelligence to all animals who feed upon it. It also cures palpitations of the heart. It helps to bring down retained after-birth. It is a valuable remedy for eye ailments. The whole plant is used. The great medieval herbalist, Paracelsus, considered that balm prolongs life of man and animals. The long-lived Welsh prince, Llewellyn of Glamorgan, drank a tea of balm daily and reached a near one hundred and ten years.

Use   Treatment of nervous and brain disorders; heart derangements; retained after-birth; uterine disorders. To promote sweating, to increase milk yield, and to prevent miscarriage.

Dose   Feed several handfuls daily, morning and night.

BARLEY (*Hordeum* species. Gramineae)   This is a first cereal, and in my opinion, the best of them all, an important wild cereal as well as a cultivated one. Distinguished by its pale grain bedded in whiskered awns. The leaves are common grass form. Stretches of wild barley denote lime-rich earth. Barley-bread was the staple food of Europe in the Middle Ages and is still the preferred cereal of many Arab nations, for themselves and their animals, especially for their Arabian horses and salukis. Among its special qualities it is blood-cooling and internally soothing. Barley-water is a long-proved remedy for ailments of kidneys and bladder. This is made by pouring water just off the boil, over the same quantity of crushed barley grains. Allow to stand over-night, and then add a further same amount of tepid water with one dessertspoon of pure lemon juice and one desertspoon of pure honey, to every cupful of this water. Strain through butter-muslin, wringing out the barley very dry. Give as a drench in fever ailments and in disorders of kidney and bladder.

Use   As a blood-cooling and tonic cereal feed, and likewise as a medicine. A famed colic remedy and a valued food for infant animals.

Planting   When the moon is middle waxing.

BED-STRAW (Yellow) (*Galium verum*. Rubiaceae)   Also commonly called lady's bed-straw. A low-growing weed, distinguished by its mass of tiny yellow flowers, making the plant look like strewn golden straw. The leaves are small, in whorls, and with downy undersides. The plant is named after the Greek for milk, on account of its special milk curdling properties. In former times when cheese-making was a more natural process, bed-straw was used both to curdle milk and colour the cheese. The famed Double Gloucester cheese of England derives its rich colour and tangy taste from the use of a mixture of yellow bed-straw and the juice of stinging nettles, added to the milk.

BEECH (*Fagus sylvatica*. Fagaceae) A well-known tree of woodland and parks. There are several varieties; the copper beech is the best known. Its fruits – nuts – are enclosed in rough, brown cups, which, as well as the nuts, are edible and much liked by deer and wild horses. The whole tree is highly medicinal, the buds, leaves, bark and nuts are all used. A brew of the leaves or bark is a remedy for ailments of liver and kidneys, also diabetics.

Use Liver diseases and jaundice, bladder and kidney ailments, diabetes, failing appetite. Very softening to hard wounds.

Dose One handful of buds, leaves or shaved bark, twice daily. Externally a brew of the buds or leaves.

BILBERRY (*Vaccinium myrtillus*. Ericaceae) This is a small, heathland shrub. Distinguished by its small green or reddish leaves and small, fleshy flowers, forming round and very juicy purple berries which are cooling and very tonic. The fruits are much sought by all wild animals. It is very astringent.

Use A wonderful remedy in prolonged diarrhoea or vomiting: a valuable mild vermifuge; a remedy for all throat ailments and an important nerve tonic.

Dose Half a pint brew of the leaves, taken fasting, morning and night. Or two handfuls of berries, pounded into milk, given twice daily.

BINDWEED (*Convolvulus arvensis*. Convolvulaceae) This is a climbing plant of the hedgerows. Distinguished by its twining growth, heart-shaped leaves and big, white, bell-shaped flowers. The name convolvo means, I climb. The Spanish gypsy children eat the flowers as a tonic. Goats and sheep like the plant.

Use A powerful antiscorbutic. Helpful in dropsy. The stem and root are used.

Dose Two tablespoonfuls of shredded herb brewed in one pint of water. One cupful taken daily.

BIRCH (*Betula pendula*. Betulaceae) This is a woodland tree distinguished by its slender form, shining, silver-hued, easily peeling bark and catkin flowers. It is the favourite tree of the Red Indians. The leaves and bark have antiseptic properties. A valuable horse tonic is made from the sap, much used by the Red Indians. To obtain the sap, holes are bored in the tree in the early spring, before the appearance of the leaves. It is preserved for use by pouring a little oil on the surface of the extracted sap, thus keeping it fresh for many months.

Use Treatment of digestive ailments, diarrhoea, general debility, weak nerves, rheumatism. As an internal and external antiseptic. The leaves increase flow of urine and expel worms. A strong brew should be made, using one handful of the leaves to one cup of water.

Dose As a tonic: four tablespoonfuls of the sap mixed into bran. As a mild vermifuge: four oz. of the crude sap. Externally: mix with one part sap to one part milk, and apply.

Note The small twigs and inner bark can be used in place of the sap.

BIRTHWORT (*Aristolochia clematitis*. Aristolochiaceae) This is a plant of old ruins and rubble. Distinguished by its creeping form, heart-shaped leaves and peculiar flowers of light yellow colour and possessing stiff internal bristles which control insect pollination. The whole plant is of use in female fertility and birth, strengthens the organs of procreation and birth. The whole herb is used, but as the bristles of the flowers are barbed and may be troublesome in internal use, this herb should be used well dried and powdered and then made into pills or used as a strained brew.

Use As a pregnancy herb and to give strength in birth (labour).

Dose Two teaspoons of the powdered herb daily, or two tablespoons of the brewed herb.

BLACK CURRANT (See Currant)

BLUE FLAG IRIS (*Iris versicolor*. Iridaceae) This is a well-known waterside plant and a plant of moist meadows. It is also much cultivated in gardens. Its leaves are lancelike, its flowers blue, bearded, showy and of sweet scent. It is often called liver lily, because of its medicinal use in liver ailments. It affords a useful general conditioner of the whole system and is also gently laxative. The root is the medicinal part used.

Use Treatment of all liver ailments, jaundice, gall bladder disorders. General tonic, appetizer, mild laxative.

Dose The root, cut small into transverse sections and made into a standard brew: one tablespoon of root to ½ pint water.

It can also be steeped in wine for half a day, and then taken as an extract. One tablespoon of either brew or wine, given twice daily.

BORAGE (*Borago officinalis*. Boraginaceae)   This is a field and woodland plant. Distinguished by its rough leaves and whorls of brilliant, blue, wheel-form, flowers. Its name is derived from 'cor' – the heart – and therefore this plant is always linked with courage. Borage is also called lungwort because of its beneficial effect on all ailments of the respiratory system, especially the lungs. A great cough remedy. The plant is also called bee-bread because its honey-rich flowers are much sought by bees. The young leaves are used as salad herbs by the North African Arabs. Their herds are driven far to pasture upon borage because of its powerful tonic properties. It is tonic and nervine. The whole plant is used. Yet it is one of the herbs now condemned in Australia!

Use   Heart ailments, rickets. Also for chest ailments and as mild laxative. Will greatly increase milk flow. Externally as an eye lotion, to cure general eye ailments, and as a ringworm remedy.

Dose   Feed two to four handfuls mixed with bran and cereals, once or twice daily. Lotion: one handful to ½ pint water.

BRAMBLE or BLACKBERRY (*Rubus fructicosus*. Rosaceae)   This is a common hedgerow and woodland plant. Distinguished by its thorny foliage and stems, and white rose-like flowers. The plant bears black edible fruits, the familiar 'blackberry'. It is one of the most important of the wild plants, being eaten with avidity by all animals. It should be encouraged to grow in every pasture. A brew of the root is an effective remedy for prolonged diarrhoea. The foliage is a famed cure for eczema, a strong brew used internally and externally.

All the species of the genus *Rubus* share most of the same medicinal properties: raspberry, dewberry, loganberry. All the fruits are refreshing and tonic. Blackberry fruits are astringent; raspberries mildly laxative, and very cooling and soothing in fevers. A tonic herb in pregnancy.

Use Treatment of all gastric weaknesses, failing appetite, diarrhoea, impoverished nerves and skin disorders. Externally: for cure of all types of eczema. The gypsies say that fresh-plucked leaves, warmed over a fire, will heal most diseased places. The white underside draws when applied to the skin, the green upper side soothes. The pulped leaves are applied to burns and to foot blisters.

Dose Two handfuls of the leaves or fruits daily. A famed Spanish gypsy tonic for horses and mules is a decoction of the young leaves in red wine. The horse is given a pint draught daily, until the required health standard is reached. Externally: a brew of one handful of leaves to 1½ pints of water. Bathe the affected areas twice daily.

BRIAR (see Rose)

BROAD BEAN (*Vicia faba*. Leguminosae) A well-known garden and farm vegetable. The whole plant with roots is exceptionally rich in nitrates and iron and is an important fodder crop. The pods, stripped of the beans are the medicinal part. They are extraordinarily useful and a premier remedy for the urinary system. Also a dropsy remedy and a cure for warts.

Use Ailments of kidneys and bladder, dropsy, anaemia. The beans fed raw, fresh or dried, increase lactation. Restrict to a handful daily.

Dose Several handfuls of the crushed, emptied pods daily.

Also feed the entire plant, including the roots, as fodder. The inner sides of the pods, rubbed and bound over warts often induce the warts to wither. Plant at full moon.

BROOKLIME (*Veronica beccabunga*. Scrophulariaceae)   This is a waterside plant. Distinguished by its bright, glossy foliage and small, round, blue flowers. The whole herb is a very important blood tonic.

Use   Treatment of skin ailments, fevers, and general blood derangements. Venereal diseases.

Dose   Two handfuls of the herb fed once daily.

BROOM (*Cytisus scoparius*. Leguminosae)   This is a shrub of heaths and commons; it likes a sandy soil. It is distinguished by its tiny leaves and bright yellow flowers of sweet-pea form. The Greek and Yugoslavian peasants use it as a winter food for sheep, cutting and storing the branches in the autumn when yet green. The Russian peasants use broom tops as a very successful remedy for rabies. It is also a mild vermifuge. The flowers infused in hot milk, one handful to one pint of milk, are used internally, and externally, to cure severe forms of skin ailments. The young twigs are mildly purgative. The twigs, crushed and boiled in oil, are a cure for lice. Some species yield a strong and good perfume.

Use   Treatments of worms; skin ailments; rabies; dropsy; constipation. A strong tea of the tops is very effective to increase flow of urine in kidney ailments. Externally: parasites.

Dose   One handful of broom tops, brewed in two pints of water. Give a small cupful, morning and evening, fasting. Externally: use the same brew.

BRYONY (White) (*Bryonia dioica*. Cucurbitaceae) This is a rapidly spreading hedgerow climber. It is of the cucumber and gourd family, and has similar leaves. The flowers are five-pointed, whitish, veined with green. Fruits are bright red berries, a typical sight of the autumn hedgerow.

Use This plant possesses a fetid juice. The very large, white roots are the part used, principally as a horse tonic. It is also a general fertility herb often taking the place of the more rare mandrake.

Dose The root, dried and powdered, one dessertspoon daily for a few weeks' period only, as an aphrodisiac for stallions and bulls.

BUCKBEAN or MARSH TREFOIL (*Menyanthes trifoliata*. Menyanthaceae) A small water-loving plant; growing in boggy places and around ponds. Distinguished by its bean-like foliage and rose and creamy flower-spikes. The bean-like foliage gives the herb its name. In times of food shortage peasants in the Arctic regions dig up the roots and feed them to cows and goats which eat them with relish. The whole plant is eaten freely by deer and goats. Sheep afflicted with rot are frequently cured when led to graze upon tracts of buckbean. The plant is a powerful tonic in common with many of the Gentian family. It is also a vermifuge, especially suitable for young or delicate animals. As a tonic the leaves are cut and mixed with bran and molasses. The molasses is necessary to make the feed palatable owing to its bitter taste. As a vermifuge the leaves are cut and made into pills with flour and honey and given fasting. The juice mixed with whey, one part of juice to three parts of whey, is a cure, internal and external, for rheumatism and cramp.

Use Treatment of all digestive ailments, nervous ailments, debility. Worms. Rheumatism, cramps, dropsy.

Dose As a tonic, one handful of leaves daily. As a ver-mifuge, a half-ounce daily, made into pilules, and given fasting.

BUCKTHORN (*Rhamnus catharticus*. Rhamnaceae) This is a hedgerow and woodland plant. Distinguished by its thorny growth, white flowers and black fruits the size of peas. The leaves are eaten readily by deer, goats and sheep. The bush is a famed purgative, especially important in veterinary medi-cine. Both berries and bark are used. But the bark must be well dried and seasoned for at least one year, otherwise it can cause vomiting and painful griping. In order to prevent its griping properties, ground ginger and honey must always be added when preparing the purge. It is best to give the juice of the ripe berries to young animals, keeping the bark prepara-tion for the adults.

Use Treatment of constipation and worms. Dropsy, leg swellings, eczema.

Dose For young animals an average dose of five ripe berries gently warmed in half a pint of water for half an hour. When cool stir in one tablespoonful of honey, quarter-teasponful of ground ginger. This is the recipe for the celebrated Buckthorn Syrup. To prepare the bark boil one ounce in a quart of water, reducing by quarter-pint in the boiling. Brew for four hours. Then add two teaspoons of ground ginger, two tablespoons molasses. Give one cupful, fasting, daily.

BURDOCK (*Arctium lappa*. Compositae) This is a plant of waste places, fields and waysides. Distinguished by its large, rhubarb-like leaves and thistle-form, plum-coloured flowers, soon replaced by prickly, very adhesive fruits. Animals will not graze this herb, with the exception of the ass; but the sliced and bruised roots are one of the finest blood cleansers known to the herbalist. The bruised leaves, applied externally, are a remedy for ringworm and scabies. The fruits and roots make an excellent lotion for treatment of burns.

Use Remedy for all blood disorders; rheumatism, cough and skin parasites. Also burns, scalds, irritation of skin.

Dose Brew two ounces of the sliced root in two pints of water. Give half a pint, morning and night, fasting. Externally: use the same brew.

BUTTERCUP (*Ranunculus repens*. Ranunculaceae) A plant of meadows, liking a rich soil. Distinguished by its divided leaves and its cupform flowers of shining yellow, rich in pollen. Credited with giving good colour to the milk and the butter produced therefrom. Old-time dairy rites were garlanding cows and goats with buttercup chains on midsummer's eve, and rubbing their udders with buttercup flowers as a blessing on the milk-yield.

Use As fodder for milch animals.

BUTTERWORT (*Pinguicula vulgaris*. Lentibulariaceae) A plant of bogs, moist heaths, pond and lakesides. Distinguished by its thick, fleshy leaves with crystalline dots, which have a greasy feel (the name of this plant being derived from grease or fat). The flowers are a beautiful blue and have ability to trap and digest insects.

Use To clot milk for butter-making, use a pulp of the leaves.

CASTOR OIL PLANT or CASTOR BEAN (*Ricinus communis*. Euphorbiaceae) This is a sort of tree plant with palm-like leaves which often span several feet. The plant produces a bean which yields the well-known pharmaceutical product, castor oil. It is often called Christ's palm, alluding to the great healing powers of its palmate leaves.

Use As a speedy and powerful purge. Of great use in poisoning, also for expelling worms (including tapeworm), and when an animal is known to have eaten a harmful substance. Externally, for treatment of skin ailments, sores, old wounds, swellings, falling hair. Both the fresh leaves and the extracted oil from the fruits are used.

Dose For an average-sized animal, such as a goat, four tablespoons. For a dog such as a spaniel, two dessertspoons. Other animals decrease or increase dose in comparison with above, according to size of animal. Castor oil usually induces constipation after use and should not be used as a regular laxative but only when a speedy and powerful cleansing is required during one or two days of treatment. Externally massage cysts, old sores, thickenings, bruises, with the oil applied hot. The fresh leaves are bound over festering wounds.

CATNIP, CATMINT (*Nepeta cataria*. Labiatae) Grown in gardens, wild in hedges. Greyish foliage, pale-blue hooded flowers, all highly minty-scented.

Use Ornamental and to please cats, who nibble and roll in it.

CELANDINE (Greater) (*Chelidonium majus*. Papaveraceae) This is a plant of waste-places. Distinguished by its yellowish foliage and bright yellow, small, poppy-like flowers. The grey-green stems, when cut, yield a very acrid, yellow juice. It is a famed eye remedy, and I have cured cataract entirely with the use of this herb used externally and garlic given internally. This herb is also called swallow-wort, as herb lore informs that swallows used this plant to unseal the eyes of their young, many of whom otherwise would have been permanently blind. The whole plant is used. It is for external use only, and contains a vital crystalline substance, *celidonia*.

Use Treatment of severe eye ailments, especially cataract. Not recommended for ulcers. Cure of warts.

Dose Make a lotion by boiling approximately two table-spoonfuls of cut herb in one pint of water. Brew well. Add two teaspoonfuls honey. When cold add one part of herb brew to one part of raw milk. Bathe the eyes thrice daily. For warts, break the main stems and apply twice daily the raw exuding acrid juice; allow the juice to dry upon the warts.

CENTAURY (*Centaurium erythraea*. Gentianaceae) This is a field and hill plant. It also inhabits sea places. Distinguished by its small, slender, smooth, tiny leaves and panicles of star-shaped pink flowers. The whole plant is very bitter tasting. It shares the fame of gentian as a stomachic. It is an ancient remedy for liver fluke. It is also antiseptic. Famed also as a female remedy, in all faintness following birth or birth infections.

Use Treatment of digestive ailments, jaundice. A vermifuge, including a liver fluke remedy. An internal and external aid for treatment of all types of wounds, and for cleansing sore mouths.

Dose A handful of the herb brewed in one pint of water. Add one tablespoonful honey. Give four tablespoonsful twice daily. The same brew to be used as an external wound lotion. For fluke make pilules of one ounce centaury, mixed into balls with fat and flour. Give one ounce daily. As a birth remedy similar pills using honey and flour and omitting fat.

CHAMOMILE (*Anthemis nobilis*. Compositae) This is a plant of waste-places and stony ground. Distinguished by its feathery leaves and small, daisy-like white flowers. It is very fragrant, carrying the scent of apples. The flowers yield an oil much praised by Arab herbalists. It is a famed blood cleanser and pain reducer. Reduces tumours. It is an equally famed remedy for female ailments. It is used to cleanse the blood, and externally to heal the aching areas of wounds and bruises, also for inflamed gums. An important poultice is made with equal parts of chamomile flowers and poppy heads (the wild red poppy can be used), well crushed. Mix with one handful of linseed meal to every two handfuls of the herbs. Stir into a paste with boiling water; place on a square of flannel. Fold, dip again in boiling water. Reduce to blood-heat temperature. Apply to the areas to be treated. In the treatment of tumours, fill a small cotton bag with the flowers. Boil well in wine (or other form of alcohol); apply hot, repeating the treatment many times daily. This herb also possesses a peculiar power of reviving wilting cut flowers, and prolonging the life of cut flowers. The crushed plant is infused in hot water, two dessertspoons of plant to a half pint water. This is then added to flower vases. Bunches of chamomile were once consistently hung in stables to deter flies.

Use Treatment of blood and skin disorders, aches and pains, inflammations internal and external, constipation; especially delayed menstruation and acid uterus, and for all female ailments.

Dose One handful of flowers brewed in two pints water. Add one tablespoonful honey. Give one cupful morning and night, fasting. It is also a very important eye lotion, soothing and healing.

CHERRY or BIRD CHERRY (*Prunus avium*. Rosaceae) This is a woodland tree. Distinguished by its frail, rose-shaped, white, flowers, and refreshing, acidulated, ruddy fruits. The bark and stalks possess tonic and astringent properties. An important cough remedy.

Use All throat ailments; also for stones in the bladder. The fruit gives malic acid, high in life-giving properties. It is the chosen fruit of that immensely powerful animal, the wild bear.

The bark loosens mucus in the throat and chest. It also strengthens the heart.

Dose Feed a handful of the fruit or two dessertspoons of the shaved bark, with meals. Or make a brew from same amount of bark or cherry fruit stalks.

CHERVIL (*Anthriscus cerefolium*. Umbelliferae) This is a fragrant species of beaked parsley, distinguished by its fragrant, smooth (not curly) parsley-like leaves and largish seed pods, which extend into beaks covered with hooked bristles. The leaves are unlike common parsley because of their strong fragrance.

Use As an appetiser for animals which are poor feeders. Also, like carrots, improves eyesight.

Dose A handful daily.

CHESTNUT (Horse) (*Aesculus hippocastanum*. Hippocastanaceae) This is a parkland tree of great height and girth. Distinguished by its wide, compound leaves, formed from brown, very resinous buds. The flowers are borne in showy, candle-like spikes of rose or white flowers, producing large brown fruits enclosed in spiny green cases. The name is derived from the greedy eating of the fruits by horses and the subsequent curing of their cough and chest ailments. The gypsies utilize the nut greatly (together with beech mast) as a food for horses. This nut was a great remedy once for broken-winded horses, the nut flour mixed with molasses and liquorice and fed several times daily over one month: another reason for the naming, horse-chestnut. Spanish peasants use the nuts for all their animals, including cows and poultry. The milk-producing animals yield a very rich milk when getting chestnuts as supplement. If the animals refuse the nuts, the bitter property should be removed by pounding the nuts with a stone, steeping for four hours in a mild solution of lime and water, washing well, and then lightly heating to form a meal. Large quantities of a highly nutritious starch are thus produced.

Use Fed to all animals as a general tonic; and a strengthener of the pulmonary areas.

Dose One to three handfuls of prepared chestnuts daily.

Warning If chestnuts are shop-bought, wash them well because, in common with many types of nuts and fruits, they are often treated with a chemical spray to deter insects and rodents from eating them.

CHICKWEED (*Stellaria media*. Caryophyllaceae) This plant grows in fields under plough and in waste places. Distinguished by its creeping nature and tiny, white, starry flowers. It is one of the few readily edible herbs containing a richness of copper. All animals should be encouraged to feed upon it; but sheep must be prevented from over-gorging themselves, especially lambs, or severe digestive upset can follow owing to the richness of this herb. It is one of the herbs most praised by Turkish gypsies, not only for its edible qualities, but also its potent medicinal properties, as it contains many of the soothing and tonic powers of slippery elm. The whole plant is used. It is a highly tonic food for the digestive system, and a remedy for all stomach ailments. Externally it makes an important eye lotion and an ointment for rheumatic inflammations and stiff joints. To make chickweed ointment: wash one pound of finely cut herb, toss it into two pounds of simmering fat (goose grease or lard are commonly used, but nut fat is preferable for the herbivorous animals), simmer gently until the herb is well absorbed. Pass through a muslin bag and pour into jars to set.

Use Treatment of all digestive ailments and weakness, diarrhoea, gastric ulcers, piles (externally); skin disorders, cramps, inflamed or swollen joints and rheumatism. An important tonic food for poultry and all birds (especially caged birds).

Dose Several handfuls per animal per day. Eye lotion: one handful brewed in three-quarter pint of water.

CHICORY (*Cichorium intybus*. Compositae) This is a plant of fields and pastures, also waste places. Distinguished by its very long taproot, and its frail, many petalled, blue flowers. The plant possesses important tonic salad properties, and being planted in leys for grazing cattle it exerts very beneficial effects upon cattle health, as well as benefiting the soil with its deep roots. It is a powerful nerve aid.

Use Treatment of general debility, including weak or failing appetite. All liver weakness, including jaundice.

Dose Two ounces of the finely shredded root given in bran mashes twice daily. In jaundice make a brew, two ounces of herb to 1½ pints water, and give a half-pint morning and night, fasting.

CHIVES (*Allium schoenoprasum*. Liliaceae)   Found by ditches, in hedgerows and in pastures. Distinguished by its reed-like dark-green leaves of short height and which are strongly onion-tasting. Flowers are in purple clusters at the head of a single stem. Roots are narrow, white, with strong onion flavour. The leaves are the part used; they are eagerly sought out by all wild animals and domestic ones, if they can get to them. Although this plant grows in wide stretches, little of it is left for human gatherers owing to the animals' appetite for this healthful, internal cleansing and tonic herb.

Chives are also cultivated in gardens and in pots. They make an attractive and very useful border plant in the farm garden.

Use   As a tonic and internally cleansing aid. Also for worm removal.

Dose   A handful daily in bran mash.

CINQUEFOIL (*Potentilla* species. Rosaceae)   This is a common weed of waste lands and roadsides. It is distinguished by five-fingered palmate leaves and single, yellow, buttercup-type flowers, of flat shape and four petals.

Use   To cure sore mouths and throats, also as a nasal douche. Treatment of thrush in horses.

Dose   A small handful daily.

CLARY or WILD SAGE (*Salvia pratensis*. Labiatae)   This is a plant of dry pastures. Distinguished by its square stems and wrinkled, brown leaves and spikes of purple or blue flowers. Its name is like mountain sage plant – *Salvia officinalis*, derived from *salvare* – to save or heal. It is an important remedy for all gassy complaints of animals, calming and purifying the stomach and expelling wind. It cures hysteria. It is an important eye medicine. The Arabs use the mucilaginous seeds in

51

the removal of sand from the eyes. They well bruise the seed, warming it in the sun to form a thick mucilage and then putting a small amount inside the eyes under the lids. After several minutes the eyes are washed out with sun-warmed water. And finally this wonderful plant is credited with giving immortality.

Use Nervine. Removal of internal gas. Eye treatments, including pink-eye, keratitis, conjunctivitis, ulcers.

Dose Two handfuls of the herb fed three times daily.

CLEAVERS (*Galium aparine.* Rubiaceae) This is a field and hedge plant. Distinguished by its slender form and climbing nature. Also it is distinguished by its adhesive, hairy stems and foliage, the hooked bristles of which cling to all objects. It is a plant very rich in minerals and silica. It gives good strong texture to the hair of animals and the shell of eggs. All animals eat it and poultry especially seek it, hence its popular name of goose-grass. It is an important blood purifier and antiscorbutic. It is famed for clearing up skin ailments. Used externally, it is a proved poultice for reducing tumours. It is also known as goose-grass.

Use Tonic. Cure of eczema. Treatment of abscesses and tumours, including cancerous growths. To cure Grease in horses, merely pound the whole herb into a paste, sprinkle with cayenne pepper, one teaspoon of pepper to every cup measure of pounded cleavers, and apply.

Dose Two handfuls of the herb fed green (not dried) and finely cut, mixed with bran and molasses. Give twice daily. For poultices make as directed in Chamomile.

CLOVER (red) (*Trifolium pratense.* Leguminosae) This is a plant of pastures. Distinguished by its trefoil leaves and globes of red flowers. It should be widely cultivated not only for its food value but also for the medicinal properties of the flower heads. The flowers are powerfully tonic and a cure for nervous twitches, wasting bodies and coughs. The whole plant is sedative. The medicinal properties of clover apply to almost all of the leguminosae family. Red clover is described in old herbals as God's greatest herbal blessing to mankind. Its trinity of leaf is considered a sign of divine powers.

Use Tonic, treatment of general debility, weak nerves, throat ailments, infertility. Proved beneficial in cancer of stomach and throat, eaten as salad, and for throat used as a gargle.

White Clover An old-fashioned but effective remedy to cleanse the blood. Used externally heals old sores.

Use (Both clovers.) tonic, cure of general debility, weak nerves, throat ailments, infertility, tumours, old sores.

Dose Two handfuls twice daily or a strong brew applied as a lotion.

COLTSFOOT (*Tussilago farfara.* Compositae) This is a sun-loving plant of banks and waste places. Especially distinguished by its habit of the blossoms long preceding the leaves. The leaves are grey-green and downy. The flowers yellow, of dandelion form, smallish, solitary, with scaly, downy stems. It is one of the first flowers of the European spring. It derives its name from the Latin word *tussis* – a cough, and *ago* – to banish, the power of the plant over the pectoral region of the body being known to the Romans. Both leaves and flowers are used in medicine.

Use Cure of coughs, pneumonia, pleurisy, asthma, tuberculosis, cramps. The herb is valued for sedative powers in epilepsy, and is so used by Italian peasants. Externally a poultice is made for cure of abscess, ulcer, and earache, toothache.

Dose One handful of cut leaves or flowers to 1½ pints water. Give one cupful morning and night. For poultice, mix a handful of the cut herb with bran, place in a cotton bag, dip into boiling beer, keep in the beer for five minutes, and then apply several times daily to the affected areas.

COMFREY (*Symphytum officinale*. Boraginaceae) This is a plant of moist and watery places, ditch-sides and by water taps, although I have found a form of it growing upon sun-baked banks in many parts of Algeria. It is distinguished by its large, prickly leaves, and creamy or blue-pink, bell-like flowers, borne in drooping clusters. It is a very important medicinal plant. It was once widely cultivated as a fodder plant. Sheep and cows seek it in the ditchside and eat it greedily. English gypsies say that a handful of comfrey roots, cleaned and fed daily to horses and cows in the spring, will rid them of all winter torpor and put them into fine bloom in one week. The young shoots of comfrey are especially nutritious. Arab peasants eat of them freely. But above all the herb is famed for its peculiar powers upon the bones and ligaments. It has the power of aiding the body in the speedy and firm uniting of fractured surfaces: one of its country names is knit-bone, and its name is in fact derived from the Greek word 'to unite'. The leaves and roots are used. The truly great herb, comfrey has recently been condemned by scientists following unnatural experiments. Ignore their baneful findings.

Use Cure of all internal haemorrhages, including uterine. To aid the reunion of wounds and the knitting of fractured and broken bones. Since ancient times comfrey has been famed as a bone-mender, especially valued in limb fractures. It encourages the natural healing process and speeds up the formation of new bone cells. Such powers are probably due to the presence of *allantoin* in comfrey, for this substance is known to promote granulation and the making of epithelial cells. Another important constituent of comfrey is *cholin*, also known to be a powerful healing agent. Treatment of internal ulcers, also ruptures. The mucilaginous content of leaves and roots makes this herb a valuable remedy for pulmonary ailments. Also a proved effective remedy for rheumatism and arthritis. Externally the leaves or bruised roots make an important poultice for all types of swellings and fistulas.

Dose　A good drench is made from one lb. of comfrey, boiled slowly in 1½ quarts of water, boiling for one hour. When boiled, a handful of ground-ivy plant should be added, and two oz. of Spanish liquorice: brew well. A half-pint drench should be given three times daily. For treatment of internal ulcers, molasses should be added, one dessertspoon per half-pint, and the drench given mixed with an equal part of raw, skimmed milk. For bone knitting, feed two handfuls of well-bruised roots daily. The gypsies bruise the roots by stamping upon them. When bone breaks are set with splints and bandages, pour over the bandages three times daily a strong brew of comfrey. Also aids binding. The foliage also possesses powerful knitting properties. For poultice take a good handful of leaves, cut finely, mix with bran, place upon a square of flannel, fold, boil in water for five minutes, wring well, and apply hot. Also for swellings, make a pulp from the fresh leaves spread over the area and hold in place with cold, wet bandages.

CORN (Indian) (*Zea mays*. Graminaceae)　Found in pastures and on hillsides. Also widely cultivated. Leaves grass-like but broad, and shiny. Flowers are white and feathery and are both male and female. The cobs formed from the female are well known and have many medicinal uses as well as providing a most valued food for man and animal. This is the only cereal which fed alone can sustain life over a long period. Corn contains a rich oil as well as starch and milk sugars. The inner 'silk' of the cobs is medicinal, being a valuable kidney and bladder remedy. Applied externally, the 'silk' is a good drawing poultice. It is also helpful for placing over difficult-to-grow seedlings to keep the soil moist and retard the growth of weeds. Dried corn 'silk' can be smoked in farmers' pipes in place of tobacco, flavoured with good tasting and aromatic herbs which are also nerve stimulants, such as anise/fennel, sage, cloves, etc. It is also known as maize.

Corn is also an important fertility aid. The ancient ritual dances in praise of the beloved corn goddess and corn maidens illustrate this.

Use As fodder and medicine. Fed raw, crushed – the cobs and leaves – or dried and milled into flour. In the Canary Islands, where corn replaces wheat as a principal food, the residue of the cobs, after removal of the kernels, is dried for cattle, horse and mule food.

CORNFLOWER (*Centaurea cyanus*. Compositae) This is a plant of the cornfields. Distinguished by its greyish foliage and brilliant, azure, thistle-form flowers. It should be cultivated in all pastures on account of its powerful nervine properties; it strengthens the nerves to a degree not excelled by any other plant. It is also a valuable tonic and digestive aid. The plant is mildly laxative. Externally it has wound curative properties and is used by North American Indians as a remedy against bites of venomous animals. The herb is also of value as an eye restorative, curing weak eyes, dimness of sight and chronic inflammation. The whole herb is used. The flowers were once cultivated for the making of ink and blue dyes.

Use   Treatment of all nerve ailments, including paralysis and chorea. Poor appetite, nervous indigestion, jaundice. Insect bites, including scorpion. Eye ailments and wounds.

Dose   Several handfuls of the whole herb daily. External. A brew, one handful of herb to a half pint water. Two table-spoons of the seed as laxative.

CORN-MARIGOLD (*Chrysanthemum segetum*. Compositae) Distinguished by its dark green toothed leaves and big yellow marguerite-form flowers of strong scent.

Use   External only. The dried flowers have insect repellant properties, when dried and finely crushed. Ants avoid this powder. Use as an egg tint and flavouring. Eggs are covered with the flowers, then water added, and all baked over-night in a warm oven. They become an attractive yellow inside and out. Likewise the Pasque-flower colours eggs a 'salad' green.

COUCH GRASS or TWITCH (*Agropyron repens*. Gramineae) Also called witch grass and dog grass. Distinguished by its tough grass-leaves, runner roots and brown flower spikes. The leaves are much sought by many kinds of animals as a spring tonic: birds and poultry eat the seeds eagerly. One of the most important herbs for the urinary system, increasing flow of urine. One of the best spring tonics for man and animals. Large amounts can be taken. Dogs eat couch leaves to promote cleansing, vomiting and also as a laxative when they semi-digest the leaves. Cats also use the couch for the same effects.

Use   Treatment of all bladder and kidney ailments, gravel and stone, jaundice, gall-stones, constipation. An important vermifuge. The high silica content strengthens hooves, teeth, beaks and claws.

Dose Six handfuls of rootstocks, well sliced, to be fed morning and night. Or a brew can be made from six roots to two pints of water, boiled for thirty minutes, and brewed for three to four hours. Add a handful of raisins and two tablespoonfuls of molasses to the made brew. Give one cupful morning and night. Give also several handfuls of the leaves, twice daily.

COWSLIP (*Primula veris*. Primulaceae) This is a plant of the meadows, liking chalk and clay soils. Distinguished by its pale oval leaves and graceful umbels of tiny, bright yellow flowers, of primrose form. Very fragrant. The plant is a favourite of the gypsies, who use it as a tonic tea as well as in medicine. Cowslip flowers give good colour and flavour to dairy produce when grazed on. It is celebrated for its safe narcotic and nervine properties. Cornflower, the other nerve flower, described previously is a tonic and excitant, whereas cowslip is narcotic and anodyne, relieving pain and calming deranged nerves. It is used as an anaesthetic in a very concentrated form. The flowers are used in medicine. The powerful and pleasant scent helps in the health restoration of sick animals and humans.

Use To quieten nervous and excitable animals. Treatment of chorea and epilepsy. To aid sleep when in pain.

Dose Two handfuls of the flowers fed twice daily, mixed with bran and molasses.

CRAB-APPLE (*Malus sylvestris*. Rosaceae) Grown in hedges and woodland as a small shrub or tree. Leaves are oval and narrow with edges serrated. Flowers are in cluster form, white-to-pinkish in colour and very honey fragrant. The crab-apple produces numerous fruits, small and round, shading from brilliant red to rose and yellow; although they blacken easily and do not keep well, they are the origin of the cultivated orchard apple species. Good odour and taste make the crab-apple popular with all animals and birds.

Being astringent, it is prescribed for wounds, internal and external, the fruits being pulped and mixed with a little corn-flour. Similar treatment for diarrhoea. A small cupful of the pulp fed midday and evening before meals, or when fasting.

Use Anti-scabies because crab-apple releases its abundant vitamins immediately. A stomach and intestinal medicine, anti-diarrhoea remedy, and to check internal bleeding. Also a good nerve and heart tonic. Gives speed to racing animals of all kinds, and to birds.

CRANESBILL (*Geranium pratense.* Geraniaceae) A plant of hedgerows and woodland areas. Stems and delicate foliage are greyish green, flowers are purple. The fruits are finely pointed and long, like the bills of cranes. The root is highly medicinal and is the part used. It is one of the best astringents known to the herbalist for internal and external use, and as it is palatable, all animals will accept it.

Use Dysentery, diarrhoea, and as a wash for inflamed mouths, throats, and for treatment of wounds.

Dose One dessertspoon of the root, cut up small, to one pint water. For wounds and throat treatment the root can be steeped in wine.

CUCKOO-FLOWER (*Cardamine pratensis.* Cruciferae) This is a plant of damp meadows and marshes. It is a small, slender plant, distinguished by its cress-like leaves and corymbs of pale pink, blue, mauve or whitish flowers. Goats and sheep eat the plant, but other animals refuse it. The plant possesses blood-cleansing and tonic properties. Like many of the early spring herbs it possesses antispasmodic properties, and is thus used in chorea and epilepsy, also for spasmodic asthma. Also called milkmaids, from the resemblance to old-fashioned milkmaids and their sun-bonnets and smocks.

Use Treatment of nervous ailments, especially convulsions of young animals. Blood disorders, skin diseases.

Dose One handful of the herbs brewed in two pints of water. Add four tablespoonsfuls molasses. Give one cupful, morning.

CURRANT (Black) (*Ribes nigrum*. Grossulariaceae) This is a shrub of the woodlands, and is commonly cultivated in gardens and orchards. Distinguished by its rose-like foliage, of peculiar scent, and drooping, very juicy, purple-black, round berries. The fruit is refrigerant and anodyne. It is celebrated for its action upon inflamed areas of the throat and mouth. It is very helpful in fevers. An important aid against miscarriage and an acknowledged excellent general tonic in pregnancy. The leaves are almost as medicinal as the fruits.

Use Treatment of all fevers, mouth and throat ailments – it is sometimes called 'quinsy berry', bladder ailments, anaemia, dysentery, and pregnancy weaknesses. Anti-abortive.

Dose In fevers and for throat treatment, give one cupful of the crushed berries twice daily; or make a brew of one handful of the leaves, well cut, to 1½ pints water. Give one cupful twice daily. In cases of animals prone to miscarriage feed handfuls of the herb – foliage and twigs, daily, mixed with bran. Or give two tablespoonfuls of the prepared purée, or crushed raw berries can be given, four tablespoonfuls twice daily.

CURRANT (Red) (*Ribes rubrum*. Grossulariaceae)   Similar to black currant in type and properties. Although this shrub is called red currant, its fruits can also be white. It is more laxative and more cooling than the black species, but does not possess its anti-abortive and throat-soothing properties.

Use   Blood disorders. All fevers. Constipation. Jaundice.

Dose   One cupful of the berries twice daily.

CYCLAMEN (*Cyclamen hederifolium*. Primulaceae)   This is a plant of rocky places. The large tuberous rootstock enables it to grow on sheer rock. Distinguished by its heart-shaped leaves, beautifully patterned with silver veining, and its flowers of five joined petals and prominent mouth, sweetly scented. Colours range from white to red. A common name for this plant is sowbread, as wild swine seek out the roots greedily, despite the protective bitter substance that they possess. This is a fertility herb much used by goats and deer who eat the flowers.

Use   The flowers eaten as a tonic.

DAISY (*Bellis perennis*. Compositae)   This is a very common field plant, of dwarf height, known to all. The leaves are tonic, and the whole plant has long been celebrated as a wound herb. Plugs of the bruised leaves pushed up the nostrils bring down foul matter from the nose and frontal areas very effectively. Spanish gypsies make peculiar use of the daisy plant. They make pills of the grated root mixed with beef dripping and give them to dogs and other animals, whose growth they wish to restrict.

Use Treatment of skin eruptions, wounds, swellings and bruises. To cleanse the head.

Dose One handful of the leaves and flowers brewed in two pints of water. Give one cupful night and morning. Also use the brew externally for bathing affected areas. Pound up the leaves into butter and apply to old wounds.

DANDELION (*Taraxacum officinale.* Compositae) This is a very common plant of open, sunny places. Distinguished by its lion-toothed foliage, profuse flowers of brilliant gold, and the white juice which the whole plant exudes. This plant, generally considered as a 'troublesome weed', is one of the most valuable known to the herbalist. The great Arabian physician and herbalist, Avicenna (all the great Arabian doctors are herbalists) praised the dandelion highly. The herb is blood-cleansing and tonic. It has an important effect upon the hepatic system and is a supreme jaundice curative herb. The leaves strengthen the enamel of the teeth. The white juice dissolves warts. The plant is grazed well by goats. Horses will take quantities of the leaves when cut and mixed with bran. I know one Yorkshire racing-stable which makes much use of the herb as a general conditioner. The Turkish gypsies eat heartily of the raw roots and also feed them to their animals. The bitter leaves, once a popular, spring bloat-tonic salad herb, are still much used on the Greek islands.

Use Treatment of skin eruptions, sluggish blood-flow, weak arteries. All liver complaints, jaundice, constipation.

Dose Five raw roots daily, finely cut and mixed with bran, or several handfuls of leaves.

DILL (*Anethum graveolens.* Umbelliferae) This plant grows in hedgerows and on waste land. Distinguished by its fine feathery leaves and umbels of pale creamy flowers, which bear winged seeds, and contain an essential oil. The whole plant is highly aromatic. It closely resembles the anise plant in medicinal properties. The plant is carminative. It increases the milk yield. The seed is the part used. It is obtainable from herbalists.

Use Treatment of all digestive ailments, including windy colic, diarrhoea, fevers. To increase milk.

Dose One handful of the seeds, fed raw, mixed with bran, twice daily. The leaves are also useful.

DITTANY (*Dictamnus* species. Rutaceae) A favourite herb of the Greek peasants to safeguard health of humans and goats.

Use Fed raw, plant and seed, as tonic and to increase appetite. A nerve stimulant and to give vigour. An ancient remedy to cure bites of snakes, scorpions and dogs. Used internally and externally.

Dose Tablespoon or more, daily.

DOCK (Red) (*Rumex sanguineus*. Polygonaceae) The plant is widely spread over waste places and fields. Some varieties of the plant grow in watery places. Distinguished by its tall, broad, shiny, leaves and spikes of red flowers. It is a supreme cooling herb for external use, soothing fevered and inflamed flesh in a remarkable way. Thus it is of much use in the treatment of inflamed udders in mastitis, and in other udder disorders. The whole herb is antiseptic. The leaves and roots are used.

Use Mainly external: as a cure for skin inflammations and fevers. To cleanse and heal wounds. Piles.

Dose One handful of the cut leaves to 1½ pints of water is a good brew. The leaves can also be well pulped, slightly warmed over a low fire, and rubbed well into inflamed surfaces of the flesh. For piles make suppositories with the pulped raw herb and a little soap, and insert into the anus three times daily. To make dock leaf ointment follow the recipe given for Adder's tongue.

EARTH-NUT (*Conopodium majus.* Umbelliferae) A plant of hill places and pastures. Distinguished by its low growth, dark ferny leaves and umbels of white-green, insignificant flowers. This plant makes a small tuber root which is edible, raw, by man and animals. Considered a delicacy similar to truffles, trained dogs (and also pigs) are used to find earth-nuts. The nuts are a general tonic and a fertility herb. The gypsies are expert at finding earth-nuts and share them with their best ponies and greyhounds to increase their speed.

Use A powerful tonic.

Dose Two or three daily, when available.

ELDER (*Sambucus nigra.* Caprifoliaceae) This is a common hedgerow shrub, widely distributed. Distinguished by its umbels of highly scented, waxy white flowers, followed by clusters of dark purple edible berries. The leaves are also highly scented, flies have an aversion to them. This is one of the most important of all herbs; it possesses the strange powers of being beneficial in the cure of almost all the common ailments of man and animal. Because of this shrub's great medicinal powers, the elder is sacred to the gypsy people, and no true gypsy will ever burn its living wood. Tradition tells that the Cross of Christ was made from an elder tree. It was a favourite herb of the Greek doctor, Hippocrates. Most animals will graze on the elder bushes. The leaves, dried and powdered, are used as an insect-repellent by the Arabs. They can also well replace tobacco for smoking, mixed with dried elder flowers and some sage leaves. All parts of the shrub are used; the blossom is the most potent part for internal use, the foliage for external treatments but the blossom makes an effective lotion for treatment of wounds and skin ailments, brewed in water or buttermilk. Very cooling. A brew of the green stalks and branches, highly concentrated, makes an excellent external application against gadfly for cattle and horses. Juice of the berries, mixed with honey, is a very good cough remedy, and mixed with egg whites is an effective salve for burns and scalds.

A brew of the finely shaved root is helpful in treatment of kidney ailments and dropsy.

Use Treatment of all gastric, hepatic and pulmonary ailments. All fevers, skin disorders, wounds. Externally as an insecticide.

Dose One handful of cut leaves or blossom to 1½ pints of water, add two dessertspoonfuls of honey or molasses. Give one cupful morning and night. For external use, omit the honey or molasses, and make the brew slightly stronger by adding more herb. The berries, slightly heated and then well pounded, are an invaluable remedy for inflamed throats and coughs. Elder blossom ointment is excellent (see formula given for adder's tongue ointment). One of the best remedies that I know for skin ailments – especially scabies, ringworm – and the one I use most frequently in my cattle work, is: three handfuls of elder leaves and stalks, one handful wild geranium plant (herb Robert), one whole root of garlic. Grate the garlic, cut the elder and geranium finely, place all in a quart of water. Bring to the boil, simmer for twenty minutes, then brew for four hours. Keep covered. Bathe affected areas twice daily. Also give a cupful internally.

ELDER (Dwarf) (*Sambucus ebulus*. Caprifoliaceae) This is a plant of waste places. Distinguished by its resemblance to a small elder; it grows close to the ground. The fruits are not edible.

Use Treatment of dropsy. All female ailments, especially inflammation of the uterus and vagina.

Dose A half-handful of leaves brewed in 1½ pints of water, mixed with a dessertspoonful of honey. Give two table-spoonsful nightly.

ELECAMPANE (Lesser) (*Inula viscosa*. Compositae) Found in fields, on hillsides, road edges. Bright green leaves, sticky and of pungent scent, which protects against grazing animals. Flowers, yellow, starry. The pungency gives fame for cure of pulmonary ailments, but as it is largely used as a vapour inhalant not applicable for animals, I concentrate on the many external uses.

Use Control of insects. Bunches placed in poultry nesting-boxes to deter fleas and mice. Hung in stalls and stables to catch flies; at night the bunches are thrust into sacks and then plunged into water to drown the flies. Dry, powdered, or strong brew, as an insecticide.

ELM (*Ulmus procera*. Ulmaceae) This is a lofty tree of park-lands, sending off strong, lateral branches. Distinguished by its reddish flowers which come before the leaves and which produce winged, one-seeded fruits known as samaras. Animals eat greedily of elm foliage which possesses many tonic virtues. The outer and inner bark are the parts used in medicine, though European peasants use the leaves for astringent purposes, both internally and externally. The bark possesses nutritive properties. This tree since olden times is credited with lightning resistant powers, and cattle and other animals notably shelter under elms in thunder storms. Elm wood makes good farming tools, gates, fences.

Use Treatment of deep-seated skin ailments, diseased mouths and throats, running ulcers. Also loose teeth and inflamed gums. The jelly-like juice which can be expressed from the inner layers of the bark has diuretic properties and is a useful remedy in treatment of kidneys and inflamed or relaxed bladder.

Dose Outer bark can be dried, powdered and fed raw in a dry bran mash with molasses. Also used externally.

ELM (Slippery) (*Ulmus rubra.* Ulmaceae) Not British. It will, however, grow in England, and is worth planting as a hedgerow tree. This is a tree mainly of North America, the finely powdered bark of which is among the most important of all herbal remedies as it possesses supreme healing properties. Slippery elm bark provides a most nutritious gruel which also possesses remarkable medicinal properties, a poultice both internally and externally.

The bark is tough and fibrous of texture, pink hued, and possesses a large quantity of antiseptic alkaline mucilage.

Use Treatment of all digestive complaints, including ulcers, for which slippery elm is a specific; invaluable for cure of scouring. All pectoral disorders, including tuberculosis, lung and bronchial haemorrhage. Wasting diseases, rickets, stunted growth. Externally: a poultice for all skin ailments, especially old wounds and hard swellings.

Dose Two tablespoonfuls of elm powder mixed into a smooth texture with one tablespoonful honey. Slowly stir in one pint of warm milk (or for scouring, use milk and water, equal parts); give one cupful morning and night. The powder can also be mixed in dry form into a bran gruel. To make a poultice merely place some powdered bark upon a square of flannel, fold carefully, dip into boiling water for five minutes, and apply. Or a paste of slippery elm powder can be made with whites of eggs and painted over the areas to be treated.

EUCALYPTUS (*Eucalyptus globulus*. Myrtaceae) This is a most valuable tree, the blue gum of Australia, found commonly planted in sub-tropical and warm and temperate climes, especially in such zones in Europe and throughout Africa. Distinguished by its tall, graceful form, delicate willow-like, shimmering foliage and aromatic properties. The tree is almost a panacea for all ills, similar to the remarkable elder tree. The various species of eucalyptus are very free from insects on account of the strong aromatic oil in the leaves and bark. The Arabs recognize that the tree has important anti-malarial powers, as its roots drain the ground well, and leaves and bark give out a volatile oil, and thus plant it extensively around their homes. Nevertheless the Arabs call this tree 'The Jews' Tree', because the Zionist settlers planted it wherever they settled in Israel. An oil, eucalyptol, is extracted from the leaves. The leaves are the part most generally used. Dried leaves, whole or pulverized, can be obtained from herbalists.

Use Treatment of all fevers, including malaria. All pulmonary ailments, including tuberculosis and pneumonia. Inflammation of the female organs and bladder, gonorrhoea. Externally a valuable antiseptic and disinfectant without injuring any tissues. A valuable local application in cancers. Also as an inhalant in treatment of diphtheria, asthma and all bronchial ailments. The dried and finely powdered leaves make a valuable insecticide when dusted into the hair. The oil, one teaspoonful to half a pint of warm water, rubbed well into the skin, is a powerful insect repellent.

Dose One handful of leaves brewed in 1½ pints water; one cupful taken fasting, morning and night. This brew can be used externally as well. Also the leaves can be made into a mulch with warm water and gentle heating and applied to the skin. The leaves as a rinse strengthen and brighten hair. In common use as a hair tonic in the Yemen, massaged into the hair. Used for manes and tails of Arab horses. For inhalation purposes, ten drops of oil to one cupful of hot water.

EVENING PRIMROSE (*Oenothera biennis.* Onograceae) This is quite a common weed, found on waste places and sand dunes. It can grow as tall as five feet. Stems and leaves are greyish, flowers are large and of primrose shape. It is night-flowering and its most sweet scent attracts moths and other night insects. Being astringent and mucilaginous, the plant has use as a cough cure, and for wounds and skin ailments.

Use Treatment of coughs, sore throat, wounds, skin irritations and all inflammations.

Dose Two tablespoons of the flowers steeped in a large cup of boiling water. Externally, pound up a small handful of flowers and mix into egg whites.

EYEBRIGHT (*Euphrasia officinalis.* Scrophulariaceae) The plant is plentiful in meadows and pastures. Distinguished by its tiny growth, and miniature, solitary, white flowerets, tinged with purple, and marked with a yellow eye. The name of the plant is derived from its remarkable eye restorative powers, even curing blindness in many cases. The whole plant is also nervine, tonic and astringent. Its use is both external and internal, strengthening greatly the eye nerves when so used. The high potassium and sulphur content of the plant make it also of value in treatment of gastric ailments, especially insufficiency of gastric juices.

Use Treatment of weak and inflamed eyes, keratitis, conjunctivitis, ulcers. Also all gastric disorders.

Dose One handful of herb brewed in one pint water. Give one cupful morning and night. Use the brew also for external bathing of the eyes.

FENNEL (*Foeniculum vulgare*. Umbelliferae) This is a perennial plant of open spaces. It prefers coastal areas. Distinguished by its finely divided, very aromatic leaves and umbels of yellow flowers. The plant smells sweetly of hay, from which its name is derived. It is a very important medicinal herb possessing highly antiseptic and tonic properties. Peasants drive their flocks to feed upon it owing to the abundance of milk that the herb produces, and the sweet odour that it imparts to the milk. However, the Arabs state that if cattle over-gorge on fennel they poison themselves. Native cattle never over-gorge, but imported cattle will do so unless watched. The white hearts of fennel shoots much resemble celery hearts, and are very popular in Arab countries as raw food for man and beast. The seeds yield a sweet oil of high medicinal value, and the stems a gum known as fennel gum. The herb has internal and external uses. As the Spanish gypsies use poultices of wild celery leaves over the stomach area to bring out foul discharge through the navel, so the Arabs use poultices of fennel stalks and leaves. They use fennel poultice also to resolve old and hard tumours. The roots are extolled by the Arabs as one of the finest of all aperient roots. The foliage, brewed, also yields a valuable eye medicine for internal and external use. I was much impressed by the remarkable use of this herb that I witnessed in Tunisia and Algeria. Gypsies say this plant protects animals from evil forces.

Use Gastric ailments, including colic and severe inflammation of the bowels; acute constipation. Fevers, cramps and worms. All eye ailments. The seeds (added to teas) cure indigestion.

Dose Two handfuls of the whole herb fed raw twice daily. Make use of the seed also. For constipation, give four raw roots daily, finely sliced and mixed with bran and molasses.

FENUGREEK (*Trigonella foenum-graecum.* Leguminosae) Not British. This is a plant of sandy soil and sunny places. It is widely cultivated by the Arabs, especially by the Egyptians, the Arabic name for the herb being helbeh. Distinguished by its clover-like foliage and pea-form flowers of yellow-white. The plant possesses highly aromatic seeds, having powerful disinfectant and emollient lubricant properties; the feeding value of these is about equal to linseed. It is one of the great fattening herbs; when fat women were prized in past ages, by the Arab countries, they were largely fattened upon fenugreek. It contains substances which make it an important appetizer, especially sugars and albuminous compounds. Its chemical composition indeed closely resembles that of cod-liver oil. It is the perfect 'sister' herb for garlic, enhancing all the latent and remarkable powers of that supreme herb, especially increasing its disinfectant properties. Very tonic and eagerly sought by all animals. It is highly rich in vitamins, including the fertility vitamin E; it also contains nitrates, calcium and phosphorus. The whole plant is used. The seed can be purchased from herbalists. This plant will grow in Britain, but because of the colder climate does not make enough size for a fodder crop. It would be very advantageous to agriculture if plant breeders would produce a hardy variety for field cultivation.

Use Treatment of all gastric weaknesses and ailments, nerves and neuralgia. Female ailments, including failing milk supply. Externally as a poultice for relief of abscess, boils and running sores.

Dose Two handfuls of plant fed daily. To obtain quicker results use the seed. Two ounces of seed daily. Use seed for making a standard poultice.

FERN (Male) (*Aspidium filix mas.* or *Nephrodium filix mas.* Filices) This is a plant of woods and shady banks. Distinguished by its curled shoots resembling shepherds' crooks, and its tall fern foliage which bear countless kidney-shaped scales on the backs, covering the spores. Another distinguishing point is that the fronds are tougher and darker than other ferns and the fern leaflets have rounded tips instead of the general pointed ones. All animals eat the foliage of the male fern. The young shoots are especially beneficial. Gypsies make horse fodder from the dried bracken, which in winter they soak in hot water and feed in place of hay. The root rhizome is the most powerful medicinal part of the plant, possessing potent vermifuge properties, and is only equalled by the pomegranate rind cure of the Arabs as a remedy for tapeworm. This root (rhizome) has a sickly bitter-sweet taste and contains a green fatty oil, gum and resin. Tapeworm capsules, made from oil of male fern, could be obtained from most chemists but are now becoming difficult to obtain as people prefer stronger chemical treatments which often do more damage than the worms. A common vermifuge is also made from an ethereal extract prepared from the root.

Use Nutritional and tonic. Vermifuge, especially against tapeworm.

Dose After fasting the animal for one day, feed one large root of about one hand's breadth, finely sliced and made into a pulp by boiling for thirty minutes, giving the pulp mixed in three-quarter pint of its own water. Follow with a strong drench of castor oil, thirty minutes later. Repeat treatment after eighteen days if necessary. Alternatively, the dried root, finely powdered, may be used. One heaped table-spoon is formed into pills, adding one teaspoon cayenne pepper and half teaspoon ginger, both in fine powder form. Add enough wheat flour and honey to bind the herbs for rolling into pills. After fasting the case for twenty-four hours, give a senna pods purge (see Senna) late at night. Next morning give the fern dose pills early, followed thirty minutes later with castor oil (see p. 44), and thirty minutes after that a warm, sloppy meal of flaked oats, bran and molasses. This treatment is for a dog, the animal most prone to tapeworm; for larger animals increase the amount of male fern, etc., in proportion to size.

FEVERFEW (*Chrysanthemum parthenium.* Compositae) This is a plant of poor soil and waste places. Distinguished by its feathery yellowish foliage, and flat, button-like, white daisy flowers. The flowers are aromatic with a pleasing scent. It is one of the most important herbal aids for female ailments, the plant exerting remarkable powers over the uterus. It is also a mild and very safe aperient. The whole plant is used.

Use Digestive aid and tonic. Treatment of all female irregularities, especially scanty or failing menses, inflamed or weak uterus and uterine and vaginal ulcers. Abortion. Difficult labour and retained afterbirth.

Dose Two handfuls of the herb fed twice daily. In treat-ment of the uterus and vagina, make into a brew, one hand-ful herb to two pints water, and give as douche in addition to internal medicine. In difficult labour and delayed expul-sion of afterbirth, make a strong drink together with rasp-berry leaves, approximately three handfuls of raspberry to

73

each one of feverfew, brewed in 1½ quarts of water, plus four dessertspoonfuls honey. Give frequent drenches from this brew.

FLAX (Linseed) (*Linum usitatissimum*. Linaceae) This is generally a cultivated plant, although as a wild plant it inhabits cornfields as an 'escape'. Distinguished by its frail, solitary flowers of intense blue, and the fine, thin character of the whole plant. Apart from the plant's industrial use for linen cloth, it is rich in nutritional and medicinal properties. The seed is the principal part used for veterinary purposes. Linseed is very demulcent and tonic and gives valuable aid in the treatment of pulmonary complaints. Linseed oil, obtained from the crushed seeds, is a very safe and effective laxative, especially for young animals; it is also a fine conditioner. The residue, left after the oil extraction, makes good cattle cake when mixed with cereals. The oil is also valuable as a rubbing lotion, especially effective when spruce fir shoots are macerated in it, and the two herbal products thus combined. Crushed linseed makes a valuable poultice, prepared in the standard way.

Use Nutritional and tonic. An important food in pregnancy. Treatment of pulmonary tuberculosis, pneumonia, bronchitis, coughs. Externally for the same ailments; and to reduce hard swellings, and cure sprains and strained ligaments. As a poultice for the same ailments, and treatment of boils and carbuncles, abscesses. The oil cures constipation and worms.

Dose Variable. An average medicinal dose is one pint of linseed brew twice daily, made by boiling two handfuls of linseed to 2½ pints of water, plus two tablespoonfuls molasses. For worms ten to fifty drops of turpentine are added to one to 1½ ounces linseed oil, plus a pinch of ground ginger.

The strength of the dose must vary with size and age of the animal being treated.

FOXGLOVE (*Digitalis purpurea*. Scrophulariaceae) This is a common wayside and woodland plant. Distinguished by its tall spikes of rose-pink, purple-freckled, bell-shaped flowers. The seed yields the drug, *digitalin*, and the bruised leaves are one of the remedies most valued by the gypsies for poulticing swellings on the udder, and also on the limbs. The plant has sedative properties, and for that use is employed internally. Also internally as a dropsy remedy. I am opposed to the use of poisonous plants in medicine and thus only mention this plant for external use.

Use External: As a crude liniment or poultice, for the cure of tumours and all types of swellings. As a cataplasm over the navel area to reduce fever. As an external pain remover.

FUMITORY (*Fumaria officinalis*. Fumariaceae) A hedgerow and wayside plant. Distinguished by its delicate, creeping, fern-like growth, of dusty-grey colour, with erect spikes of pinkish flowers. The plant's appearance has gained it the name of 'earth-smoke'. The Turkish gypsies extol the plant's properties as a skin cure, and for treatment for all forms of liver ailments. It is mildly aperient and a powerful, bitter tonic. This is also a chosen herb of the American Indians – and mine.

Cows and sheep seek it out greedily. The whole plant is used.

Use Treatment of skin eruptions, eczema, wounds, ulcerated mouth. Inflamed liver, jaundice and biliousness. Also to curdle milk mildly.

Dose One handful of herb brewed in two pints water. Give

one cupful every morning, fasting. Use the brew as an external lotion as well. Or can be fed raw internally, and used raw, crushed externally.

GARLIC (*Allium* species. Liliaceae) A woodland plant, preferring damp places. Widely cultivated in the Eastern world. Distinguished by its shining oval-shaped leaves and tall umbels of white, starry flowers. The whole plant possesses a very distinctive and pungent odour. The modern farmer is apt to look upon this supreme medicinal plant as a 'troublesome weed', because cattle, recognizing its beneficial and medicinal properties, have a craving for it, and are apt to gorge themselves and affect the flavour of their milk. The plant is rich in a volatile oil and sulphur and is worshipped by the gypsies who uphold that it possesses magic properties on account of its being able to cure the majority of ailments which afflict man and the animals he has domesticated. Their secret name for this herb is *moly*. It is highly antiseptic. Russian scientists have acclaimed garlic as an internal purifier of the greatest importance and that 'garlic, onions and horseradish contain powerful anti-toxic elements essential for good health.' Throughout the history of mankind garlic is credited with great anti-plague powers. In the Great Plague of London, it was the principal remedy for protection and cure and fetched more than gold in price. In Yorkshire, England, I saved many thousands of hill sheep condemned as incurable, by using garlic. Gorillas often plant areas of garlic where they have their colonies. Because of its remarkable penetrative disinfectant and mucus-expellent powers, garlic is a valuable basic remedy for the treatment of all ailments in which the cleansing of the blood-stream and expulsion of mucus accumulations are required. It is supreme in the cure of all infectious ailments of the blood-stream, lung and digestive areas. American scientists discovered that garlic contains a substance – crotonaldehyde – which is excellent for diseases of the nose, throat and intestine. It is also of especial use as a febrifuge and vermifuge. And it is a fertility herb for both sexes. Wild animals seek out all species of garlic not only as a general protective and cleansing herb, but also to increase their sexual powers. Externally, for the disinfecting and healing of all types of sores and wounds, also parasitical infections.

Use Treatment of all fevers, pulmonary, gastric and skin complaints, rheumatism, all worms, also liver-fluke, mange, ringworm, ticks, lice. The supreme immunizer of stock against infectious diseases. Garlic, as medicine, is the most famed cancer curative herb.

Dose Garlic roots are composed of many small sections called cloves, held together by a thin skin. For dogs and cats an average dose is four cloves, finely minced, mixed into food, or crushed and pushed down the throat. Or powdered dried garlic made into pills with flour and honey, one teaspoon. Other vegetable-eating animals – goats, sheep, horses, etc. – can be dosed more easily. When available, use the leaves as well as the roots, shredded and mixed into a mash of bran and molassses. On average, a handful of leaves and several whole roots for sheep and goats, and double the dose for horses and cattle.

Note Feed garlic to milk-producing animals at milking time so that the garlic will have left the milk-stream by the time of the next milking and thus not taint the taste of the milk.

Externally: make a strong brew from a handful of minced cloves to a pint of cold water. Keep covered, bring to boiling point, then simmer gently for several hours. Allow to stand and brew. Do not strain; apply where needed. A famed skin ailment remedy, including parasitical mange.

A Spanish gypsy remedy of renown, for treatment of inflamed joints and rheumatism, is made from a dozen garlic cloves, well minced, put into a tin large enough to hold half a pint of olive oil. Tie a thick piece of cloth over the top of the tin. Then place the tin in a pan of hot water and keep the water simmering for several hours. Allow to stand and steep; do not strain. Reheat before use and rub affected parts. A few drops into the ears is a good remedy for ear-ache. Crushed spice cloves added to the oil further improves this remedy.

An agricultural note Dried, powdered garlic, as a dust or in solution in water, is becoming a popular agricultural insect pest deterrent. I invented and used this, in dust form, when in Mexico, to prevent small birds and insects from devouring seedlings.

Note Avoid popular, commercial garlic oil capsules. The concentration of oil is an internal irritant.

GENTIAN or FIELD GENTIAN (*Gentiana campestris*. Gentian-aceae) This is a plant of the marshes. Distinguished by its four-petalled flowers of intense blue. This is a beloved plant of the Red Indian herbalists: 'blue blossom medicine' they call gentian extract, although the root is the medicinal part used. The gentian is one of the most important tonic herbs, being considered the prince of bitters. It will quell vomiting when all other herbs fail. The Arabs value the herb highly in treatment of malaria in cattle. The name gentian came to the herb in respect of the Greek King, Gentius, a skilled herbalist. A yellow variety, *Gentiana lutea*, yields bigger roots and is in more popular use in medicine.

Use Treatment of all forms of digestive weakness; vomiting; nervous ailments, including hysteria; malaria. To improve appetite of all poor feeders.

Dose One ounce shaved root brewed in one pint water. Add one tablespoonful honey. Give one cupful twice daily before feeding. Or one root, shaved, mixed into a mash of bran and molasses.

GOLDEN ROD (*Solidago virgaurea*. Compositae) This is a plant of plains or woodlands. It is very common in North America (*S. lanceolata*) where it is the unofficial national flower. Distinguished by its tall rods of glowing, golden, tiny, daisy flowers. It is a famed wound herb, being distributed by the Saracens, who always took golden rod into battle areas with them. The Red Indians make great use of it. It is an important remedy for female disorders. All cattle eat it; it brings them into good appetite and gives bloom, the whole plant used. The garden variety can be used in medicine.

Use A powerful digestive aid. Treatment of jaundice, kidney ailments. Used internally and externally to induce perspiration.

Dose Three handfuls of herb once daily, or as a drink, using one tablespoon of the herb to one cupful of water. The warming, aromatic and pleasant taste of golden rod makes it useful to mix with other herbs of disagreeable taste to disguise them.

GROUND IVY (*Glechoma hederacea* or *Nepeta glechoma*. Labiatae) A woodland or hedgerow plant. Distinguished by its ground-creeping nature, and small, pale-blue, hooded flowers. Cattle and sheep seek out the herb and it provides an excellent tonic for them. The plant is tonic and slightly aperient. It is a useful colic herb. Its chief value is as a poultice aid, being used especially in combination with other herbs, which depend upon ground ivy to draw out their medicinal properties. Two important combinations are: ground ivy with equal parts of ragwort and groundsel, to form a poultice for treatment of all skin gatherings and tumours; ground ivy, yarrow and chamomile, to form a poultice for treatment of skin diseases, abscesses and boils. Used with liquorice and honey it is a powerful aid for pulmonary ailments, including tuberculosis.

Use Treatment of cough and tuberculosis. Ulcers, abscesses, boils, inflamed glands, retention of afterbirth. As a nasal douche.

Dose One handful or more ground ivy chopped up in a bran mash, or as a brew, one handful to 1½ pints water, one tablespoonful honey. Give one cupful three times daily.

GROUND-PINE (*Ajuga chamaepitys*. Labiatae) This is a plant of chalky places. Distinguished by square, reddish, hairy stems and yellowish hairy leaves having the scent of pine-tree resin. The flowers are lipped, bright yellow and faintly spotted with red. An old name for the plant was arthritic ivy, on account of the herb's great powers in cure of joint ailments. Excellent for the swollen limbs of lambs. It is a rich blood tonic. The whole herb is used.

Use Treatment of all forms of rheumatism, arthritis, and all weaknesses of the joints. North African Arabs use the herb to cure paralysed animals, also in treatment of hysteria in horses.

Dose One handful ground-pine, finely cut, mixed with bran, brewed in 1½ pints water. Give one cupful morning and night. Use internally and externally.

GROUNDSEL (*Senecio vulgaris*. Compositae) A common plant of waste places and pastures. Erect growth, greyish-green leaves, branching with jagged lobes. Flower-heads in close terminal clusters, the individual flowerets being of tubular shape, solid, yellow, like minute candles, and possessing no ray petals. The herb is rich in minerals, especially iron. Animals seek it out as a tonic, especially poultry. The herb possesses powerful drawing and antiseptic properties. Mixed with ground ivy it makes an important poultice. It strengthens the eyes and reduces inflammation.

Use Treatment of general debility, impoverished nerves, jaundice. Externally: all wounds, especially old ones; inflamed areas, gatherings, poisoned limbs, sore breasts. Eye ailments.

Dose Three handfuls of herb fed daily. Externally: a strong brew of several handfuls cut herb to two pints water. Or make a poultice by bruising fresh leaves and adding bread boiled in milk.

HART'S-TONGUE (*Scolopendrium vulgare*. Filices) A woodland fern. Distinguished by the fronds shaped like the tongue of a deer. A favourite herb of the North African Arabs. Much used in cure of bowel fevers, including dysentery. Also for treatment of enlarged spleen.

Use Treatment of colic, dysentery, diarrhoea. Enlarged spleen. All wounds.

Dose One handful of finely cut herb brewed in two pints water. Add half an ounce ground ginger and one tablespoon honey. Give one cupful three times daily.

HAWKWEED (*Pilosella officinarum*. Compositae) Also called hawkbeard, hawkbit, hawkseye. Under whichever name, it is a herb for the poultry family, including turkeys and geese. A plant of dry places, rocky terrain and waysides. Leaves are oval-form, have downy undersides and uppersides green with white hairs. Flowers are the Compositae type and can be mistaken for dandelion, though they are generally more orange of hue and often tinged with red (not seen on the dandelion). Again like the dandelion, the stems possess a white, bitter juice. The seeds form typical round, downy 'clocks' for wind dispersal and are very medicinal.

This herb, eaten by the hawk, especially the young leaves and later the seeds, is said to giver the bird its wonderfully keen sight. Eaten raw, the herb is good for the eyesight, especially when combined with raw, flaked carrot. It is also an important remedy for all disorders of the liver and gall bladder; a jaundice remedy.

Use As described above.

Dose A small handful daily, cut small and mixed with bran, etc. Give seeds also.

HAWTHORN (*Crataegus oxycantha*. Rosaceae) Found in hedges, on commons and in woodlands. Distinguished by its dark, small, shiny, toothed leaves, and pinkish, roseform flowers of easily shed petals and very fragrant scent. It is a thorny bush or small tree and bears small, hard, dark red, fruits called 'haws'.

Its name comes from the word for strength, and this is referring to the extreme hardness of hawthorn wood, which makes everlasting staves and crooks and is also highly valued for farm implements. A tree known for its powerful magic forces, it is therefore pinned (branches – especially flowering ones) to farmhouse doors, stables, barns and byres, and hay-ricks, to protect from lightning strikes. The sprouting buds called 'salt and pepper' by countryfolks, because of their tangy taste, are eaten raw by children and make an excellent tonic food for young animals of all kinds when being weaned from their mother's milk.

A poultice of the leaves or the pulped raw fruits are of high repute as a drawing remedy for deeply embedded splinters and thorns and for whitlows. The fruits are also given against miscarriage.

Dose A handful of the sprouting buds or the leaves, fed daily, or a handful of the berries, also daily.

HAZEL (*Corylus avellana*. Corylaceae) This is a small nut-tree of hedges and woods. Distinguished by its shiny, crisp round leaves and attractive flower catkins of yellow-green touched with red, and its autumn nuts contained in green 'bonnets' with cut edges, from which this tree-name, meaning 'a cap' is derived. Known as a tree of special magic, it is the one which gives the famed (and much used) water-divining rod, *virgula devinata*. Head bands of woven hazel twigs were put on farm and coach horses to protect them from ill-luck of all kinds, including theft and poison. Hazel sprigs nailed to cow-sheds guarded against fire and flood.

Use A general tonic. The foliage fed to milk animals increases their milk yield. The nuts fatten. Bark shavings are used to treat fevers.

HEATHER (*Erica* species. Ericaceae) A well-known plant of moorlands and mountain slopes, distinguished by minute bell flowers usually of purple or pink colour and possessing rich honey scent. Foliage is greyish and very small. Is associated with good spirits. Heather flowers, crushed finely and made into balls with honey, are used to dissolve bladder stones.

Use All the heathers are nerve and heart tonic. Heather flowers crushed finely and made into balls with honey, are used to dissolve bladder stones. Heather is also a remedy for stomach-ache. Scottish Highlanders use the flowers as a cough remedy, in a strong brew with honey. The flowers are also used to flavour beer. A good tonic for all animals, especially horses, goats and poultry. Cut and dried – dries easily – makes a good fodder for all animals.

Dose Several handfuls daily of the shoots, either in leaf or flower, chopped fine and mixed into bran.

HEDGE-MUSTARD (*Sisymbrium officinale.* Cruciferae) Found by hedges and waysides. Distinguished by its pale green toothed leaves, small yellow cross-form flowers, needle-thin leaves. The whole plant is biting hot and very tonic.

Use Tonic and digestive stimulant, and to curdle milk.

Dose A handful, cut up and mixed into bran.

HEMP-AGRIMONY (*Eupatorium cannabinum.* Compositae) A plant of moist places. Distinguished by its cylindrical reddish stems filled with a white pith and its corymbs of multitudes of rose-purple florets. It is named after King Eupator Mithrid-'ates, a herbalist, who discovered the healing powers of hemp-agrimony. The plant possesses a powerful scent. It is much famed for the curing of swollen feet in horses and cows, being used both internally and externally.

Use Treatments of all foot ailments, including swellings and rot. Also tumours, ulcers and jaundice.

Dose One handful of herb, twice daily. Finely cut and mixed with a mash of bran and molasses. Externally make a poultice by standard method: the mixing of hemp-agrimony with bran aids the curative powers of the poultice.

HERB-ROBERT (*Geranium robertianum.* Geraniaceae) This is a

plant of hedgerows, waysides and woodlands. Distinguished by its resemblance to garden geranium, and having the same powerful odour. It bears small, rose-coloured flowers. It is much liked by horses, goats and deer. This is a long-famed veterinary herb, for cure of internal haemorrhages in cattle, and red water ailment, also mastitis. It is a very important wound herb; also possesses insecticide properties. The whole plant is used. All geraniums are wound herbs and leaves of the garden geranium, with stalks removed, dipped in cold water and bound over wounds, have powerful healing powers.

Use Treatment of haemorrhage, kidney and bladder complaints, tuberculosis. Externally for wounds. Dried and powdered, it forms a useful insecticide. As a remedy for cure of scab and ringworm see the recipe given under Elder herb.

Dose Four plants given twice daily.

HOLLY (*Ilex aquifolium*. Aquifoliaceae) This is a hedgerow or woodland tree of small stature. Distinguished by its spiked leaves and white four-petalled blossoms which produce round berries of brilliant red. The berries are emetic and laxative. The leaves possess bone-knitting properties. The inner bark yields a sticky substance from which bird-lime is produced. This lime makes a good paste for applying to hard tumours; also for mixing into plaster casts for the binding of broken limbs. The leaves have to be scissor trimmed of their spiked edges. Planted by farms, protects against storms, fires, thieves and witches.

Use Treatment of limb fractures and breakages. Constipation and colic (the berries). Tumours, carbuncles, spavins.

Dose One handful of well-cut leaves brewed in one pint water. Give one cupful three times daily. Twelve berries make a good average laxative, or give relief in colic. Give twice daily in bran and molasses.

HOLLYHOCK (*Althea rosea*. Malvaceae) This is a well-known garden plant. It also grows wild in many parts of the world, the wild variety usually having a single pinkish flower. This plant is distinguished by its tall height, greyish foliage, and attractive mallow-shaped flowers of many colours, single and double.

It possesses powerful soothing properties, and in its medicinal powers is close to marshmallow of the same family. Goats graze its foliage eagerly. When boiled it becomes a useful worm remedy for children and animals, and is much used for this purpose by Bedouin Arabs. Boiled in wine it is given to prevent miscarriage when threatened. The flowers are also similar in medicinal virtues.

Use To soothe the digestive tract. Worm treatment. Female ailments, including miscarriage. Inflammation of mouth and throat.

Dose A handful of the leaves either brewed and given as a drench, or fed raw, chopped finely and mixed with cereals.

HONEYSUCKLE (*Lonicera periclymenum*. Caprifoliaceae) This is a hedgerow and woodland shrub of twining nature. Distinguished by its clusters of wonderfully fragrant honey-coloured flowers, which give bright red berries. Most animals eat its foliage, especially goats, the French name for this herb being goat's-foliage. The whole plant is medicinal. The flowers have heart tonic properties, and form an old English gypsy remedy for asthma when pounded and mixed with black treacle. The bruised leaves exert curative powers upon the skin. The bark is an aid in rheumatism and most joint ills. French gypsies use the inner part of the honeysuckle root as a conditioner and vermifuge for horses. They make balls of walnut size, with flour and fat, and give two daily.

Use Treatment of heart weakness, asthma, cough. Skin ailments, including ulcers and fistulas. Rheumatic complaints, paralysis, sprains. Worms.

Dose One handful of chopped leaves or flowers, mixed with bran, given once daily. A brew of two ounces of flaked bark to two pints of water. Give one cupful morning and night.

HOP (*Humulus lupulus*. Cannabinaceae) This is a climbing plant of rich, moist earth. It is named after 'rich earth' which it needs. Distinguished by its vine-like leaves and peculiar, green-yellow, scaly buds. The fruits, called 'strobiles' carry a yellow, resinous dust, called lupulin, giving the hop most of its medicinal properties. The young spring shoots of hops have much the delicate taste of asparagus. French and English gypsies eat quantities of 'hop-tops' and condition their young colts with them. The hop plant is famed for its tonic and nervine properties; it is also a pain reliever, sleep inducer and hypnotic. It is antiseptic and a vermifuge. Several handfuls of ripe hop flowers fed to cows daily in the heat of summer are a fine tonic and milk stimulant.

Use Treatment of all digestive ailments, general debility, failing appetite, wasting; fevers; eczema; all worms. Also fed mixed with fodder, to quieten restless animals. Externally the crushed flowers make a good plaster for giving pain relief and curing eczema. As a rub for congested lungs or general chills, steep a handful of hops in half a pint of hot vinegar or ale, then reheat and use hot.

Dose Five handfuls of hop flowers given once daily, early morning.

HOREHOUND (White) (*Marrubium vulgare*. Labiatae)   This is a plant of dry, waste places. Distinguished by its wrinkled, grey-green, somewhat woolly leaves, which exude a wine-like odour. The small white flowers encircle the stem in whorls. The plant possesses a peculiar anti-febrile principle – *marrubin*. It is one of the most important pectoral herbs, a famed cough and throat remedy. It is highly expectorant. The whole plant is used.

Use   Treatment of cough, pneumonia, pleurisy, bronchitis, tuberculosis, atrophy of the lungs. Ear disorders, canker. Diarrhoea, inflammation of the liver, jaundice. And externally mixed with powdered charcoal to cure bites of dogs and wolves.

Dose   Two handfuls of the herb made into a strong brew with 1½ pints water. Give one cupful morning and night, fasting.

HORSERADISH (*Armoracia rusticana*. Cruciferae)   Grows wild in waste places and is cultivated in gardens. It has rough leaves and a white or pink rootstock, with a stringy end. Its 'hot' properties make it valuable in expelling worms, stimulating appetite and as a general tonic. It is an internal antiseptic. It helps to remove excess urine from the system and stones from the bladder. It is a warming plant, good to feed to animals in cold weather. All parts, root, leaves and flowers are used. The freshly taken and grated root has the most powerful effects.

Use   Worm and kidney treatment. To reduce tumours including cancerous ones: used internally and externally. To remedy lack of appetite, and overthinness. Externally as a poultice for swellings.

Dose   One or two roots, grated and mixed with bran, given

twice daily, or the grated roots stirred into hot water. One
heaped teaspoon to a half cup water.

HORSETAIL (*Equisetum arvense.* Equisetaceae) This is a herb
of roadsides and waste ground. Distinguished by its
resemblance to a horse's tail. The stems are hollow-jointed
and the leaves reduced to mere scales at the points. The plant
bears no flowers, but produces brown spores from the fertile
stem. The goat eats the plant but it is not a good food for
cows. It is highly medicinal. It is an old-fashioned scourer for
milk-pails and other dairy implements, having the action of
emery paper owing to its high silica content. It is still in
general use with gypsies for such purposes. It disinfects as it
cleanses. Horsetail has manifold medicinal uses. It is, however, foremost a wound herb.

Use Treatment of nasal haemorrhage, laryngitis, ear pains
(externally). Intestinal ulcer, Hodgkin's disease, inflammation of the uterus, vagina, bladder. To cure internal wounds
of the bowels, dysentery, enlarged anal glands. Obesity,
dropsy; and in a strong brew to dissolve stones in bladder.

Dose This is a potent herb. Make a half-handful of herb into
a brew with 1½ pints water. Give one small cupful twice
daily. Externally: gently heat several handfuls of the herb,
well dissolve in a pint of vinegar, and apply. For wounds
dilute with two parts of raw milk.

HOUND'S-TONGUE (*Cynoglossum officinale.* Boraginaceae) A
plant of sunny places, roadsides, banks and open wasteland.
Distinguished by its rough, tongue-shaped leaves, which
give this plant its name, and by bugle-shaped flowers of
blue-purple or pink. All animals enjoy honey-rich flowers: a
bee favourite. A tonic and general nervine herb. Externally
for wounds.

Dose   A handful of whole plant daily.

HOUSELEEK (*Sempervivum tectorum.* Crassulaceae)   This is a plant of old walls, house-tops, rubble heaps. Distinguished by its habitat on buildings, its rosettes of fleshy, green leaves and spikes of rosy, starry flowers. Goats and sheep eat this herb. Its use is mainly external, being very powerful as a remedy against bruises and chronic ulcers. Also used as a remedy for stings, itching skin and warts. Treatment of burns. It is valuable in the treatment of weak and fading sight. The foliage, well pounded, and made into pills with flour and grease, is a vermifuge.

Dose   Externally: one handful of the plant brewed in 1½ pints water, applied as a lotion. The plant can also be applied on flannel, pulped up, raw, as a poultice. For worm pills, two balls of the pulped plant, the size of beans, given before the morning feed.

HYDRANGEA (*Hydrangea arborescens.* Hydrangeaceae)   A shrub of woodlands and banks of streams. Also much cultivated in gardens. Ovate leaves with serrated edges. Flowers are conspicuous, borne in large, flat clusters, white, blue or pinkish. The stem bark peels freely, reputedly in seven successive layers, giving the shrub its further common name of seven barks. It was a favourite remedy of American Cherokee Indians. It is a mild and soothing remedy for urinary ailments, rheumatism and dropsy.

Use   Treatment of bladder and kidney ailments, for removal of stones, rheumatism, arthritis, dropsy.

Dose   One handful of leaves twice daily.

HYSSOP (*Hyssopus officinalis.* Labiatae)   This is a hill-loving plant, of shrub type. Distinguished by its beauty and fragrance, the long leaves being highly aromatic. The hooded flowers are pale blue, growing in the axils of the higher foliage. Hyssop is a very ancient herb, having been celebrated in the Bible. It is an important plant in pectoral complaints, because it both removes mucus accumulations and also tones up the membranes and fortifies the whole system. It possesses mild vermifugal powers, and is used much in the Nordic countries as a vermifuge for delicate lambs and kids. It is a cure for inflamed and blood-suffused eyes.

Use Treatment of cough, sore throat, pneumonia, pleurisy, tuberculosis; worms. Eye disorders, conjunctivitis.

Dose Two handfuls of the herb given twice daily in bran. Externally for eye treatment, a handful of herb is well bruised, then tied in muslin, the whole is then dipped in hot water, submerged several minutes, then applied to the eyes in a form of eye poultice.

ICELAND MOSS (*Cetraria icelandica*) This plant is a native of Britain and northern countries of Europe, and naturally of Iceland. It grows from two to four inches high and is usually brownish or greyish of colour although sometimes also of a red shade. This lichen plant is dry and cartilaginous and dries up into a grey-white powder. It swells up when put into water and when boiled and cooled it becomes a fine jelly. This plant is immensely life-giving and nutritious and will sustain life where little else grows. It is a favourite with reindeer. It contains a special substance called *cetrarin*, which is highly tonic.

Use To remedy malnutrition, rickets, tuberculosis, bronchitis.

Dose One teaspoonful stirred into one large cup of boiling water. Or a half cup of water can be used and then a further half cup of milk added when the mixture has cooled to tepid. For young animals add honey or molasses.

IVY (*Hedera helix*. Araliaceae) This is a well-known evergreen climbing plant. Distinguished by its peculiarly shaped leaves, small, honey-coloured, sticky flowers, which develop into succulent black berries of pea size. The berries are a famed cure for fevers; they are also used to induce perspiration. They possess mild purgative and emetic properties. They are an excellent tonic for poultry. The leaves are a valuable external aid for poulticing enlarged glands. Sheep, goats and deer eat ivy greedily. The Greek peasants say that the woodland gods gave the ivy to the animals to guard them against starvation in times of heavy snow. Many people have the belief that ivy is a totally poisonous herb – all parts. But one has only to observe how the bees crowd to its flowers, and the birds to the berries, and how animals seek out its leaves, to discredit this idea. I think that the name of that dangerous plant poison ivy, which is not of the same plant family as true ivy at all – indeed a totally alien plant – gave the poison belief to common ivy. Overeating of true ivy, however, will cause discomfort and sickness. This is especially true when ewes are pregnant. Ivy is one of the best herbs for complete internal cleansing after birth. Feed one handful to sheep and goats immediately after giving birth. Larger quantities for cows and mares. In treatment of retained afterbirth make a strong brew, one handful leaves to one pint water. Give half-pint drenches every three hours. Use ivy brew also in difficult birth, same dose; fortify with southernwood. This has saved many animals from birthing loss.

Use Treatment of all fevers. Loss of appetite, dropsy, constipation. Inflamed joints, enlarged glands, chilblains, birth.

Dose Two tablespoonfuls of fresh leaves finely cut and mixed into bran, or brewed in 1½ pints water, two dessertspoonfuls honey added. Give one small cupful daily. Externally: make a standard poultice from the bruised leaves and berries. Interesting and effective ivy treatment for warts and horny growths, is a pulp of fresh ivy leaves packed over the area and bound with strips of cloth soaked in vine sap.

JUNIPER (*Juniperus communis*. Cupressaceae) This is a medium-sized evergreen shrub, liking chalky districts. Distinguished by its red woody stems, dark-hued needle leaves and the blue-black berries that it bears. This shrub is considered as a blessing to the world. The young shoots are very beneficial to animals, and are sought by horses, goats, sheep and deer. The whole plant is tonic and a nerve stimulant. The bark and berries are used. From the interior reddish wood of trunk and branches, healing juniper 'tar' is made. Oil of juniper (called oil of cades in the Balearic Islands, where it is much used for animal injuries of all kinds) is made by heat-infusing one large handful of berries, crushed in a half litre of pure olive oil.

Use The bark: treatment of inflamed liver and kidney, gallstones, jaundice and obesity. Sciatica and rheumatism. The berries: blood ailments, acid milk, malaria, and miscarriage.

Dose Two ounces of flaked bark given in bran and molasses, once daily, early morning. A small handful of berries, fresh or dried (less if dried) made into a paste with molasses and bran, given morning and night. An old treatment for miscarriage in cows.

External, for fumigation of farm buildings, dog kennels, etc. Damp branches are burnt slowly and will overcome or drive out insect pests, rodents, weasels. The pungent fumes are especially used against mosquitoes; used also indoors in farmhouses.

KNAPWEED or BLACK KNAPWEED (*Centaurea nigra*. Compositae) This is a field and wayside plant. Distinguished by its narrow, greyish foliage and hard heads of dark purple flowers of thistle form. The plant is as valuable as gentian for its tonic properties and its curative powers in all digestive disorders. The flowers are used.

Use Treatment of dysentery, gastritis, sour stomach, failing appetite. To arrest all bleedings from nose, mouth and internal haemorrhages. Swollen neck glands. Bruises and running sores, wounds. Gypsies extol its use in treatment of glanders in horses.

Dose Two handfuls of flower heads fed daily. For external use make a brew of one handful of flowers to one pint water and add two dessertspoonfuls of vinegar.

KNOT-GRASS (*Polygonium aviculare*. Polygonaceae) This plant grows in waste places and likes damp areas. It is distinguished by its jointed and loosely knotted and wiry stems, often reclining on the ground at the base, its small, fleshy leaves and small pinkish flowers. The whole plant is cooling and is used externally for abrasions, wounds, inflamed skin and ear ailments. It also has a veterinary use in diarrhoea as it is very binding. Its botanical name is derived from *aves*, birds, likely because birds are known to eat pieces of the stems of this herb to harden their droppings. Peasants then adapted the birds' example and fed knot-grass to farm animals and poultry when they had loose bowels and dysentery.

Use A small handful daily of the whole plant mixed into the food. External, for treatment of ailments and skin and ears, particularly for running ears. For ears make a standard lotion of the herb and drop a teaspoon of this into each ear.

Massage gently, then dry out with dampened cotton wool wound around tweezers.

Dose A handful daily, mixed into the feed. Also a handful of the finely cut herb brewed in one cupful of water. Externally as a raw pulp for massage into enlarged veins.

LADY'S BED-STRAW (see BED-STRAW)

LADY'S-MANTLE (*Alchemilla vulgaris*. Rosaceae) This is a plant of moist pastures and woods. Distinguished by the cloak-like shape and pleatings of its leaves, which have given the plant its name of lady's-mantle. The flowers are numerous, minute, yellow, borne in corymbs at the tips of the stems. The dew which gathers in the leaf folds is a rare eye remedy. The real name of the plant is Arabic – *alkemelych*, from the alchemists, forebears of the chemists. The herb is greatly esteemed by Arab herbalists and herdsmen. Horses, goats and sheep seek out the herb. The plant is tonic, an important fortifier of the blood and the walls of the arteries. It is an old herbal remedy for diabetes.

Alchemilla arvensis is also known as parsley peart. It is famed among gypsies for curing stone, and as an after-tonic in the treatment of colic. The herb taken on Midsummer's Eve, was said to give invisibility to man and animal.

Use Treatment of lack of appetite, wasting. Weak blood, sluggish blood, all weaknesses of the arteries. Heart disease, diabetes. Taken from one period to the other it is reputed to aid conception in barren animals.

Dose Two handfuls twice daily.

LAMB'S-QUARTERS (*Chenopodium album*. Chenopodaceae) A herb of waste places and pastures of rather poor soil.

Distinguished by its grey-green leaves, toothed at tips, with pale, silvery undersides, giving the name *album*, from white, also giving a dusty look. Flowers are in small, crowded spikes resembling clusters of small balls. On good ground the herb can grow many feet tall. The whole plant is acrid and bitter, but nevertheless is an esteemed salad herb.

This is a plant of many country names, signifying its beneficial effect on creatures which eat of it, in addition to lambs: it is called also fat-hen, fat-goose, hog's delight, pigweed.

Use As a pasture tonic herb. Improves the digestion and is a great tonic for the whole digestive system. An anaemia remedy.

Dose The whole plant cut up small and given in bran, several handfuls daily.

LAUREL (*Laurus nobilis*. Lauraceae) This evergreen bush and small tree is a native of Asia Minor, but found in many lands as a garden shrub. Its leaves are oval and shiny, sometimes speckled with yellow. Laurel leaves are much used by peasants to flavour food. It is an important stomach remedy, aromatic, warming, tonic and stimulating for the digestive juices. Good for horses prone to colic. Laurel is astringent and therefore good in dropsical conditions. Its pulped leaves are a remedy for treatment of burns and swellings. A laurel wreath was always associated with victory, and heroes were crowned with laurel. It was also used in dairy shows to crown winning cattle.

Use Stomach tonic, treatment of ailments of digestion. To remedy lack of appetite. Externally for burns, swellings, bruises, soft tumours and as a good-tasting preservative for olives and pickles. Packed around dried figs to protect them from moths.

Dose Six leaves twice daily. Externally: a handful of the leaves, pulped and warmed over hot water.

LAVENDER (*Lavandula vera.* Labiatae) This is a plant of sandy soil. It is distinguished by its shrubby growth, grey, fine-leaved foliage, and spikes of blue, very fragrant flowers. The whole plant is a powerful fortifier and nerve tonic. It is eaten eagerly by sheep and goats on the Mediterranean mountains where the plant abounds; it gives a sweet flavour to the milk and cheese, and prevents rapid souring of the milk, lavender being antiseptic. The whole plant is used, but especially the flowers, which yield a valuable oil, stimulating and warming.

Use Treatment of vomiting, faintness, sunstroke, headache. All nervous ailments, including paralysis. As a douche for all female ailments. A lotion for foul mouths and loose teeth. Add leaves to food, to make it more palatable.

Dose Two handfuls of herb brewed in 1½ pints water. Give one cupful three times daily. External: make a similar brew, using the flowers only. Pack dried fruit between layers of lavender leaves to protect the fruits from destructive moths and weevils. Rub teeth and gums with lavender sprigs to clean them.

LEMON (*Citrus limonum.* Rutaceae) The lemon tree, notable for its sweet-scented blossom and popular lemon fruits, is too well known to need description. It originated in Eastern Asia, but its cultivation is now widespread and its fruits are available world wide. The lemon fruit has extraordinary healing powers, it is also one of the most efficient blood-cleansers available to man and animals. During the internal cleansing fast, an essential part of many disease treatments, there is nothing better to give man or animal for drink, than diluted lemon juice, two teaspoons lemon juice to a small cup of water.

Use The fruit: to cleanse the system of mucus and to cool the blood. To heal sore throats and internal ulcers. Treatment of diarrhoea, eczema, all fevers, diabetes, worms. The leaves can also be used for all these purposes but are much milder and less effective in action. The seeds, crushed in honey, are a mild vermifuge for young animals, one tablespoon given early every morning. Externally: to cleanse sores (the raw juice), abscesses (ditto), toothache (ditto), discharging ears (ditto), ringworm (ditto), mange (juice and peel of the fruit): see Mange treatment (dog section), and as a general poultice (the leaves). Very diluted lemon juice, a quarter teaspoon to a cup of tepid water is a good general eye treatment. For discharging ears a half teaspoon raw juice to one and half teaspoons tepid water. In fevers sweeten with honey.

LETTUCE (*Lactuca sativa*. Compositae) A well-known garden salad vegetable. Its medicinal property is in its white, sticky juice, present in stem and leaves and in the upper root. The juice is a sedative. The whole plant is a milk stimulant, and therefore increases lactation, and is much enjoyed by all animals. The seeds are a tonic poultry and bird food.

Dose The whole plant in quantity, as available.

LILY-OF-THE-VALLEY (*Convallaris majalis*. Liliaceae) A woodland plant. Distinguished by its oval leaves, from a brace of which comes the flowering stem of white, waxen, bell-like flowers possessing exquisite scent which gain for this lily the lovely name of 'Tears of the Virgin Mary'. The plant is eaten by goats and sheep. It is a supreme heart herb, far more important than the digitalis-yielding fox glove, the lily-of-the-valley being also a safe herb, unlike the fox-glove, which, unless used with care, can have some danger-ous effects. All parts of this remarkable plant are medicinal, although the flower is the most potent and celebrated part. The flower is used for all heart disorders; bringing quietness to the heart as well as improving its condition. Gently nar-cotic, it is useful in all fits, including epilepsy, also for hys-terical conditions. The leaves cool skin inflammation. The fruits cure fevers and have vermifuge properties. The roots soothe the bowels and are mildly aperient.

Use Treatment of cardiac debility, all valvular heart ail-ments, high blood-pressure, rapid pulse. Dropsy and all lymph irregularities. Skin eruptions, bruises and sprains. Mild fevers. Round and thread worms. Inflamed bowels, constipation, piles.

Dose Two handfuls of flowers in a brew of 1½ pints water; add one tablespoonful honey. Give one cupful morning and night, fasting. Or use two small roots to 1½ pints water. Do not overdose with this lily because it is a strong herb.

LIQUORICE (*Glycyrrhiza glabra.* Leguminosae) Also spelt licorice. This plant grows wild in many parts of Europe. It is also largely cultivated as a medicinal and nutritive plant. It is distinguished by its perennial nature, woody roots, pale green laburnum-like foliage and pea-like flowers of pale blue. This is rightly one of the world's most famous herbs. It is praised by all of the ancient great herbalists, such as Hip-pocrates, Avicenna, Paracelsus. The root is the part used, possessing unique pectoral and emollient properties; it is also nutritive and slightly laxative. It has been found to contain important female sex hormones. Either the whole root is employed, or the extracted solidified juice, obtained in black sticks. The root, finely powdered, is much used by the Arabs to sprinkle over discharging parts of the skin, to disinfect and also absorb the watery fluid.

Use Treatment of cough, inflamed throat, pneumonia, pleurisy, tuberculosis, and all catarrhal conditions. Gallstones, chronic constipation, mild worms in young animals. Female infertility. Also to still the pains of colic. External use: skin ailments. Also the steeped (i.e. softened in hot water) leaves are applied to the ears when there is sign of pain (earache). The Red Indians make a poultice for use on sore backs of horses, by first chewing the leaves to a pulp and then applying them warm from the mouth to the sore places and binding into position.

Dose The solid juice is the most practical form for veterinary medicine. Give two to four inches of stick, dissolved in halfpint milk-water, morning and night.

LIME (*Tilia x europaea*. Tiliaceae) This is a parkland tree. It is distinguished by its abundance of yellow-green, bracted blossoms of sweet and pungent fragrance. The flowers yield a volatile oil, sugar, a large amount of gum, chlorophyll and tannin. They possess powerful nervine and blood-cleansing properties. Lime blossom is a famed treatment for fits and nervous twitchings of all kinds, including epilepsy. In Spain I met with epileptic horses and they got nosebags of lime blossom and foliage. Linden blossom is a great tonic for bees, and lime trees should be planted by apiarists. The foliage is eaten with avidity by all animals, and in France the foliage is often dried like hay and stored as winter feed. The whole tree is very rich in mucilage, especially the inner bark, which is employed as a liniment to reduce inflamed areas, swellings and soft tumours. The leaves are also medicinal.

Use Treatment of all nervous ailments, especially epilepsy, twitchings, vertigo. Good for colds and to remove slime and mucus from the system. Treatment of vomiting, heart pains, fevers. To soothe inflamed eyes and as a gargle for sore throats. Treatment of tumours by poultice.

Dose Two handfuls of the flowers fed twice daily, or leaves. Externally: make a brew from flower and/or the inner bark.

LOBELIA (*Lobelia inflata*. Campanulaceae) This is a field plant, native mainly to North America. Distinguished by its racemes of brilliant blue flowers, one of its names being blue cardinal flower. This is one of the most important herbs of the Red Indian herbalist, and is one of the most remarkable of all herbs, sharing with garlic the powers of being able to cure nearly every ailment which afflicts the human and animal body. It is a famed remedy for all chest ailments, for removal of obstructions in all organs and tissues. One species, *Lobelia syphilitica*, is used by the Canadian Indians in the treatment of all types of venereal disease in man and animals, very successful results being obtained. The foliage and the seeds are used generally, but in venereal disease a decoction of the roots is employed.

Use Treatment of pneumonia, pleurisy, bronchitis, asthma. Liver, bladder and stomach inflammations or obstructions. Venereal diseases. Externally as a poultice or lotion for all inflammations, swellings, ulcers and running sores.

Dose Two handfuls of the herb brewed in 1½ pints water. Add two dessertspoonfuls honey. Give one cupful morning and night, fasting. External use: apply the brew without the honey or make a standard poultice. The roots: four to six roots are sliced and boiled for two hours in one quart water, give half a pint dose twice daily in venereal ailments; also use the brew externally, as a douche, once daily.

LUISA HERB (*Lippia citriodora*. Verbenaceae)   Also known as reina Luisa. A garden herb, given the name of 'royal' in many lands because it is so beloved and valued. Luisa often reaches shrub proportions and is frequently trained as a climber to give fragrant shade as well as medicine. Leaves are narrow and of dark green or greyish hues, dotted with glands which give Luisa its special fragrance, which rather resembles lemon and has given this herb its botanical name of *citri* from citrus, but the odour is sweeter and more pungent and penetrating. Luisa is certainly a favourite of mine and I make much use of it. The flowers are insignificant, greyish silver, borne in slender spikes. It is also known as lemon verbena.

Luisa is used as a peasant medicine to provide a nerve-calming and sleep-encouraging tea, also as a digestive aid and tonic. In the Balearic Islands it is an official veterinary remedy against digestive ailments in animals of all kinds, and to soothe colic.

Use   General tonic, nerve remedy, also cure of nerve spasms.

Dose   One handful fresh herbs, less when dried.

MAIDENHAIR FERN (*Adiantum capillus veneris*. Filices)   A fern of moist woodlands and rocky places. Distinguished by its frail appearance, fine shining stems and tiny, fan-shaped leaves which shimmer in the wind and always remain very dry. It is eaten by animals. It is of value as a hair tonic and strengthener, both internal and external use, and it is employed by the Turkish peasants for producing high quality hair in mohair goats. It has useful lung-cleansing properties and is further tonic, and cheering to the temperament. It is most soothing for sore throats and in treatment of coughs.

Use   For loss of hair or poor hair. Chest ailments, coughs.

Dose One handful of the fern fed twice daily mixed with bran and molasses. Or make the leaves into a sweet brew with honey, one handful of leaves to one pint water. Give two tablespoons three times daily. Externally: standard brew used as friction.

MALLOW (MARSH) (*Althea officinalis.* Malvaceae) A plant of waste places, but especially common on sea marshes. Distinguished by its greyish foliage, mauve-coloured, red-veined flowers. The whole plant order of the Mallows is one of the most benevolent known to the herbalist, and their growth should be encouraged on all farms. The foliage of the mallow is eaten by all animals. The roots are the part most used in internal medicine, but externally the flowers, stems and foliage are all used. The leaves also heal internally, especially inflammation of stomach and bowels. The leaves are eaten raw in quantities as a blood-cooling salad, by Bedouin Arabs and others. The root contains a quantity of gummy matter, starch, asparagin, albumen, crystallizable sugar and a fixed oil. It contains over half of its weight in a sweet-tasting mucilage, which gives the plant its well-justified fame, the mucilage possessing unique properties of lubricating, soothing and healing. The fresh-gathered roots, crushed or pulverized, make an important poultice for relief of all inflammatory conditions and are an acclaimed prevention of mortification, one ancient name for mallow being mortification plant. The stalks and leaves make an important ointment for all skin rashes, inflamed surfaces, abrasions, bruises; (for recipe see Adder's tongue). Gypsy herbalists chew the stalks to a pulp, mixing very well with their saliva; the pulp is then applied warm from the mouth to inflamed and sore areas.

Use Treatment of sore throats, pulmonary catarrhs, pleurisy. Diarrhoea, dysentery, bowel inflammations and haemorrhage. Externally: all skin eruptions, abrasions, swellings, inflammations, bruises. Sore or inflamed udders. All eye ailments. Internally and externally in venereal ailments. Externally fresh leaves, pulped, bound over bruises and sprains of all kinds.

Dose Three to four sliced roots boiled for one hour in two pints of water. Add two tablespoonfuls honey, raisins and a half dozen cloves. Give one large cupful three times daily. Use also externally, without the honey. The pulped leaves and blossoms, slightly heated, make an excellent rubbing lotion and application for external injuries. The roots, fresh or dried, make good fodder for they are soothing and nutritious. I use mallow root in my gruel for feeding young (and sick) animals.

MAIZE (Sweet-corn, Indian-corn) (see Corn)

MANDRAKE (*Podophyllum peltatum*. Berberidaceae) This plant is famed for its root which is supposed to possess magical properties and to scream when pulled from the ground. But apart from this the root is highly medicinal and greatly esteemed by the American Indians who make much use of it for themselves and their animals. The plant has yellowish-green leaves and solitary, large, white, flowers, of quite fragrant scent, borne in forks of the stem. The fruits are known as may apples and are lemon colour and fleshy. The medicinal part is the root which yields a substance known as podophyllin which has powerful effects upon the liver. The root is jointed and dark brown and grows in peculiar shapes. Time for collection of root is soon after the fruits have ripened.

Use Constipation (this herb acts upon the bowels without causing later constiveness, a fault of many laxatives), worm remedy, liver ailments, jaundice, liver fluke.

Dose One teaspoon of the root cut small to three-quarter pint of water. Give one tablespoon three times daily.

MARIGOLD (*Calendula officinalis*. Compositae) This is a plant of cultivated fields, especially vineyards. Distinguished by its brilliant golden, aromatic, marguerite-like flowers. A 'Herb of the sun', possessing important medicinal properties. Goats and sheep seek it out. The flowers are tonic and a good heart medicine. They possess important restorative powers over the arteries and veins, and thus are much fed by the Arabs to their racing horses. The flowers are fed also to make miserable and fretting animals cheerful. The whole plant is useful in inducing perspiration. The leaves are useful in treatment of warts and to reduce tumours. Both the flowers and leaves contain mucilage.

Use Treatment of vomiting, internal ulcers, fevers. All ailments of arteries and veins, heart diseases. All skin ailments, eczema, warts.

Dose Three handfuls of flowers, mixed into bran, twice daily. For external use make a strong brew of the flowers. For warts use the raw leaves. An excellent healing lotion or cream, can be made: (lotion) by boiling finely cut flowers and leaves in milk; (cream) by placing finely cut leaves or flowers in melted cold cream or mixing into ordinary milk cream or unsalted butter. Marigold flowers soaked in vinegar, and applied, take the pain and swelling from stings, especially bee and wasp.

MARJORAM (*Origanum onites*. Labiatae) This is a plant of sunny slopes and dry, sandy earth. Distinguished by its panicled spike-heads of purple-rose flowers, very honey-sweet. The whole plant is highly aromatic: marjoram – 'joy of the mountain', being the translation of its name. The plant possesses an aromatic oil. It is well liked by goats and sheep, and imparts a sweet taste to their milk. The whole plant is highly tonic, nervine and blood purifying. A British species, *O. vulgaris*, has much the same properties and can be used. Marjoram has the enviable reputation among the herbs of curing all aches and pains.

Use Treatment of digestive ailments, especially flatulence, colic, catarrh of the stomach, obstructions. Nervous ailments, hysteria. Fevers. Externally: wounds and tumours.

Dose Four handfuls of the herb fed twice daily in bran mash. Externally: cut finely, place in linen bag, infuse in hot wine, and then apply to inflamed areas, swollen glands, wounds and tumours: a Spanish gypsy remedy.

MEADOWSWEET (*Filipendula ulmaria*. Rosaceae) This is a plant of damp places and ditch sides. Distinguished by its rose-like leaves, plumes of creamy flowers of rare and lovely scent. An important fever and diarrhoea herb. Much used by gypsies as a spring tonic for their animals including their lurcher dogs. Eaten plentifully by goats and sheep. The flowers are used.

Use Treatment of fevers, blood disorders, diarrhoea, dropsy.

Dose Two handfuls of flowers cut up small and mixed with food, or brewed in two pints water. Add two dessertspoonfuls honey. Give one cupful, morning and night, fasting.

MELILOT or YELLOW MELILOT (*Melilotus officinalis*. Leguminosae) This is a plant of pastureland. Distinguished by its pea-like trefoil foliage, and spikes of pea-like, creamy yellow flowers of sweet scent. The whole plant is highly scented, smelling like new-mown hay. Melilotic acid is found in the flowers. This is an important milk maker also a tonic herb, and anti-colic. It is liked by animals and should be encouraged in all pastures. It is used as an enema in colic of cows and horses. The macerated flowers and seeds of this plant are used to flavour Gruyère cheeses. The whole herb is used. Blue melilot (curd herb) is a well-known milk producer much used by the Arabs. The seed is the most potent part. Melilot, all types, should be planted widely as a fodder plant.

Use Treatment of colic and most stomach and intestinal disorders; flatulence, swelling. Externally as a poultice for aching and bruised areas; skin disease, also as an eye salve (mixed with honey).

Dose Two handfuls of herb given three times daily. In enemata: one handful of herb brewed in two pints water. A melilot plaster, of much use in chronic eczema: one handful melilot pounded into two ounces each of beeswax and resin and one ounce olive oil.

MILKWORT (*Polygala vulgaris.* Polygalaceae) This is a tiny plant of heaths and sandy meadows. Distinguished by its small stature, small narrow leaves, and flat flowers of pale or dark blue. The plant has long been famed for its powers in giving increased milk flow in animals. It should be in every pasture. In North Africa peasants cultivate patches as fodder for their cows and goats. The plant is mildly laxative. It removes mucus accumulations from the pectoral regions and digestive tract.

Use To increase milk yield. Treatment of catarrh ailments.

Dose Four handfuls daily, fed with cereals at milking times, twice or thrice daily.

MINT (*Mentha aquatica*. Labiatae) This is a plant of moist places. Distinguished by its hairy foliage and terminal spikes of pale purple flowers. The whole plant is highly aromatic and possesses the peculiar mint scent due to menthol in the foliage. This is an important herb. As wild water-mint it grows widely alongside ditches; all grazing animals should be given access to it. It is one of the supreme herbal tonics and digestive aids. It is an important aphrodisiac tonic for male animals, especially effective for bulls and stallions. Its only negative quality as an agricultural herb is that if eaten in large amounts it decreases the milk flow. Recognizing that quality in mint, the Arabs use it freely to dry off animals before the latter months of pregnancy. It has been observed that new milk into which the finely cut leaves of mint are introduced curdles far more slowly than untreated milk. Other important forms of mint are: *Mentha piperita* (peppermint), *Mentha rotundi* (apple mint), and *Mentha arvensis* (the wild corn mint). The mints are strewing herbs, giving healthful scents when strewn and trodden on floors of farm buildings and stables of favoured animals.

Use Treatment of all head pains, gastritis, hyperacidity, flatulence, vomiting, colic. Inflammation of the liver, stricture of the rectum. Abscess, asthma, udder ailments, including too free flow of milk for fertility. Dried mint tea to cure diarrhoea: a little brandy may be added, half teaspoon to cup of tea. Externally: a rub for rheumatic and arthritic pains.

Dose Two handfuls fed twice daily. In udder treatment feed at milking time. Externally: pulp several handfuls of the herb, heat gently for a few minutes, add one to two tablespoonfuls of vinegar; rub well into the pain areas.

MISTLETOE (*Viscum album*. Loranthaceae) This is a parasitical plant of woodlands. Distinguished by its yellowish horse-shoe leaves, and round, white berries, which are very viscid. Herbalists understand that the medicinal properties of mistletoe differ with the host tree on which it is parasitical. Mistletoe taken from thorn trees is the most potent medicinally. Sheep seek out the foliage of mistletoe and shepherds believe that it gives the animals protection against rot. The berries are a famed herbal epilepsy cure.

Use Treatment of nervous ailments, epilepsy, hysteria, chorea. Uterine and vaginal haemorrhages. Joint ailments.

Dose Six berries, pounded into half a pint of milk, twice daily, given in a bran mash. Externally: as a rubbing, emollient agent, for stiff or inflamed joints.

MOTHERWORT (*Leonurus cardiaca.* Labiatae) Found on wastelands, waysides and hedgerows. Distinguished by its tubed leaves, whorls of whitish pink tinged flowers, with toothed calyx. The plant is named after the tail of a lion which shape it sometimes resembles. The toothed quality of the calyx necessitates this plant being used only as a strained brew. Motherwort is considered a life-giving plant, beneficial for all female disorders. Also a general heart tonic. A sacred herb of ancient China because of its healing powers.

Dose A cupful of standard brew (strained) twice daily.

MOUNTAIN FLAX or CATHARTIC FLAX (*Linum cartharticum.* Linaceae) A plant of meadows and pastures, preferring chalk soils. Distinguished by its tiny size, spidery form and diminutive, starry, white flowers. It is an important laxative, being very similar to senna in its purging powers without any of the griping properties of that herb. It is known as purging flax, and is much sought by animals for that purpose. The plant should be introduced into all pastures for the grazing animals to avail themselves of it as they desire. The whole plant is used.

Use Treatment of constipation, piles, catarrh of bowels. Worms, dropsy.

Dose Two to four handfuls of herb 1½ pints water, two dessertspoons of honey added. Early morning, fasting (before meal).

MOUSE EAR (*Gnaphalium uliginosum.* Compositae) This is a plant of dry pastures. Its greyish leaves have a silky hair over them and in shape resemble the ears of a mouse. Flowers are round, composite and whitish: sometimes yellow. The whole herb is used, it promotes sweating, also is a remedy for bladder and kidney ailments. Also known as marsh cudweed.

Use Treatment of fevers, rheumatic ailments. Urinary ailments.

MULBERRY (*Morus alba, nigra, rubra,* Moraceae) A well-known fruit tree, distinguished by its big and shiny leaves, a principal food of silkworms, and by its fleshy, juicy, many-seeded and pendulous fruits of a rich purple colour or whitish-green. The fruits and bark are medicinal being very blood-cooling, cleansing and tonic; likewise the young shoots.

Use Treatment of worms, blood disorders, infections of mouth and throat, swollen glands, also as a laxative.

Dose Several handfuls of the fruit twice daily. Or one dessertspoon of the cut bark, grated finely and mixed with bran. (As a dye.) Mulberry fruits yield a useful, fast-holding dye. The white fruits yield a brown stain, the dark fruits a red-purple colour.

MULLEIN (*Verbascum thapsus*. Scrophulariaceae) This is a plant of dry places, banks and waste ground. Distinguished by its tall shape, very downy grey leaves, spike-form racemes of yellow, rose-like flowers. The herb is famed for its powers in pulmonary ailments, being much used in lung ailments of cattle, one of its names being cow lungwort. The powdered roots are used to fatten poultry. The whole plant is used, but the flowers must be stored in tin canisters because they turn black if exposed to light. The down from the soft leaves of mullein can be scraped off and compressed for use as wicks in candles and lamps. Another name for this plant being candlewick, from such use in farmhouses of former times.

Use Treatment of cough, pneumonia, pleurisy, bronchitis, tuberculosis, asthma. Diarrhoea, internal bleedings of the bowels and lungs. Externally as a poultice for neuralgia pains and cramps: the downy leaves especially are used.

Dose One handful brewed in 1½ pints water. Give morning and night. Externally: make a standard poultice.

MUSTARD (Black) (*Brassica nigra*. Cruciferae) This is a plant of pastures and wasteground. Distinguished by its bitter-tasting cress-like leaves and seeds, and racemes of bright yellow flowers. Animals eat the herb and it is an important tonic. It also possesses disinfectant properties both for the animal body and the earth itself. The plant promotes appetite, stimulates salivation and excretion of the digestive juices. Its seeds provide a useful worm expellant. Also when chewed are a toothache remedy. It is one of the most important of all poultice and plaster herbs. Its property as an external agent is irritant and excitant, making it valuable in the treatment of paralysis and pectoral complaints. (*Sinapis alba*, the white mustard, is of similar value. *S. arvensis*, charlock, of lesser merit.)

Use Treatment of poor appetite, flatulence, emaciation, poisoning. Externally: it is used as a poultice or as a rubbing remedy (the latter with or without vinegar) to relieve internal inflammations, paralysis, arthritis, rheumatic pains and all pectoral ailments, toothache and chilblains.

Dose Four handfuls of the whole plant or two handfuls of the seed, given in bran mash, add two dessertspoonfuls molasses, twice daily. Externally: make a hot poultice with mustard flour, or make a lotion with mustard flour and rub into the affected areas. Vinegar can be added.

NASTURTIUM (*Tropaeolum majus*. Tropaeolaceae) This is a well-known garden annual, notable for its running or climbing habits, its brilliant green umbrella-shaped leaves, its brightly coloured, spurred flowers. The whole plant has a hot, biting character, especially the seeds which were once a popular pickle. Animals eat the whole plant greedily. It is richly medicinal, being strongly antiseptic, highly tonic, cleansing and vermifuge – especially the seeds, which should be collected and fed to poultry for this purpose. The seeds can be preserved in vinegar to provide a tonic and anti-worm remedy. Crushed fresh leaves, sprinkled with salt, for treatment of tumours external.

Use General antiseptic, tonic, appetizer, for nervous ailments, depression, poor sight. A fertility herb. Treatment of all worms. Externally: a poultice of the seeds crushed and placed on flannel wrung out in boiling water, applied to abscess, old sores.

Dose Several handfuls of the leaves, fed daily. For worms, one dessertspoon of the seeds.

NETTLE, BLIND (*Lamium album*. Labiatae) This plant, commonly known also as stingless nettle and white nettle, is a common weed of woodlands, waste places and gardens. Its leaves resemble common nettle but are more hairy. The flowers are creamy and in whorls. Also known as dead-nettle.

Use To stem copious bleeding; also an important vaginal douche.

Dose The whole plant steeped as a brew, one handful to one large cup of water. Applied externally to wounds and internally as a douche.

NETTLE, COMMON (*Urtica dioica.* Urticaceae) This is a plant of waste places and hedgerows. Distinguished by its hairy, stinging leaves and white-green clusters of flowers, which are male and female. This is an important herb. It is one of the richest sources of chlorophyll in the vegetable kingdom. The dried herb is excellent forage for cattle and horses, being very rich in such minerals as iron, lime, sodium, chlorine, and containing much protein. It is a preventative against many contagious ailments, also worm preventive, and increases milk yield. Raw nettle juice is used in the dairy to curdle milk for cheese-making. An old peasant remedy for round and thread worms is nettles boiled in whey and given as a drench. It is a long-famed fattener for poultry, the young leaves given raw, cut small, the old tough leaves boiled and made into a mash with cereals. Give also nettle seed. The gypsies make much use of nettle as a scourge – nerve and tissue excitant – in chronic rheumatism, paralysis, or failing muscular strength: they bind fresh-cut plants into a brush and flog the affected areas with the brush. The fibre of nettle is used for spinning twine and cords by the Red Indians, who especially value such for the safe hobbling of their horses.

Use Treatment of wasting diseases, poor appetite, heart diseases, lung disorders. Blood impurities. Worms. Externally: paralysis, rheumatism, arthritis, loss of muscular power. Nettle seed, which this plant produces in abundance, when mixed into horse etc. feed, is an excellent appetizer. Nettle juice mixed with nettle seed is a valuable hair tonic. This mixture used internally and externally gives bloom to animal coats and encourages beautiful dappling and shine on horses. It is also said to make them more spirited. Important for racehorses.

OAK (*Quercus robur*. Fagaceae) This is a tree of woodland and parkland. It is distinguished by its powerful size, long, horizontal, spreading branches, and its peculiar, oval fruits of yellow-brown contained in green cups and known as acorns. The name of the tree is derived from the Latin *robur* – strength. Many of the individual parts of the tree are used in herbal medicine and animal husbandry. The bark, the leaves, the acorn fruits and the green cups that contain them – all are valuable. The bark is highly astringent, with a high tannin content. When prepared by thorough bruising it is known as 'tan'. This substance is used to check bleeding and as enemata in prolonged severe diarrhoea. The young foliage is eaten by all animals; it is tonic and astringent. Its astringency is important in the spring diet of animals as it helps to balance the sometimes over-laxative nature of the spring herbage which animals graze. The acorn fruits are tonic and feeding; but must be eaten fully ripe, not when green. They require some preparation in order to remove their bitter principle which makes them unpalatable to many animals. When prepared they yield an important tonic flour. However, their over-use can cause digestive upsets to animals which do not feed upon them habitually. When pigs eat acorns they consume only the kernels, discarding the husks which contain the bitter element. The Turkish peasants bury acorns in the ground for them to ripen and for their bitterness to be diminished. They then utilize them as *raccahoun* – which is a form of nutritious starch meal. The French gypsies use large quantities for themselves and their horses. To remove the bitter property they place the acorns on a good thickness of newspaper, to absorb the juices, which they drive out of the acorns by pounding them with heavy, flat stones. They then dry the residue in the sun, reduce to a powder, mix with equal parts of wheat flour and make a nourishing gruel. The green cups of the acorns are highly astringent. They are used to check bleeding, being made into a strong brew and used internally and externally. The oak is another of the magic trees and is known to possess benevolent powers. Ancient oaks near farmhouses owe their presence there to the belief that this tree protects against lightning and witches' evils. The growth of oak makes hollows and such are chosen nesting places of owls of many species. The bird which is the farmer's best friend, keeping territory free of rodents.

Use Treatment of loss of condition, rickets, enteritis, diarrhoea, dysentery, intestinal ulcers, bronchial haemorrhage. Hodgkin's disease. External treatment of haemorrhage, prolapsed organs.

Dose Two ounces of bark brewed in two pints water. Give one cupful morning and night. For treatment of loss of condition and rickets, give one pint acorn gruel daily. External: use the bark brew, or a brew of two handfuls shredded acorn cups to 1½ pints water.

OATS (*Avena sativa*. Graminae) Found in corn-fields and on banksides and under cultivation in pastures. Leaves are typical grass-form, darkish, brittle spikelets are drooping and frail, the grains are awned and turn dark gold when ripe.

Oats are a strength-giving cereal. Low in starch, high in mineral content (especially potassium and phosphorus, also magnesium and calcium). Particularly rich in vitamin B, with some of the rare E and G also. Highly nerve-tonic and bone-building, and a contribution to speed in racing horses and greyhounds. Since ancient times, a basic food of the hardy Scottish Highlanders, who shared their oatmeal with their border collies, collies and sheep-dogs.

Use As a nutritive food. Remedy and cure for rickets. Important for *strong* teeth, hooves, horns, nails and hair.

Dose As required. Whole oats for general use for farmstock, rolled oats for young stock and for dogs. An oats tonic drink can be made for sick animals, prepared in the same way as barley water, using oats in place of barley and omitting the lemon juice.

Planting When the moon is middle waxing.

ONION (Wild) (*Allium ampeloprasum*. Liliaceae) Mostly found as an escape from gardens or from cultivated fields. Distinguished by the long thin highly-scented leaves of burning taste. Flowers in large round balls of purple colour. The edible root is a single fleshy bulb, also of burning taste. The name of the onion, garlic and leek comes from the Celtic 'all', meaning hot or burning. Onion is a plant long and rightfully famed for its healthful properties, being strongly nutritious, soothing, antiseptic and vermifuge.

Use As a general cleansing medicine and tonic for all catarrhal disorders and for feverish colds. External, in crushed form, for cure of bruises and sprains (Greek islands).

Dose As a blood-cleanser, one or more raw onions sliced up freshly and given in bran mixed with molasses. For bad coughs and colds, slice up several raw onions and place in a basin. Pour over them enough fresh, warmed milk to cover the onions well. Then add a small teaspoon cayenne pepper and half dozen crushed cloves. Cover with a lid and allow to stand for several hours. Then give two tablespoon doses morning and night. In congestion of nostrils, slice raw onions, place on a piece of heated metal and hold close as possible to the nostrils as an inhalation. Cover the eyes to protect against the smarting onion fumes.

ORCHID (Early Purple) (*Orchis mascula*. Orchidaceae) A meadow and pastureland herb, preferring moist places. Distinguished by its shining elliptical leaves, usually dark spotted, and spikes of rose-purple flowers of the peculiar orchid form. The tubers are the important part of this plant, and give to it its Arabic name of *sahleb* – and the Turkish – *salep*. In the Orient the orchid root furnishes an important medicinal and nutritional article for man and animals, salep meal being widely used. The tubers are dug up after the flowering of the plant. They are then sun-dried to ripen well, then crushed and fed raw. Or for use of sick animals they are made into a flour, mixed well with honey and boiled in water, milk then being added to form a thick brew. In Turkey, Arabia and Persia, *salep* is highly prized as a restorative for aged people and animals; to restore strength to female animals during and after difficult labour, and as a powerful aphrodisiac. Highly prized in treatment of digestive weakness and ailments, stunted growth, poor nerves and fevers. This herb is extremely rich in readily assimilable iron.

Use Treatment of general weakness, sterility, abortion. Diarrhoea, dysentery. Nervous twitchings and lack of tone, nervous fevers exhaustion.

Dose Two ounces of salep flour mixed into 1½ pints milk.

Add one dessertspoonful honey. Give half a pint morning and night, fasting. Give half-pint restoratives during difficult labour.

PANSY (*Viola tricolor*. Violaceae)   This is a plant of moorlands. It is distinguished by its bright, viola-shaped, purple flowers, marked with yellow. It has a popular name of heart'sease, due to its tonic and pain-relieving effects on the heart. The leaves and flowers are the part used. Especially valuable for all racing creatures such as horses, dogs, pigeons.

Use   Treatment of heart weakness and pain. Skin ailments, eczema, scurf. Fits in young animals. Inflamed udder.

Dose   Two handfuls of the herb brewed in 1½ pints of water. Add honey. Give one cupful twice daily. Externally without honey.

PARSLEY (*Petroselinum crispum*. Umbelliferae)   This is a plant liking dry, rocky places. It is distinguished by its curled leaves of an intense green and umbels of small, yellow flowers. This is an important herb. The foliage is well liked by sheep and goats. It improves their milk yield and keeps them free from foot ills. It is a great enricher of the blood, being very rich in iron and copper. The plant yields apiol, which possesses carminative properties. This substance is important in the treatment of all ailments of the urinary system, also female ailments, rheumatic complaints and dropsy. Parsley roots are one of the most famed aperient roots known to the herbalist. All parts of the plant are used, including the seed. The seed is highly tonic, also is credited with magic powers giving both supernatural strength and invisibility.

Use   Treatment of all disorders of the kidneys and bladder, gravel, stone, congestion, cystitis, jaundice, obesity, dropsy, worms. Rheumatism, sciatica, neuritis, arthritis, swellings of the joints. The leaves in lotion for fevers and as an eye lotion. The root: constipation, obstructions of the intestines, fevers. The seed: colic, fevers.

Dose Three handfuls of the herb fed twice daily, or three roots daily, or two ounces of seed daily. Fresh leaves, well steeped in vinegar, soothe all types of sting.

PEANUT (*Arachis hypogea.* Leguminosae) Also called groundnut. This is a peculiar plant, beginning as a typical pea-type plant with fertilized seeds in the regular legume-shaped pod. But then the pod stem reaches over to the ground to enable the fruit pods to go subterranean where they then become the familiar groundnuts, which require digging-up and air-drying. The drying is important because if the nuts remain damp they produce a mould harmful to all which may eat them.

Peanuts are one of the most nutritious of all plant foods on account of their high vitamin content, also minerals and oil (arachnis). They provide an excellent flour, readily digestible raw, and eaten with enjoyment by all animals, including dogs and cats. (Dogs, foxes and jackals dig up peanuts for themselves.) They also provide a valuable poultry food, which stimulates egg production. Fire heat spoils the nuts, rendering them indigestible, but for young animals light sun-roasting makes the nuts more digestible, but only natural sun. The residue from peanuts in factories after oil extraction yields a valuable cattle and poultry food.

PENNYROYAL (*Mentha pulegium.* Labiatae) This is a plant of moist soil, damp commons and brooksides. Distinguished by its tiny growth, pointed, stalkless leaves and clusters of lilac flowers. The name *pulegium* is derived from the Latin word for flea, denoting the plant's powers as an insecticide. It is also a powerful mosquito repellant, and is much used for that purpose by the Arabs, the leaves being well pulped and rubbed on the skin. It is the forerunner of the cultivated mints. Animals seek it for its tonic and stimulating properties; it is accepted by herdsmen as an important after-calving stimulant and restorative for the cow. The distilled oil of pennyroyal possesses soothing and warming powers and is beneficial in the treatment of pulmonary ailments.

Use Treatment of digestive ailments, including failing appetite, sour stomach and intestinal gas. Cough, pneumonia, bronchitis and pleurisy. After-birth exhaustion. Female complaints, including uterine ulcers.

Dose Two handfuls of the herb brewed in two pints of water. Give half a pint daily. Pennyroyal is excellent when brewed in whey.

PEONY (*Paeonia officinalis*. Ranunculaceae) This is an attractive wayside and hillside plant. Distinguished by its thick, reddish stems, wide, winged, green leaves and large, solitary, red-petalled flowers. In Britain it is purely a garden plant. The plant possesses important medicinal properties, its name coming from Paeon, the great god herbalist of the Greeks. The flowers are male and female; they yield a syrupy extract. The seeds have purgative and emetic properties. The root is the part chiefly employed by herbalists. It possesses important nervine properties, and is especially famed as a remedy in epilepsy. It is also purgative. If the garden variety is used, then the common double red peony is best; the more modern hybrids are crossed with the garden variety and are not so powerfully medicinal.

Use Treatment of all nervous disorders, notably those of

convulsive or spasmodic nature, chorea, epilepsy, twitchings. Rheumatism, dropsy.

Dose One root, finely sliced, brewed in 1½ pints water, add one tablespoonful molasses. Give one cupful three times daily, or infuse two ounces of the shaved root in one pint hot liquid, made of one part wine, two parts water. Give two tablespoons morning and night.

PEPPERMINT (*Mentha piperita*. Labiatae) Found in damp meadows, sides of streams, and cultivated in gardens. Distinguished by its small, grey leaves, and plumes of purple flowers. The whole plant is highly aromatic. The plant possesses a warming volatile oil which is highly medicinal.

Use Colic, all internal aches and pains, indigestion and gas.

Dose A handful of the whole plant, cut up, in bran, or a standard brew of same, twice daily. Oil of peppermint six drops, essence of peppermint three drops, spread out on lumps of sugar or cubes of raw carrot: a great colic cure.

PERIWINKLE (*Vinca minor*. Apocynaceae) A plant of woodlands and shady banks. Distinguished by trailing stems, glossy, oval, evergreen leaves and solitary, violet-blue flowers with pale centres. It is an important herb, nervine and astringent. It is much used by peasants to dry up an over-abundant milk flow and to dry off animals when in the late stages of pregnancy. The leaves and flowers are used.

Use Treatment of haemorrhages, to arrest bleeding from deep wounds, the nostrils and vagina. Prolonged chronic diarrhoea. Excess of milk, dripping teats. Slack muscles. Nerve debility. Externally as an ointment for wounds and sores. (See Adder's tongue for recipe.)

Dose One and a half handfuls brewed in two pints of water. Give one cupful, morning and night, fasting. Use the brew also externally.

PIMPERNEL (Scarlet) (*Anagallis arvensis*. Primulaceae) This is a plant of fields and waste places. Distinguished by its tiny, thread-like growth, and solitary, round flowers of intense red, which open only in sunlight. The plant is sought by animals, being especially relished by sheep, to which it gives protection against gid. This herb has important medical powers quite out of keeping with its insignificant growth. A strong brew of the herb quietens enraged or hysterical animals. It is an ancient peasant cure for the bites of serpents and rabid animals: the herb is used both internally and externally for such treatments. It is beneficial in jaundice and ailments of a dropsical nature.

Use Treatment of gid, hysteria, epilepsy. Inflamed liver, jaundice, dropsy, kidney diseases.

Dose Two handfuls, twice daily.

PINE (*Pinus* species. Pinaceae) Though pines or firs differ botanically the substances they contain are so similar that most species can be used, so long as the species has long needles and has not the 'Christmas tree' shape of the spruce. The Scots pine (*P. sylvestris*), the Corsican pine (*P. caricio*), the black pine (*P. austrica*), the cluster pine (*P. pinaster*), can all be used. In general the species *Pinus* is a lofty tree of the hill country or sandy places. Distinguished by its great height, rough, reddish bark, evergreen, needle-form foliage and brown cones. All parts of the tree yield a valuable resin. In countries where the tree is very abundant the young shoots are fed to animals to replace hay when that is in short supply. Flour can be made from the inner bark, which must be slightly treated by heat, then ground into flour. Animals fatten well upon it. The valuable substance, turpentine, is obtained from trees of the *Pinus* order. This substance is obtained by tapping the trees for their sap and collecting this in vessels. It is an oleo-resin, the oil when distilled being known as spirit of turpentine, the residue being the resin. The resin is highly irritating, and it is the resin-free spirit that is used in medicine. Gypsies are adept at this, and use the sap thus obtained both for medicine, especially for their horses, and to kindle their wood fires. Turpentine makes a valuable vermifuge for animals; but needs to be administered with care owing to its pungent properties which could cause choking if swallowed over-rapidly: mixing with fine meal is one method or dissolving into lumps of sugar is another. Natural tree turpentine was a common and praised vermifuge in the era of natural medicine. A WARNING is again repeated, that synthetic turpentine sold in hardware shops, etc., is often made from petrol and could kill if used internally. Take care to use only pure medicinal turpentine sold in pharmacies. The same applies for external use. (Read carefully the *Important Note* below.) It is also a good external embrocation when combined with other healing herbs, such as chickweed, comfrey, mallow and plantain; it possesses powerful antiseptic properties. The cones, crushed and well boiled, also yield turpentine. Tar is also obtained from the *Pinus* species, through distillation or by slow burning of pieces of wood and roots piled into a pit and covered with turf, a channel being cut at the base of the kindled pile, into which the tar runs, and can then be collected. These peasant methods of tar and turpentine manufacture are primitive, and those who wish to distil their own will find clear instructions in any forestry book written over fifty years ago, or in an old encyclopaedia. Tar forms a valuable dressing for the diseased feet of animals; it also makes a good skin dressing, especially when combined with the healing herbs mentioned. Tar water is much used by the gypsies as a rubbing lotion for verminous animals and as a hair tonic: they mix the leaves of wild daffodil into this for the purpose of hair growth, or blend with melted animal fat. All parts of the pine are medicinal, including the cones. Pine sap is the base of retsina, a tonic wine traditional in Greece, and used also, added to bran, as a tonic for animals.

Important Note   When turpentine is advised in the veterinary treatments in this book it must be the genuine pine turpentine, not the chemical sold nowadays as 'Turps Substitute', which, in common with most chemicals in veterinary medicine, is *harmful*. When using tar, the genuine pine tar is to be used, not the substitute gas tar. Purchase from pharmacies only.

Use   Treatment of all pectoral ailments, especially cough, asthma and tuberculosis. All urinary complaints. Worms. Externally: as an embrocation for old sores, hard tumours and swellings, sprained limbs. As tar: for application to diseased hooves.

Dose   Two handfuls of the shoots or two ounces of finely shaved bark, brewed in 1½ pints water. Add one tablespoonful molasses. Give one cupful morning and night. For catarrh and excess mucus, give a handful of buds, in bran, daily.

Turpentine was once used as a vermifuge, but owing to dangers from types of turpentine sold now, I prefer to use pungent tabasco sauce, which is quite safe.

PLANTAIN (*Plantago major*. Plantaginaceae)   This is a plant of pastureland and waste places. It is distinguished by its flat rosettes of oval-shaped, olive-green leaves and unusual flowering spike, resembling a thin bulrush in its narrow form and its brownish-hued flowers. The name is derived from *planta* – foot, owing to the flat growth of the broad leaves over the ground. Goats and sheep enjoy the foliage, and poultry seek its seeds. This is an important herb, the whole plant yields a soothing mucilage somewhat similar to linseed. Plantain is used internally and externally. The leaves make a powerful healing ointment, also good as a poultice.

Use Treatment of dysentery, haemorrhages, internal obstructions and ulcers, fevers. Externally: wounds, sores, ulcers and all bites – insect, snake, scorpion and dog: eye disorders. The root is also used as a brew in treatment of fevers. To make an ointment see Adder's tongue recipe.

Dose Two handfuls of the leaves brewed in two pints water. Give one cupful three times daily.

PLUM TREE (*Prunus domestica*. Rosaceae) A small tree of gardens and orchards, though there are many allied wild types. Leaves are oval, bright green, but turning rapidly to yellow. Flowers are small, white fragrant and very numerous. All the species have their fruits of different types and colours, going from the most typical black to gold, through red and rose.

The dark plums are the most medicinally rich and this kind provides the popular 'prune', used through the ages as a valuable laxative, digestive and nerve tonic, beneficial for man and animal, and an important source of minerals, especially iron.

The whole tree is exceedingly medicinal, including the flowers and the bark.

Use The fruits, fresh or as prunes, as described above. The flowers as a fever remedy and astringent in dysentery; the bark similar use but more strongly astringent.

Dose Fruits or flowers, one handful twice daily raw, or rather less if dried. Bark infused in white wine, one ounce to one standard wineglass of wine.

POPLAR (Black) (*Populus nigra*. Salicaceae) This is a tree of the fields and waysides. It is distinguished by its tall, slender, and oval form of growth, and its dark-leaved, willow-like foliage. The buds of the tree are an important wound remedy possessing both curative and antihaemorrhoidal powers. They form the basis of the famed poplar ointment. The bark, leaves and roots of the black and common poplar (*P. tremula*), contain a peculiar substance called *populin*, together with *salicin*, and an essential oil, a yellow matter, called *chrysin*. The bark and leaves (especially the buds) are used.

Use Treatment of all forms of debility, failing appetite, wasting, indigestion, diabetes, and rheumatism. Tuberculosis. Venereal diseases. Externally: all types of wounds, sores, ulcers, fistulas.

Dose Three handfuls of the leaves or buds fed daily. Black poplar buds pounded in wine and milk are an important Spanish gypsy tonic for horses. Externally, brew two handfuls to 1½ pints water. For poplar ointment take several handfuls of young buds, pound well, gently heat in a little vinegar (one tablespoonful vinegar to each handful of crushed buds) then prepare as for Adder's tongue ointment (see recipe).

POPPY (Red) (*Papaver rhoeas*. Papaveraceae) This is a plant of cornfields and waste land. Distinguished by its delicate growth, hairy nature, and very showy, scarlet, solitary flowers, the heads of which droop when in bud. The plant is a long-famed anodyne. All parts are medicinal, including the seed capsules and the seeds. Poppy petals form an ancient and famed cough remedy, and are beneficial for cure of inflamed throat and lungs. Also much used in persistent catarrh. It promotes sweating in fevers and lung diseases. Soothes the nervous system.

The leaves are edible and acceptable to all animals; the seeds are much used by the Arabs and Turks as a horse tonic. A quantity of seeds, mixed with olive oil and honey, and pounded into cakes, is given to horses which are fretful or not sleeping well. Also handfuls of the flowers are fed to over-excitable horses (English gypsy). The seed-capsules make an important eye lotion and are used with benefit in all eye ailments.

Use Treatment of pectoral complaints, including pneumonia, pleurisy, asthma. Restlessness and over-excitability of the nerves. Eye ailments, especially ulcers and pink-eye disease.

Dose Two handfuls of the whole plant (except the roots), given twice daily. One handful poppy seed is a good daily tonic. Externally: four seed-capsules brewed in one pint water. Add one part milk to three parts of poppy brew, to make the eye lotion.

POPPY (White) or OPIUM POPPY (*Papaver somniferum*. Papaveraceae) Not British. A plant of hillsides or waste ground. Found in Britain as a garden plant. Greyish-green foliage and distinguished by its large, terminal, round flowers, of bluish-purple or white. The seeds and the seed-capsules are the most important medicinal part. The crushed seed yields an important oil of high nutritional value, the residue making a very tonic cattle and poultry food. The whole seeds are fed to racing horses to increase their stamina. The poppy-heads (seed-capsules) are used as a sedative brew and to quell pain. They are beneficial in severe colic. Opium, for which the poppy is prized above all narcotic herbs, is derived by making slits in the unripe capsules, when fully green, and collecting the milky juice, which is then formed into cakes and baked in the sun until it has turned a deep brown hue. The cakes are then coated with dried poppy leaves and seeds and can be stored. It is the most powerful narcotic available in herbal medicine. It produces opium and laudanum. It is used in veterinary work to allay severe pain, to calm over-excitability and to soothe the intestines in severe colic and prolonged dysentery and vomiting. The Turks use tincture of opium in the feeding of young calves, adding small amounts to the milk of those animals which are fretting for the parent cow during weaning and thus are not growing well. When prepared as a drug by chemists it becomes highly poisonous (although beneficial when properly used). The natural plant is harmless, taken in small quantities.

Use To allay pain. To soothe inflamed areas internally and externally, colic, dysentery, vomiting. Excitability, hysteria and sleeplessness. Eye ailments.

Dose Four green poppy-heads brewed in three-quarter pint water. Add two tablespoonfuls brown sugar to make a syrup. External: for eye lotion omit the sugar, use quite hot, three times daily.

POTATO (*Solanum tuberosum.* Solanaceae) A well-known garden and farm vegetable. Its firm, white/yellow tubers are the part used as the leaves and flowers have poisonous properties and should not be given to any animal. The potato is too fermentative and watery to be a suitable food for dogs and cats because they require solid, concentrated foods to prevent distension of their small stomach capacity. This applies to all the Solanaceae family, including tomatoes and egg-plant (aubergine). I use them very rarely as food, but I do use potato as a medicine as, being very alkaline, it is both cooling and healing.

Use Internally, the raw juice, to expel worms. Fresh juice only, two tablespoons morning (fasting) and night for ten days. Add a pinch of powdered ginger. Externally, a pulp of the peeled, grated, raw tuber applied to burns and scalds (immensely effective). Also, the same, in a cold flannel poultice, to cure inflamed areas and for dogs' feet in hard-pad disease.

Planting When the moon is waning very low.

PRIMROSE (*Primula vulgaris*. Primulaceae) This is a plant of fields and banks. Distinguished by its upgrowing rosettes of oblong, much-wrinkled leaves and frail, sulphur-hued, solitary flowers. All parts are used. This is an important tonic plant, and important for removing excess acid from the system.

Use Treatment of fits, paralysis, rheumatism, sciatica. Also gallstones and worms. The dried seed heads taken when fully ripe in the autumn, are a good emetic.

Dose Two handfuls of the flowers, or leaves and flowers, once daily.

PUFFBALL (Fungus) When crushed is applied to wounds to stem bleeding and promote healing. A French gypsy remedy.

PURSLANE (*Portulaca oleracea*. Portulaceae) Found in damp pastures, irrigated orchards and places where there is irrigation. A popular pot-herb in peasant dwellings. Distinguished by its fleshy leaves of bright green, and small yellow flowers which yield an abundance of small, black seeds. An important fodder herb and should be grown for its blood-cooling properties. Keeps green and cool even in very hot weather and torrid climates.

Use As a blood-cleanser and to refresh the digestive system. The seeds, after drying and pounding, yield a piquant meal which can be added to bread flour. Also a vermifuge. Allow the plants to seed so that animals and birds can help themselves.

Dose Ad lib., raw.

QUINCE (*Cydonia oblonga*. Rosaceae) This is an orchard tree. Distinguished by its grey-green foliage, shell-pink, rose-form blossoms and big, yellow-skinned fruits. The flowers are notable for appearing at the same time as the leaves, unusual in fruit trees of the Rosaceae family. The tree is easy to grow and should be more widely cultivated in farm gardens and orchards. The fruits possess important medicinal properties; they are much used by the Turks and Arabs. The fruit, when prepared as a pulp, is an excellent remedy for the soothing and toning of inflamed or relaxed intestines. The inner side of the peel is excellent for rubbing over sore places. It is brewed and used as a hair tonic for the manes and tails of Arabian horses. The seeds hold a mucilage which forms a valuable eye lotion or salve when brewed. This soothing lotion is also of value in treatment of discharging reproductive organs.

Use Treatment of diarrhoea, dysentery, bowel haemorrhage, gonorrhoea (used internally and externally). Externally: hair tonic. The seeds: all forms of eye inflammations and ailments.

Dose Five fruits, sliced and gently heated in 1½ pints cold water for thirty minutes, or until the fruit is soft. Give a heaped cupful of the pulped fruit, morning and night, fasting. To prepare the seeds, two tablespoonfuls of seeds to half pint water. Externally: for eye lotion, add one part milk to three parts brew from the seeds.

RADISH (Common)   See Horseradish

RAGWORT (*Senecio jacobaea*. Compositae)   This is a plant of the fields, loving the sun. Distinguished by its feathered leaves, and clusters of brilliant yellow, tiny, marguerite-form flowers, which are much frequented by butterflies. The whole plant possesses a very pungent, rather acrid smell. Animals do not find this plant attractive eating; indeed it can cause severe digestive disorders. Its use is purely external, and it has important properties for drawing out impurities and dissolving gatherings. The flowers are used.

Use   External: treatment of all skin ailments, especially gatherings, tumours, fistulas, inflamed areas.

Dose   External: two handfuls of the herb brewed in 1½ pints water.

RASPBERRY (*Rubus idaeus*. Rosaceae)   This is a plant of the woodlands. It likes to grow near water. Distinguished by its rose-form leaves with silver undersides, and small, white flowers, and thorny nature. The fruits are a brilliant red and are very juicy. The cultivated plant can be used, but care must be taken that no foliage affected by mosaic disease be used. The plant is a very important one in medicine, mainly on account of its influence on the female organs of reproduction. The foliage and fruits are enjoyed by all animals. The foliage of the raspberry shrub possesses a very active principle called *fragrine*, which exerts a powerful influence on the muscles of the pelvic girdle, especially when administered during parturition. The foliage is also highly tonic and cleansing, improving the condition of the organism during pregnancy, ensuring speedy and strong expulsion of the foetus at birth. It is of much use as a drench in retained afterbirth. It is also an acclaimed tonic for all male animals. It is a cure for sterility. Raspberry herb becomes especially potent for female use when blended with feverfew plant. Use three parts of raspberry to one of feverfew.

Use Prevention and treatment of all female ailments, retained afterbirth. Digestive ailments, including diarrhoea. Externally: treatment of throat and mouth ailments, old wounds and ulcers.

Dose Two handfuls of the herb given daily throughout the later half of pregnancy. During birth, and to bring down delayed afterbirth, make a strong brew of two handfuls of leaves to one pint water, with two dessertspoonfuls honey. Give a cupful of the brew frequently. A similar brew for treatment of diarrhoea.

REED (GREAT REED) (*Arundo phragmites: Arundo donax*. Graminae) Found by rivers, lakes, ponds and in ditches. The culms (blades) of the great reed commonly reach six foot and more in height. The blades possess an inner white pith which is very medicinal and is especially curative for ailments of the urinary system. A very effective treatment for disorders of bladder and kidneys, and a dropsy remedy. In the Canary Islands the reeds are cut in quantity for farm fencing, bound with wire, and the leaves are stripped off to provide excellent fodder particularly valued for dairy cattle. Immature reeds are also much used for floor strewing in stables and byres.

Use Treatment of all urinary ailments and disorders of the lymph glands, also for dropsy, bloat and goitre.

Dose Several handfuls to be fed daily, the leaves and two tablespoons of the extracted pith, every morning.

REST-HARROW (*Ononis arvensis*. Leguminosae) This is a plant of dry pastures and sand dunes. Distinguished by its somewhat hairy, greyish, ovate leaves and solitary, axillary, pink, pea-form flowers. The foliage has a pungent smell. The relish with which asses eat this herb has given it its generic name – asses' delight. The name rest-harrow is derived from its widespread, much tangled roots, which arrest the ploughman's harrow. Asses, goats and sheep eat the herb; peasants use the young shoots as a tonic vegetable. The herb is exceptionally rich in minerals. The whole plant is used; the roots are especially potent in medicinal virtues.

Use Treatment of obstructions and stone in kidneys and bladders. Glandular deficiencies and swellings. Loss of hair.

Dose Two handfuls of the whole herb, or two well-sliced roots, brewed in 1½ pints water. Give one cupful morning and night. Use the brew internally and externally, but for external friction to promote hair growth, add one dessertspoonful castor oil.

RHUBARB or WILD RHUBARB (*Rheum palmatum* or *R. rhaponticum*. Polygonaceae) This is a waste-land herb. Distinguished by its very large leaves of somewhat rough texture, of umbrella form, solitary and borne on very thick, fleshy, rose-hued, edible stalks. The leaves are rank and are not edible. They possess some poisonous properties. The root is highly medicinal and provides one of the most important aperients known to the herbalist. The aperient action of the root is both effective and simple, being free of griping and other unpleasant effects. In small doses it will cure diarrhoea. It is also highly tonic. The root contains a substance *bimalate of potassium*, also a peculiar substance *rhabarbarin*. The cultivated plant can be used in all cases.

Use Treatment of chronic constipation, diarrhoea, lassitude, impure blood, gastritis. Anaemia, nervousness, lack of appetite.

Dose One or two rhubarb roots, finely sliced in bran, given in the morning, fasting. Rhubarb root is not an easy herb from which to extract medicinal properties. Rhubarb pills prepared by a skilled herbalist are recommended as a reliable aperient; they are especially effective when blended with the juice of aloes.

ROCK-ROSE (*Helianthemum* species. Cistaceae) A plant of rocky places. Distinguished by its small, dark leaves and frail, rose-form flowers, which drop petals by midday. Differing from 'true rose' in having square petals. Colours vary from white, rose to dark reds. The plant contains a valuable oil. The whole plant is used against cancers and venereal diseases. It is also a carminative for highly-strung and nervous animals, and to reduce trembling. Also a cure for shock of all kinds. Preserve rock-rose flowers in sweet, red wine, for use against shock.

Dose A handful daily of the whole plant. Two spoonfuls daily of the wine.

ROSE (BRIAR) (*Rosa* species. Rosaceae) This is a plant of hedgerows and woodlands. Distinguished by its compound leaves of many leaflets, its solitary, showy, pale pink, fragrant flowers, brilliant red, smooth-fleshed berries, known as hips, and its thorny nature. Rose foliage, including that of the cultivated species, is enjoyed by all animals. The flowers are tonic and astringent. The fruits slightly aperient and good in treatment of female ailments; they are very rich in vitamin C. The root is used as a rabies cure – hence the likely origin of the name of one of the most common species of rose: *Rosa canina*, dog rose.

Use The flowers, leaves and fruits. Treatment of catarrh, diarrhoea, haemorrhages. Tuberculosis. Eye ailments. The fruits: all female ailments including leucorrhoea, metritis, miscarriage. The essential oil of roses: is an active stimulant of the nervous system and the uterus; it is an important nerve, heart and brain tonic, and is also a tonic for the ovaries and uterus. Petals of white rose for sore and inflamed eyes.

Dose Two handfuls of rose flowers once daily, pounded into two tablespoonfuls honey. Fruits: fifteen to twenty hips daily, topped and sliced, and fed in bran. Oil: five drops in one cupful of warm milk.

ROSEMARY (*Rosmarinus officinalis*. Labiatae) This is a plant of sandy and rocky places, mountain slopes and sea cliffs. Distinguished by its small, dark, shiny leaves, which are highly aromatic; the grey-blue flowers are small and hooded. The sea has given rosemary its name – *Ros Marinus*, dew of the sea, it is also a popular plant of cultivation found in gardens everywhere, and is further readily obtainable from herbalists. The whole plant exudes a camphorated odour. It is one of the most important of the aromatic herbs. It imparts a fine fragrance and tonic properties to the milk of goat and sheep which graze it eagerly. The Arabs sprinkle powdered rosemary on the umbilical cord of young animals and infants as an antiseptic. The Spanish peasants pound rosemary into salt, and consider the compound as the finest of all wound remedies. They also use a salt and rosemary brew, internally and externally, for the cure of rheumatism. The Arabs also extol this cure. Rosemary is also a nerve tonic and carminative. It is an effective insecticide.

Use Treatment of all ailments of the heart; rheumatism, fits, epilepsy, chorea, paralysis. Impure blood, gastritis, diarrhoea, dysentery, obesity and torpid liver. Wounds. Externally: falling hair and nervous spasms. A hot, strong brew for massage of rheumatic and arthritic areas of the body and limbs.

Dose Three handfuls of herb, given finely cut in a mash of bran and molasses, daily. Bags of the dried herbs, dipped into hot water and rubbed into bruises and watery gatherings, are an effective treatment. A strong brew for insecticide use, or infused in oil.

ROWAN or MOUNTAIN ASH (*Sorbus aucuparia*. Rosaceae) Found on hills, mountains and fringes of woods. Distinguished by its finely cut shining leaves. Corymbs of white flowers which yield red berries. The tree is named after 'a flame'. It is considered a fortunate tree, and therefore used for farmhouse rafters, herdsmen's staves, churn staves, driving whips and hunting crops. Also for farm implements of endurance. Rowan berries are a purge for poultry. An approximate half-dozen berries per dose.

RUE (*Ruta graveolens*. Rutaceae) Not British. This is a plant of mountainous and barren places. It is a common garden plant and can also be obtained from herbalists. Distinguished by its much divided, flat leaves and flat, yellow flowers. The whole plant is highly aromatic and bitter tasting. The essential principle of the plant is rutin, which possesses most potent powers, strengthening weakened bloodvessels, toning the nerves and glands, and imparting hardness to the bones, teeth and nails. The herb is highly antiseptic and is also an insecticide. It is one of the most favoured herbs of the Arabs. It was blessed by Mahomet, who, it is told, was cured of a fatal illness, by the aid of rue, brought to him by gypsies, when all other remedies of his doctors had failed. It is also an old remedy for prevention and cure of rabies.

Use   Treatment of fevers, hysteria, epilepsy, neuralgia, heart disease, ailments of the arteries and veins; worms. Externally (in powder or as a wash): all skin parasites including scabies and ringworm. The bruised leaves are put into horses' ears to cure staggers. A lotion for ear and eye ailments.

Dose   The herb is a potent one; dosage is small. Do not over-dose. A half-handful of herb to 1½ pints water. Give one cupful twice daily, or a half handful chopped small, given in bran. For eye ailments, including cataracts, dissolve the rue flowers by placing in a shallow vessel in the sunlight (or in warm water if no sunlight is available). Bathe eyes several times daily with the yellow water produced by squeezing the soaked blossoms. Externally: apply juice from the unripe fruits to reduce warts and cysts.

RYE (*Lolium perenne*. Gramineae)   From this wild cereal grass the domestic species are derived, found on wasteland and roadsides and in pastures. Distinguished by the dark colour of its glumes (berries) and the dark flour obtained from their crushing. A very mineral-rich cereal, also high in protein.

Use   Tonic, nervine. For feeding stock which are unhealthily over-fat, to help weight control, being nutritious but low in carbohydrates.

Planting   When the moon is full.

SAGE (*Salvia officinalis*. Labiatae)   This is a shrub of the plains and hills. Distinguished by grey, rather woolly, aromatic foliage, and whorls of blue-grey, fragrant flowers. It is an important medicinal herb. Its name is derived from the Latin *salvere*, to be well. Sage is well liked by animals, and in common with other aromatics, makes the milk refreshing and tonic; it increases the milk yield. It is nervine, digestive and blood cleansing. A first-rate remedy for treatment of all disorders of throat, lungs and ears. Externally it is an effective application for bruises, watery swellings and tumours. The Mexicans make brushes from branches of the herb, using them to cleanse and dry off the sweating bodies of their horses and cattle, the leaves being both absorbent and invigorating to tired flesh. The Mexican wild sage is *S. azurea grandiflora*, with deep blue flowers, and is powerfully medicinal. Sage grown among vegetable crops and vines, gives protection against insects and mice.

Use Treatment of nerve debility, paralysis, all heart ailments. All gastric ailments, constipation, obesity and female ailments. Blood-cleansing, eczema, fevers, wound infections. Scanty milk yield and loss of milk. Externally: wounds, bruises, swellings and tumours. Falling hair and scurf. Sore mouths and throat ailments: give mixed with honey. It is a proved fertility herb.

Dose A strong tea can be made, one teaspoon of herb to two small cups of water, or two handfuls of herb finely cut, made into a mash with bran and molasses, daily. Externally: one big handful of herb brewed in 1½ pints water.

ST. JOHN'S WORT (*Hypericum perforatum*. Hypericaceae) This is a plant of the wayside and woodlands. Distinguished by its foliage, which is peculiar, the leaves containing numerous bright specks, which are the oil glands. The flowers are terminal, held in leafy panicles; they are bright yellow and notable for their abundance of fine stamens. The plant contains an important medicinal resin, gum and acids. The herb is astringent, and is much used as a pectoral, wound herb and in rheumatic complaints. The fresh flowers steeped in olive oil make the famed oil of St. John's wort, a treatment for all wounds and skin complaints. The herb, combined with chamomile, is made into an ointment which is renowned for its pain-quelling and soothing qualities. The whole plant is well liked by cattle, goats and sheep. A thorny species, which grows in Eastern countries, is pickled in vinegar (the flower buds) and used as a digestive tonic.

Use Treatment of coughs, inflammations of the chest and lungs, pulmonary ulcers. Rheumatism, jaundice. Hodgkin's disease, dropsy, earache and inflammation. Worms. Externally: treatment of all wounds, eruptions, ulcers, swellings and skin inflammations.

Dose One handful of herb to two pints water. Give one cupful morning and night. Externally: use a stronger brew, two handfuls of herb to two pints water. The oil: two handfuls of the flowers, finely cut, immersed in a half-pint bottle of olive oil: the bottle tied up in a piece of cloth. Place the bottle in a pan of cold water. Bring slowly to a high temperature, keeping below boiling-point, and allow to simmer for one hour. Leave the flowers to steep in the warm oil for several hours after removal from the pan of water. The oil is then ready for use. The ointment: pound the flowers into a pulp, mix with chamomile flowers, likewise pounded, two parts St. John to one of chamomile. Melt lanolin into a hot, fluid state, then mix in the flowers, half flowers, half lanolin.

SANICLE (*Sanicula europaea*. Umbelliferae) An interesting all-green plant of woodlands and thickets. Foliage is dark and shiny of finely cut type. The flowers are unusual, very pale green in the umbel type of this plant group. The barren flowerlets of the umbels are stalkless. The plant is such an important healing one that the Crusaders painted this herb on their shields and banners as a symbol of protection for themselves and their war-horses. Also provides a very well-liked fodder, eaten with relish by all farm animals, especially goats and sheep, and by wild deer and ponies.

Quite similar in type and properties is the sea samphire, which is also an Umbelliferae with grey-white flowers. Samphire is much eaten by goats and sheep and all the wild animals of the sea cliffs, especially rabbits. Makes an excellent pickle for the farmhouse, raw shoots, with buds, in vinegar.

Use Particularly effective for internal wounds and bleeding, for ulcers, haemorrhages, inflammation of stomach and intestines. Externally, as a strong lotion with some honey added, for all types of sores, wounds, rashes, and ailments of the mouth and throat.

Dose Several handfuls daily, the whole plant.

SANTOLINA (*Diotis maritima*. Compositae) As its name denotes it is a plant of sea areas in its wild form, sea cliffs and windy slopes, but it is also found inland on waste areas. Also cultivated in farm gardens where it is grown as a border plant, popular for its tangy scent and for its use as a warming tea for man and animals. Distinguished by its ferny, grey, rather woolly leaves of very strong odour. Flowers are rayless and resemble small, round, hard, yellow buttons; also of strong scent and much used as a tea herb in the Balearics, in inns and in the homes, where it is given to their animals as a soothing tonic.

Use As a cure for high fever. Also as a remedy for all types of worms. Externally, as a rheumatism remedy and as a rub for painful joints and ligaments; also in clothes closets as a moth repellent (good protection for horse blankets). In solution to repel biting insects.

Dose For fevers as a strong brew, given cold, several tablespoons three times daily. For worms the flowers are finely minced and made into balls with thick honey to bind them. One dessertspoon of the flowers in pill form is given night and morning. As an external rub, the whole plant is cut small, pounded and then infused in equal parts of vinegar and olive oil. Applied hot, several times daily.

SAUCE-ALONE (hedge garlic) (*Erysimum allaria.* Cruciferae) This is a common hedgerow and bankside plant. Distinguished by its cordate leaves, tiny, white cruciform flowers and long, brownish fruit pods of nearly two inches in length. The plant possesses an onion smell, and in a slight degree imparts this to the milk of the animals that consume it. Animals seek it for its highly tonic properties. It increases the milk yield. It is an important anti-colic herb and should be encouraged in all pastures. It derives its name from its piquant foliage, which tastes of combined garlic, mustard, pepper and salt.

Use Treatment of colic, flatulence, dew-blow. Scanty milk yield. It is also used to curdle milk for cheese-making.

Dose Two handfuls of herb fed twice daily.

SCABIOUS (Field) (*Scabiosa arvensis,* also *Knautia arvensis.* Dipsaceae) This is a plant of fields and banksides. Distinguished by its handsome, pale-lilac, many-stamened, solitary flowers born on round, slender stems. It is a plant beloved by the gypsies, one name for it being gypsy rose. Its properties are highly cleansing and antiseptic. The whole herb is used.

Use Treatment of all skin ailments, all female ailments. Heart diseases, venereal diseases. Externally: a brew of the roots will cure bruised, weak sinews, old sores and gatherings. A brew of the herb and root, thickened with borax, will remove dandruff and old sores from the head and body.

Dose   One handful of flowers and foliage brewed in 1½ pints water. Give one cupful morning and night. Externally: two handfuls of herb and/or three or four finely cut roots. Brew in 1½ pints water. When the brew is still hot, after removal from the fire, stir in 1½ tablespoonsful of borax powder.

SCURVY-GRASS (*Cochlearia officinalis*. Cruciferae)   This is a plant of the seashore and mountainous places. Distinguished by the spoon-like form of its concave, kidney-shaped leaves (one name for the herb being spoonwort), and racemes of small white flowers. It is an important medicinal herb, being a most powerful blood cleanser and tonic, and highly antiseptic. The leaves distilled in water yield a sulphurous essence. It has been found that a brew of the plant quickens the healing of wounds. It is one of the most potent herbs for vitamin content, and for that reason its place of growth, on the seashore, makes it invaluable for grazing animals where green food is scarce. It is of the same group as the horseradish – *Cochlearia armoracia*.

Use   Treatment of all skin ailments and bladder disorders. Rickets, rheumatism, sciatica.

Dose   One handful of herb every morning.

SEA-HOLLY (*Eryngium maritimum*. Umbelliferae)   This is a plant of the seashore. Distinguished by its blue-tinted, spiky foliage, and dense, rounded, terminal flower-heads of deep blue. It is rich in minerals, especially iron and magnesium, and also silica; its iodine content is important. It possesses nervine and tonic properties. The young shoots are agreeable to animals who seek them eagerly despite their spiky nature.

Arabs eat the shoots cooked. The roots are very nutritious. Arabs candy them for their own use and to feed as titbits to their favourite horses as award for good conduct.

Use Treatment of liver complaints, chest pains and inflammation, glandular deficiencies and disorders, constipation.

Dose One root, finely sliced and mixed into a mash with bran and molasses, once daily. Or one handful of finely cut leaves, fed fresh, also given in bran and molasses.

SENNA (*Cassia acutifolia*. Leguminosae)   Not British. This is a plant of open plains. Distinguished by its bean-like foliage, loose clusters of yellow flowers and flat seed pods. It is the laxative most used by the herbalist. It contains acids, gums and sugars. It is one of the most important laxatives, being also a cleanser and restorative of the entire digestive system. The griping tendency is diminished by the addition of powdered ginger. As heat destroys the properties of this herb it should be prepared by cold water infusion, steeping the pods or leaves for a minimum of four hours. Both pods and leaves are readily obtainable from herbalists and pharmacy shops. Use the large Alexandrian kind.

Use Treatment of constipation, catarrhal ailments, jaundice, obesity, worms of all kinds.

Dose Five large senna pods for an average-size dog, seven for sheep, eight for goat, twenty for horse, twenty-four for cow, soaked in cold water for a minimum of four hours, preferably seven hours. Use one teaspoon cold water to every pod. About a half saltspoon of powdered ginger. Before use, squeeze all moisture from the pods, then add a little honey. The honey will usually tempt the case to drink the senna. Add ginger in powder form: a pinch to six pods, ditto to ten, a half teaspoon to twenty and twenty-four. Give the senna dose last thing at night at least two hours after food has been taken; can also be given early morning.

SHEEP SORREL (*Rumex acetosella*. Polygonaceae)   This plant is also called sour grass and red sorrel. It is a common weed of waste lands and pastures. Its leaves are yellowish in colour and arrow-shaped and have a distinctive sour taste. The plant is much enjoyed by grazing animals. It also makes a good addition to table salads. The leaves contain acids of potassium, oxalate and tartaric and are very cooling to the whole system and good also for the kidneys.

Use   Blood ailments, fevers, kidney ailments. Externally: skin irritations.

Dose   One handful of the leaves twice daily. Externally extract the juice by grating the leaves and then pouring fresh milk over them. The resultant green lotion is applied fresh to the skin.

SHEPHERD'S PURSE (*Capsella bursa-pastoris*. Cruciferae)   This is a plant of waste places and fields. Identifiable from its insignificant form, narrow leaved foliage, tiny, white, cruciform-shaped flowers, and seed pods which resemble the old-fashioned leathern purses of shepherds. It possesses important astringent properties. All animals like this herb, and poultry seek it eagerly.

Use   Treatment of haemorrhages, internal and external, profuse bleeding of deep wounds, kidney ailments, general debility, dropsy. All ear ailments and afterbirth haemorrhage.

Dose   Two handfuls twice daily. Externally: bathe wounds with a strong brew made from three handfuls of herb to three-quarter pint of water. French gypsies complete the treatment by plugging the wounds with fresh spiders' webs.

SKULLCAP (*Scutellaria galericulata*. Labiatae) Not British. This is a plant of damp places, distinguished by its square stems, opposite, short-stalked leaves and hooded, pale-blue flowers. One species is found wild in Cambridgeshire, but it is rare. It is a supreme nerve herb, and has restored many cases of nervous disorders considered beyond cure by non-herbal treatments. All parts are used.

Use Treatment of all nervous complaints, especially hysteria, fits, chorea, meningitis, nervous spasms, gastro-enteritis. Lack of appetite, sterility. An old cure for rabies.

Dose One handful of herbs brewed in 1½ pints water; add one tablespoonful of honey. Give one cupful three times daily.

SLOE (*Prunus spinosa*. Rosaceae) This is a shrub of the hedgerows and woodlands. Distinguished by its spiny growth, white, rose-form flowers, and dark-purple plum fruits, very bitter tasting and astringent. The leaves of the 'blackthorn' are enjoyed by all animals, also the bark. The flowers are laxative and vermifuge. The fruits are astringent. It is a good fever cure. Gypsies prepare the fruits by burying them for several months in straw-lined pits in the ground to ripen well; this further increases their medicinal properties. The bark is antispasmodic and sedative.

Use Treatment of fevers, nervous debility, dropsy. Skin ailments. Nervous disorders. In the making of gin – a medicinal drink.

Dose One handful of flowers daily or eight fruits, destoned, pounded in bran and molasses mash. Add sufficient honey or molasses as sweetener to make palatable. One teaspoon of shaved bark added to food.

SORREL (*Rumex acetosa*. Polygonaceae) This is a plant of fields and waste places. Distinguished by its long, arrow-shaped leaves and tall spikes of small flowers of red, brown or green colour. The whole plant is very acid-tasting. It is famed for its cooling and soothing qualities. All animals eat this herb, including the seed. French farmers feed sorrel seed to their cattle as a tonic. The leaves are used to curdle milk, for junket-making and medicine, by squeezing their acid juice therein, or making strong decoction of the leaves.

Use Treatment of all fevers, sweating, overheated blood. Externally: the pulped leaves are curative for skin eruptions, festering ulcers, gangrenous conditions.

Dose Several handfuls. For dairy use, milk curdling, etc., one tablespoon of the herb, finely cut, to every two cups of fresh milk.

SOUTHERNWOOD (*Artemisia* species. Compositae) This is a conspicuous plant of sunny hillsides. Distinguished by its hoary, feathery, grey-green leaves of sweet, pungent scent, and slender racemes of round, green-yellow flowers. It is commonly found in herb gardens and plant nurseries. This is a powerful herb; its nauseous, bitter-tasting brew is an important vermifuge. As with most bitters, it is also very tonic. It is of great help in difficult birth problems, given as a drench, a dessertspoon of the herb, finely cut, fortified with one teaspoon sage herb and six spice cloves. Add a large cup of cold water and make a brew. When cool, sweeten with honey and give at two-hourly intervals. It is an excellent wash for skin parasites. It is a tonic for the hair. The chief medicinal property of the herb is an essential oil, absinthol, which is a worm expellant, antiseptic, tonic and insect repellant. Spanish farmers wishing to preserve the skins of lambs for commerce, place southernwood amongst them as a moth repellant.

Use Treatment of worms, digestive ailments, obstructions, udder ailments, kidney and bladder complaints. In difficult labour. Externally: as a rub or wash to cleanse the skin and hair of parasites and their ova, especially fleas.

Dose One handful of herb brewed in two pints water. Add one tablespoonful honey. Give one cupful morning and night. Externally: use the crushed leaves, or the brew, omitting the honey. It is excellent in difficult births.

SOW-THISTLE (*Sonchus arvensis*. Compositae) This is a common plant of wasteland and ploughed fields. Of medium height, distinguished by its triangular-lobed leaves and small, prickly teeth. The flower-heads are bright yellow, of thistle form, borne in loose terminal panicles. The whole plant is very refrigerant. It is rich in minerals. It is internally antiseptic and fever reducing, and remedies palpitations of the heart. All animals eat it with relish. It will increase milk yield. Hares, when hard pressed by hounds, given the opportunity will snatch bites of the foliage to cool off their running heat and succour their hearts. A country name for this herb is hare's-lettuce. The herb is eaten as a salad by peasants of the French alps and Switzerland; also by Arabs.

Use Treatment of fevers, skin eruptions, acid stomach and intestines. Heart palpitations, high blood-pressure.

Dose Four handfuls twice daily.

SPEEDWELL (*Veronica officinalis*. Scrophulariaceae) This is a plant of pastures and copses. Distinguished by its frail growth, rough, serrated leaves and round, very frail, pale blue flowers, usually marked with a white 'eye'. The leaves are eaten by all animals, for their tonic properties; they impart a good flavour to the milk of cows and goats. The plant is remarkably medicinal, out of keeping with its frail form. It is an excellent mucus expellant, and for that reason is much employed as a pectoral and anti-catarrhal. It is used in dysentery, jaundice, skin and eye ailments.

Use Treatment of cough, bronchial asthma and catarrh, pleurisy, tuberculosis, ulcerated lungs. Dysentery, gastric insufficiency, jaundice, impure blood and eczema. Externally: skin eruptions, ulcers and rashes. All eye ailments and weakness.

Dose Three handfuls of the herb to be given daily. Externally: brew one handful of the herb to one pint water.

SPHAGNUM MOSS (*Sphagnum cymbifolium*. Musci) This is a plant of damp places, especially peaty moors. Distinguished by its growth in closely knitted tufts, to form a spongy mass. The cells of the leaves are water-storing: their colour greenish yellow, sometimes stained a bright orange. The formation of the moss much resembles that of edelweiss. It is of the plant group *Bryophyta*, between the ferns and the seaweeds. It is the best absorbent material known to the herbalist, being able to absorb many times its own weight in fluids, and is much used in surgical dressings and skin treatments. Absorbent bandages were made from sphagnum during the two World Wars. It is very refrigerant and antiseptic, and yields some iodine. Sphagnum moss, partly dried, and then saturated in garlic brew, is one of the most popular external wound and skin treatments of the Hungarian gypsies. The moss is eaten by moorland sheep and by deer. It has the highest economic value of the mosses for apart from its medicinal value it is largely responsible for that important substance, peat.

Use Externally, as a surgical and antiseptic dressing. It is also put in the drinking-troughs of sheep and cattle to render the water tonic.

SPRUCE (Norway spruce – commonly known as Christmas tree) (*Picea abies*, formerly *Abies excelsa*. Pinaceae) This is a tree of forests and mountain spaces. Distinguished by its triangular form and great height. It has a red-tinted, scaly bark. A coniferous tree. The young shoots, cut and mixed with cereals, make a good winter tonic for horses. Also the young shoots, well bruised, are used as a rubbing liniment for stiff joints and bruised or aching limbs. A brew made from spruce shoots is good for all throat and pulmonary ailments. A form of pitch made from the inner layers of the wood is excellent for treatment of foot-rot in sheep.

Use Nutritive and tonic. Treatment of sore throat, cough, bronchitis, pneumonia, tuberculosis. Externally: for all forms of limb injuries or ailments.

Dose One handful of finely cut shoots to two pints water, add two dessertspoonfuls molasses. Give half a pint morning and evening, fasting.

STONECROP or BITING STONECROP (*Sedum acre*. Crassulaceae) This is a plant of rocky and sandy places favouring coastal areas. It is much found on old walls. Distinguished by its rosettes of smooth, very succulent, upstanding leaves and starry, yellow flowers. The generic name of the plant, *Sedum*, is derived from *sedo* – to sit, signifying the growth of the plant upon rocks and walls. It is a very useful herb, beneficial in treatment of all nervous ailments, and externally for cure of fistulas, tumours and cancers. Its presence on farm buildings is welcomed as a protector against fire and lightning.

Use Treatment of chorea and epilepsy. Externally: skin

ailments of obstinate form, especially fistulas, tumours, cancerous growths and boils.

Dose This herb is very pungent and should be used only in small doses internally and for short periods externally. Half a handful brewed in 1½ pints water. Give two tablespoonfuls morning and night.

STRAWBERRY or WILD STRAWBERRY (*Fragaria vesca*. Rosaceae) This is a plant of shady banks and woodlands. Also cultivated in gardens. Distinguished by its grey-green, rose-form leaves, rounded, white flowers and soft fleshed, round, red, very juicy berries. The whole plant is very refrigerant. It is much liked by goats and sheep. It is a valuable herb, being highly rich in minerals and antiseptic. The fruits are valued above all others by the Red Indian people. The leaves and root are mildly aperient and very cooling. They are used in fevers and as a summer blood cleanser. They are antidiarrhoea and wound curative, stemming bleeding. The leaves are a good remedy to prevent abortion, and to check over-prolonged menstruation. They are exceptionally rich in easily assimilable iron; stock-owners would do well to obtain sackfuls of leaves from market gardeners at the end of the fruit season and feed as a tonic to any backward or nervous animals; strawberry foliage is extra good for racehorses. The berries are very tonic, blood cooling, and a mild vermifuge. If using garden (non-wild) foliage, ensure that no chemical spray has been used.

Use Treatment of impure blood, acid blood, lowered vitality, fevers, diarrhoea, jaundice, obstructions of the viscera. Abortion, menstrual irregularities.

Dose Two handfuls of leaves, or leaves and root, once daily. Or one handful of berries once daily. Externally: juice from the berries or pulped and slightly heated foliage, for treatment of inflamed areas, skin rashes, ulcers, inflamed or discharging eyes.

SWEET CICELY (*Myrrhis odorata*. Umbelliferae) This is a plant of the wayside and of mountainous places. Distinguished by its feathery leaves, or aromatic, sweet myrrh scent, and large umbels of white flowers. It is very tonic, and is beloved by goats and horses. The Red Indians say that horses are so fond of the roots, that if some roots are bruised and held in the hands, and one stands in a position so that wild horses get their scent, they will come running to eat the roots and then can be caught easily. The leaves and root are used.

Use Treatment of all digestive ailments, general debility, constipation. Cough, catarrh.

Dose One handful of leaves or sliced roots, once daily.

SWEET FLAG (*Acorus calamus*. Araceae) Also commonly called sweet sedge. This is a plant of marshy places and banks of streams; it grows also in the water, and is not to be confused with the common flag or yellow water-iris (*I. pseudoacorus*). Distinguished by its reed-like growth, wave-like form of the leaf edges, and rush-like, blunt spikes of yellow-brown flowers. The foliage is much liked by animals, especially cows and sheep. The root-rhizome is a powerful medicine. The interior tissue is of pinkish white colour and of spongy texture, very sweet scented and aromatic: this is the famed calamus root. It is highly nutritive and is most beneficial in treatment of all digestive disorders and wasting conditions. It corrects over-acid condition of the body.

Use Treatment of gastritis, dysentery, colic, chronic constipation, lack of appetite. Fevers, cramps.

Dose   Two roots twice daily, finely flaked, and mixed into a mash with bran and molasses.

SWEET GALE (*Myrica gale*. Myricaceae)   This is a plant of moorlands and boggy wastes. It grows several-feet-high greyish leaves, sweetly scented. The plant is a general tonic and wound herb. It is much used by New Forest gypsies and sought by wild deer and ponies. It is also called bog myrtle.

Use   A general tonic, to remedy lack of appetite. Nerve cure. Externally: the leaves as a hot poultice applied to wounds.

Dose   One handful of leaves several times daily.

TANSY (*Chrysanthemum vulgare*. Compositae)   This is a plant of the wayside and waste places. Distinguished by its dark, fern-like leaves and small, bright yellow, disk-like flowers, born in clusters. Both foliage and flowers have a very pungent, camphorous odour and hot, aromatic taste. Cows and sheep eat the herb. The plant is a powerful worm expellant, especially the seeds, although the flowers are most commonly used. The young leaves are made into a brew and used as a preventative against abortion. Externally it is used as a skin remedy and in treatment of sprains. The whole herb is highly prized as a tonic by gypsy tribes.

Use   Treatment of all types of worms. Debility, hysteria, abortion, fevers and dropsy.

Dose   One handful of leaves and flowers brewed in two pints water, with two tablespoonfuls of honey. Give one cupful twice daily, fasting. Externally: use as a poultice in linen bags. Two ounces of seeds act as a worm expellant.

TEA PLANT (Common tea, Indian tea, China tea.) (*Thea sinensis*.)   'Common' tea is found in packets in most farmhouses.

It is rich in tannic acid and therefore is of great use as a cooling agent to reduce the heat in fire burns and burns from the sun, also sunstroke and head pains. Taken internally it is over-astringent and habit-forming because of its high tannic content. It is best used as an external remedy, but can be of service for severe colic pains when no other remedy is available. A strong solution in vinegar will deter biting insects.

Use As stated above. Externally: in sunstroke (to which goats are prone) apply in very strong solution, two parts to one of vinegar. Soak cotton cloth in this mixture and apply to the head. Also apply hot, on cloths, to the belly area of horses in grass fever.

Dose One level tablespoon of tea to one cup hot water spiced with cinnamon and cloves. Give cold in sunstroke, adding one teaspoon of vinegar to every three dessertspoons of the tea mixture.

THISTLE (*Carduus* species. Compositae) This is a plant of waste places. It is distinguished by its spiny foliage, and its round thistle-heads of purple flowers in a spiny calyx, which produce down-plumed seeds. The plant, cut when young and dried, makes a tonic fodder for cattle, one of its names being milk-thistle. It is the only thistle which can be killed by hoeing. The roots, when young, are also edible and very tonic. The seeds are used in rabies and epilepsy; also in chest complaints. The juice expressed from the leaves is used externally in skin ailments and swellings. It is comparatively rare except as a weed of cultivation. But seeds can be obtained from nurserymen who usually call it *Silybum marianum*, its alternative name.

There are other species of thistle closely related to the artichoke species. These are of yet greater value to the farmer because, also possessing the same tonic and nervine properties as the thistle above, they further have the power to curdle milk as strongly as rennet (and giving a far nicer taste to the cheese than rennet) and this thistle-curdled milk can be made into long-keeping cheeses. The richer milk of ewe and goat is required. I first met with the cheese thistle in the Spanish Balearic Islands and have since met it again in the smaller of the Canary Islands. These thistles are of the Cynara group and are *Cynara lumilis*, of the Balearics, and *Cynara marinaris* and the more common *Cynara cardunculus*. All can be used to curdle milk for cheese, as also can the globe artichoke plant already described under Artichoke. In all cases the ray flowerets of the composite thistle flower-heads are used, either fresh or dried. Usual proportion is one heaped teaspoon of the flowerets to 1½ pints of milk. Crush the flowers well, then place in a piece of muslin cloth, press out the juice into the milk and leave the muslin within the milk until curdled.

Use   Treatment of debility and female complaints. The seeds: rabies, epilepsy, pleurisy, catarrh. Externally: eczema, ulcers and tumours, including cancerous types. Thistle is associated with endurance and promotes this.

Dose   Two handfuls of leaves, well crushed, given in a mash of bran and molasses, once daily. The seeds: one ounce boiled in one cupful water. Add one cupful milk to the brew, when cold. Give as a drench, once daily. Externally: make a pulp of the leaves trimmed of prickle edges, and massage into the affected areas.

THORN-APPLE (*Datura stramonium.* Solanaceae) This is a plant of dry ground and waste places. Distinguished by its showy appearance, broad, glossy leaves of an unpleasant, narcotic odour and big, white, solitary trumpet-shaped flowers. The seed vessel resembles a small round prickly cucumber. The plant yields valuable narcotic drugs, especially atropine and hyoscine. It is a semi-poisonous plant of the *Belladonna* group. The Red Indians burn the dried fruits and foliage, and use it as a smoke treatment in chronic asthma conditions. The Arabs use the pulped fruits in jaundice treatment, pushing the fruits up the nostrils and then making poultice bags of the fruits and placing over the stomach regions. The fruits are brewed, and a narcotic is extracted. Because of the plant's semi-poisonous nature I prescribe it only for external use.

Use   (External only.) Treatment of asthmatic conditions, to relieve pain. Jaundice.

THYME (*Thymus serpyllum*. Labiatae)   This is a plant of hills, heathlands and dry, sunny banks. Distinguished by its creeping, rooting stems (which give the plant its specific name – *serpyllum*), tiny, flat, dark green, very aromatic leaves and whorls of small, lilac-pink flowers of very sweet and pungent scent. The plant is eaten by sheep and goats; it is a milk tonic for them. The whole herb is highly tonic and antiseptic. The expressed oil yields the important antiseptic and worm-expellant substance, thymol. The whole plant is used. Dried and powdered thyme, called za'atar by the Arabs, is a well-known tonic condiment, eaten sprinkled on bread. It is a favourite bee herb and should be planted by apiarists. In the Balearic Islands thyme is used to protect dried fruit against moth and weevils. Dried thyme is sprinkled on them.

Use   Treatment of all digestive complaints, including colic, inflammation of the liver, rickets. All pectoral ailments. Hysteria, nervousness, nervous indigestion, sciatica. Retention of afterbirth, inflamed or diseased uterus, metritis. Worms – including hookworm.

Dose One handful of the plant brewed, finely cut, mixed in the food. Give one cupful morning and night. Thymol is given in small controlled doses of twenty to thirty grains in capsule form. It is also used externally to cure local severe irritations of the skin, and as a scabies remedy. An infusion in vinegar against biting insects.

TOAD-FLAX (*Linaria vulgaris.* Scrophulariaceae) This is a plant of fields and waste places. Distinguished by its upright growth, small, flat leaves and erect racemes of yellow and white flowers of familiar snapdragon form. Cows and horses eat the foliage. The plant is powerfully dissolvent and penetrative, and forms one of the best jaundice remedies known to the herbalist. The whole herb is used.

Use Treatment of jaundice. Affections of the kidneys and bladder, dropsy.

Dose One handful of the herb brewed in 1½ pints water. Give one cupful three times daily.

TORMENTIL (*Potentilla erecta* or *Tormentilla officinalis.* Rosaceae) This is a plant of heathland and dry pastures. It is distinguished by rose-form foliage, and sparse, rose-like yellow flowers. The name, *Tormentilla*, is derived from *tormine*, the sense of which is 'a griping', and refers to the popular employment of this herb in dysentery, for cure of which it is famed. The root is highly astringent, containing tannin and quinovic acid. It is an important wound herb, its powerful astringency arresting over-profuse bleeding. The foliage is eaten by animals. The root is praised by herbalists on account of its powerful and peculiar effect upon the stomach and bowels, expelling rapidly accumulations of slimy mucus. Cloth, soaked in a strong decoction of the foliage, applied very frequently, removes warts.

Use Treatment of gastritis, dysentery, colic, diarrhoea, bowel haemorrhages, sour stomach and intestines, cramps. Externally: treatment of all wounds and bleeding, ulcers, sores and warts.

Dose One handful of foliage, mixed with two finely sliced roots, brewed in 1½ pints water. Give one cupful morning and night. Externally: make a pulp of the foliage or roots, and place in cotton bags, apply warm as poultice to the affected areas. For wounds, make a strong brew of the roots, and bathe the wounds, or apply on pads of sphagnum moss.

VALERIAN (*Valeriana officinalis.* Valerianaceae) This is a plant of banksides and old walls. Distinguished by its opposite, compound leaves, and its abundant terminal corymbs of rose or white flowers. The root is the medicinal part of this important herb, and has earned the plant its popular name of all-heal. The root contains a volatile oil, a resin, and valeric acid. The roots, which are perennial, are allowed to reach at least two years before being lifted. The medicinal properties are powerfully nervine and sedative without being narcotic. It is also febrifuge and vermifuge. Valerian is one of the supreme remedies for epilepsy. Red Indian herbalists state that if epileptic fits resist valerian treatment, they are incurable. Cats have a great desire for valerian plant and will chew all parts including the roots.

Use Treatment of epilepsy, hysteria, chorea. Acute constipation, worms, malaria. Externally: the expressed oil is used as a rub for paralysed limbs, cramps, swollen arteries and veins. The root washed, and thin shavings cut, infused in water for one day, soothe greatly the nerves of the eyes, used as an eye lotion.

Dose Four roots, finely sliced, in one quart water; half pint dose morning and night. Or the powdered herb (sold at most herbalists) may be used; two dessertspoonfuls morning and night mixed into honey balls. Give more frequently in cases of severe fits. Owing to the unpleasant odour of valerian, several pinches of powdered ginger can be added with advantage to each tablespoonful dose.

VERVAIN (*Verbena officinalis.* Verbenaceae) This is a plant of dry, barren places. Distinguished by its insignificant appearance, spare foliage of opposite leaves growing on square stems, and spikes of frail, closely growing, pale lilac flowers. The herbalists of Greece and Italy placed vervain among the small group of all-curing herbs. It was a favourite of Hippocrates – the father of all medicine; also a favourite of the Druids. It is valuable in every type of fever, also nervous disorders and eye ailments. Renowned as a plague remedy in ancient times. The American Indians extol vervain as a general cure-all herb.

Use Treatment of all fevers, fits, convulsions, hysteria, chorea. Liver complaints, gall-stones. Externally: weak and inflamed eyes, inflamed throats, sore and ulcerated mouths.

Dose Feed two handfuls of the whole plant twice daily. Externally: one handful of herb brewed in one pint of water. For eye treatment add one teaspoonful of raw milk to each two tablespoonfuls of herbal brew used.

VETCH (Common vetch) (*Vicia sativa.* Leguminosae) Found wild in pastures, also planted as an early crop for all the farm animals. Vetch is often planted as a companion crop to rye, the early cereal. Vetch is a climbing plant and binds itself around the rye cereal grass. The whole crop is then cut as one, formed into stooks for drying and used fresh or stored, a valuable fodder contribution. Vetch is a small, wiry plant with small, oval, pointed leaves, climbing spiralling stems and small bluish or yellow pea-form flowers. It makes slender, fat pods.

Use To provide a fodder rich in nitrates and vitamins.

VINE (*Vitis vinifera*. Viniferaceae) A well-known garden shrub, cultivated since the dawn of civilization. No crop is more use to man and his animals than this king plant of agriculture, the grapevine. All parts are used and all parts are vitally medicinal. Grape residue from the wine-presses provides a rich food for all animals and poultry.

Use The leaves: a nerve tonic and mineral-rich food, also deeply healing when bound over wounds, burns, tumours. The tendrils: used as a food are considered anti-cancerous. The fruits and their juice are extremely nutritious, refreshing and restorative. The seeds, well crushed, are very mineral rich. The criterion for the successful use of the vine and all its parts is that it is not ruined by irrigation (the vine needs to be grown dry to tap the deep soil layers for minerals) and also that it is never harmed by chemical spraying.

VIOLET (Sweet) (*Viola odorata*. Violaceae) This is a plant of hedge-banks and woodland. Distinguished by its small stature, heart-shaped, dark green leaves and deep purple, very fragrant flowers of typical violet shape. All parts are used. The flowers and leaves are expectorant and antiseptic; the flowers very mucilaginous. Both are used to reduce and cure cancerous growths. Being emollient they are used in skin lotions and ointments. The root is mildly aperient.

Use Used internally and externally for treatment of tumours, cancerous growths, swollen glands, boils. Internally:

inflammations of the liver, kidneys and bladder, gall-stones.

Dose Two handfuls of the herb given twice daily. Externally: a brew of two handfuls of the herb in 1½ pints water.

VIPER'S-BUGLOSS (*Echium vulgare.* Boraginaceae) Found on wastelands, banks, old walls. Distinguished by its greyish, rough leaves, freckled with light dots. Flowers are purple or pink – both colours on same spike. It is a tonic plant as fodder or medicine, especially the flowers. The whole plant is an instant remedy against the bite of vipers. Also a dog-bite remedy.

Use As a tonic and a viper cure.

Dose Crush up a whole fresh plant (including root) and apply to the bite.

WALNUT (*Juglans nigra.* Juglandaceae) This is a tree of parkland and woodland. Distinguished by its handsome appearance, its grey trunk and lofty branches, large, compound leaves, and its oval nuts for which it is famed. The nuts are enclosed in green, fleshy cases. All parts of the tree are medicinal. The leaves, bitter and astringent, are valuable in treatment of scurvy, skin ailments, rickets, venereal diseases, worms and skin parasites. The nut's green pericarp possesses the same properties as the leaves, but it induces more powerful contractions of the digestive tract, and thus is yet more efficient as a worm cure. The oily embryo of the nut is highly rich in minerals and vitamins; the Arabs say that it is a supreme food for fertility in female animals and women, as in the same degree almonds give fertility to the male. The residue, after expression of the oil, is a favoured tonic food for cattle and horses. Applied externally it is healing and is also a hair tonic. The flowers have astringent properties; they are valuable in wound treatments and to cure warts.

Use   Treatment of worms, skin parasites and ringworm, all skin ailments, abscesses, venereal diseases, constipation, acidity, throat and mouth ulcers, discharging ears. Externally: the leaves make an effective douche in female ailments.

Dose   Two handfuls of the leaves or six green nut cases fed pulped, or brewed in two pints of water, then add two dessertspoonfuls of honey. Give one cupful three times daily. For external use, omit the honey. External also: walnut leaves, cut small and strewn on floors of farm buildings and in outdoor pens and dog kennels, deter parasite such as ticks, lice and fleas.

WATER AVENS (*Geum rivale*. Rosaceae)   This is a plant of streams and riversides. The foliage is deep green, the flowers are droopy and resemble wine-glasses held in green calyx. There are many colourful garden varieties of geum. The whole herb contains medicinal properties, but the root is the most powerful part. It is a favourite tonic herb of American Indians and of herbalists the world over.

Use   To increase appetite, soothe the stomach, dry up mucus and diarrhoea.

Dose   One teaspoon of the shaved root twice daily in bran, or one handful of the whole herb.

WATERCRESS (*Nasturtium officinale*. Cruciferae)   This is a plant of brooks and ditches, growing in the water. Distinguished by its slender, compound leaves of brilliant green and biting taste and corymbs of small white flowers followed by long, narrow, brownish seed-pods. It is an important tonic and cleansing herb. Watercress is very rich in minerals, and provides an effective cure for anaemia. It is one of the best blood herbs, and should be available to all animals: it increases the milk yield. Cows, horses and sheep greatly relish its foliage. One plant of the species, possessing large-size foliage, is eaten so avidly by cattle that it has acquired the name of cow-cress.

Use   Treatment of anaemia, eczema, scurvy, failing appetite, scanty milk yield. Heart weakness and ailments, rheumatism, rickets.

Dose   Two handfuls given twice daily. It is also excellent chopped finely, and given in cold milk.

WATER LILY (*Nymphaea alba.* Nymphaeaceae) The well-known white lily of ponds and lakes: sweetly scented. Its trailing roots are the part used. Lily root is soothing, cooling and astringent.

Use   Treatment of soreness and irritations of mouth and throat; all dropsical conditions. Vaginal douche.

Dose   One length of root, about twelve inches, cut fine and steeped in one pint boiling water.

WHEAT (*Triticum* species. Gramineae) The great cereal, esteemed in the Bible. It has many varieties both wild and cultivated. It has been proved that the 'mother-of-wheat', the true first wheat plant from which the hundred-fold wheat varieties descended, came from the lands of Rosh Pinna, in Galilee, Israel (where I myself have worked in agriculture). Wheat is a nutritious and strengthening cereal. Its germ is rich in the fertility and nerve vitamins E and B. The outer skin 'bran' has cleansing and drawing properties.

Use   As a strengthening food for all animals and poultry. As a source of natural vitamins and minerals. Externally the bran as a cleansing rub and general poultice.

Planting   When the moon is waxing full.

WILLOW (White) (*Salix alba*. Salicaceae)   This is a tree of moist places and riversides. Distinguished by its straight form, narrow leaves, shining, green-white and silky under-surface; it is catkin bearing, male and female. Cattle and horses eat the young shoots and foliage. It is a refrigerant herb, valuable in fevers. Tonic, astringent and antiseptic. The bark contains a crystalline substance, *salicin*, valuable in the treatment of intestinal inflammations. Beloved by bees; they use willow blossom as an after-winter purge.

Use   Treatment of all fevers, debility, enteritis, colic. Pleurisy, rheumatism, sciatica. Externally: rickets, cramps.

Dose   Three handfuls of foliage or two ounces flaked bark, brewed in two pints of water. Give one cupful three times daily. Externally: use the same brew; use hot and massage well.

WILLOW (Sallow) (*Salix caprea*)   If one wants to please goats, grow this tree for them. The word *caprea* is an ancient one for goat. The whole tree, leaves, twigs and bark, is highly tonic and medicinal, iron rich and blood cooling, calming the hot tempers of goats. Old prints and wood carvings depict goats eating from this tree.

WITCH HAZEL (*Hamamelis virginiana*. Hamamelidaceae)   This is a beautiful shrub of woodlands and watersides, from North America. Distinguished by leaves which are like the common hazel, but smaller and more deeply veined. It bears yellow flowers, like spidery, slender, incurved chrysanthemums. It is another of the sacred herbs of the Red Indians, who claim magical healing properties for the witch hazel. The whole shrub is medicinal, but the bark is the most potent part. The chief medicinal properties of the herb are antiseptic and powerful astringency: it is also very refrigerant. It is sold in most pharmacy shops, and in all herbalists, mixed with alcohol – extract of witch hazel. It is one of the supreme wound herbs and also reduces bruising.

Use Internally to heal ulcerated and burnt tissues in cases of poisoning. Also for stomach and intestinal ulcers. Externally: wounds, sores, bruises, ulcers, inflammation of the organs of reproduction, torn udders resulting in milk leakage, inflamed udders and glands, sore eyes and inflamed ears.

Dose One or two dessertspoonfuls of the extract of witch hazel twice daily. Externally: apply neat on swabs of cotton wool.

WOODRUFF (*Galium odoratum*. Rubiaceae) This is a woodland plant. Distinguished by its small, delicate growth, whorls of small, narrow leaves and terminal corymbs of tiny, white flowers, which are very sweetly scented. The whole herb is aromatic, the scent increasing on drying. All grazing animals relish woodruff, which increases their milk yield, being especially good for cows, and should be encouraged in all hedgerows. It is tonic and nervine.

Use Treatment of nervous debility, failing appetite, hysteria, chronic constipation, jaundice, fevers. Externally: wounds, ringworm, scabies. To strengthen wasted limbs.

Dose Four handfuls of the herb given twice daily. Externally: make a pulp of the herb by well pounding, gently heating in a little water and adding one part vinegar to four parts herb. Its good fragrance helps to protect wool against moths.

WOOD BETONY (*Betonica officinalis*. Labiatae)   This is a plant of hedgerows and woodland. Distinguished by its rough stems and foliage, spikes of red-purple hooded flowers. The whole plant possesses a pungent and peculiar aroma, especially noticeable when trampled on. This herb is soothing to the animal body, being warming and resolvent. It is of much benefit in the treatment of digestive disturbances and rheumatism. Externally: treatment of hard tumours and swellings, warts, corns.

Use Treatment of debility, gastritis, acidity, glandular deficiency. Rheumatism, arthritis, sciatica. Externally: rheumatism, sciatica, rickets, tumours, swellings, boils, abscess, corns, warts, blisters.

Dose Two handfuls made into a syrup by simmering in 1½ pints water to which has been added quarter-pound brown sugar. Externally: make an ointment with the foliage and flower spikes. (See Adder's tongue recipe.)

WOOD SAGE (*Teucrium scorodonia*. Labiatae)   This is a plant of shady places, woods and hedgerows. Distinguished by its rough, downy, very dark leaves and spikes of greenish yellow, hooded flowers. The plant possesses a distinctive aroma, somewhat resembling hops; it is very bitter tasting. Animals eat it. The herb exerts a powerful influence over the udder, and combined with garlic dosage it is a specific for mastitis. The name of wood-sage, *scorodonia*, is developed from the Greek word of 'garlic'. The herb is also very blood cleansing and mucus expellent. It is used in cleansing treatments for the blood, colds and fevers. The whole herb is used.

Use Treatment of mastitis, udder tumours and inflammations, obstructed menstruation. Internal inflammations, fevers, skin ailments, boils, catarrh, rheumatism.

Dose Two handfuls of the herb fed raw daily, or brewed in half-pint water, with one tablespoonful honey added. Give one cupful morning and night, fasting.

WOOD SORREL (*Oxalis acetosella*. Oxalidaceae) This is a plant of the woodlands. Distinguished by its frail appearance, shamrock-like leaves, purplish underneath, and delicate, white, solitary flowers, bell-shaped and purple-veined. The plant has an acid taste and contains oxalic acid – this acid property giving the herb its generic name, acid or sharp. Goats and sheep seek its foliage, enjoying its refrigerant properties. Red Indian horsemen pound up the roots and feed them to their horses to give them swiftness.

The herb possesses important medicinal properties, out of keeping with its delicate form. It is highly antiseptic, also possessing much refrigerant power which makes it of service in treatment of all fevers and inflammations. It increases the flow of urine, and together with its other properties is thus an excellent herb for treatment of urinary complaints. Externally it is used in eye treatments and scrofulous ulcers. One peasant method of preparation for external use is to wrap a handful of herb in a cabbage leaf and macerate in warm ashes until reduced to a pulp.

Use Treatment of all fevers, urinary complaints, haemorrhages, menstrual irregularities, catarrh, venereal diseases. Externally: scrofulous ulcers, eye ailments, piles, skin eruptions, wounds.

Dose Two handfuls of herb brewed in 1½ pints water, add one tablespoonful honey. Give one cupful three times daily. Externally: use the brew without the honey. Or make a pulp of the leaves by gently heating.

WORMSEED (*Chenopodium ambrosioides anthelmiticum*. Chenopodaceae) This is a plant of waysides and waste places. Distinguished by its grey-hued, profuse, smooth, rather cut-up foliage, but especially by its spikes of small, ball-shaped, grey-green flowers, which the Spanish say resemble a swarm of ants, and therefore call this plant the ant herb. The whole plant exudes an acrid smell when pressed and leaves a bitter taste on the hands. The bitterness is due to the presence of a bitter substance called *chenopodium*. This is extracted and sold bottled or in capsule form as a very effective worm remedy, particularly for thread and round worms. The botanical name *anthelmiticum* comes from the word for worms. In Spain it is a common pot plant, seen outside many a farmhouse, where it is employed as a blood-cleansing tea, and the leaves and flower spikes are minced up and put into a mash of corn and wheat for infants, puppies and poultry to expel worms.

Use As above, and to soothe stomach pains.

Dose One handful, cut small, given before any food, early morning.

WORMWOOD (*Artemisia absinthium*. Compositae) This is a plant of waste places and dry hillsides. Distinguished by its downy stems, greyish, fringed foliage, covered with short, silken down and leafy, erect, panicles of flowers, small, yellowish and globular of form. Its greyness and bitterness have given it a folk name of old woman whereas the brother herb, southernwood, closely allied to wormwood, is called old man and also Crusader herb, so esteemed by the Crusaders to prevent and cure plague. The whole herb exudes a very strong penetrating odour, and is extremely bitter tasting. The pungency and the bitterness are due to the presence of absinthate of potassium, and a quantity of a green, camphorated, volatile oil, both found in the leaves and flower spikes. The herb owes most of its potent medicinal powers to those two substances. In antiquity wormwood herb was made a symbol of health. The foliage is eaten by horses, cows and sheep. Its chief merit is worm expellent and tonic. It protects against contagious diseases and plagues. Is also insecticide and hair tonic. An important herb for all female ailments. The goddess Artemisia, after whom many plant species are named, was the protector of women and all female creatures. Therefore all the Artemisia group have special curative powers for female troubles and are eaten by pregnant animals despite their extreme bitterness. The Artemisia group includes mugwort and tarragon. Their bitterness provides famed use as worms remedy. It is an important aid in difficult birth. Give as a brew with sage herb and honey water.

Use Treatment of all worms, failing appetite, gastritis, gastric ulcers, acidity, enteritis, constipation, jaundice. Tuberculosis, tumours, pneumonia, pleurisy. Obesity, dropsy, paralysis. All female ailments, also bladder troubles. Externally: prevention of falling hair. Insecticide, especially lice, verminous sores, mange (for which it makes an excellent lotion when fortified with a little ammonia), inflammation of the ear, corneal ulcer, conjunctivitis.

Dose One handful of herb brewed in 1½ pints water, add one tablespoonful honey. Give one cupful twice daily. Or pound the herb into a pulp, and make into pills. Externally: use the brew, without honey.

YARROW (*Achillea millefolium*. Compositae) This is a plant of pastures and waysides. Distinguished by its finely feathered leaves, and corymbs of white or pinkish disc-form flowers. The plant has an aromatic odour, and is pungent and bitter tasting. It is a famed wound herb, for staunching excess bleeding, and derives its name from the Greek warrior, Achilles, who healed his wounds and those of his soldiers, with yarrow blossoms. The herb is also one of the most important febrifuges known to the herbalist, opening the skin pores and inducing lavish perspiration. The gypsies make much use of the herb, one peculiar use being to induce nose bleeding of animals which are feverish; yarrow leaves being introduced far up the nose, where their short hairs act as a mechanical irritant and cause bleeding: it needs skill to achieve this. Sheep seek out the herb on dry ground as food and tonic. It dries well as a fodder herb. Used as fodder by Dutch farmers.

Use Treatment of all fevers. Pneumonia, pleurisy, inflamed throat, haemorrhages, uterine haemorrhages, dysentery. Hysteria, epilepsy, rheumatism, colic. Externally: wounds, skin eruptions, abscess, earache, baldness (for which the flowers are made into an ointment). See Elder recipe.

Dose Two handfuls of herb, raw, finely cut, or brewed in 1½ pints water. Give one cupful morning and night, fasting, Externally: use a stronger brew, three handfuls to 1½ pints. A wad of crushed and gently warmed leaves is placed in the ears for earache. The brew can also be used as an ear lotion.

YEW (*Taxus baccata*. Taxaceae) A towering tree found in mountainous woods, and cultivated in parklands and cemeteries. It is distinguished by its great height and often nearly conical form, with foliage of very dark colour, filiated. Its strange looking fleshy, coral-coloured cup-form fruits hold a solitary horny seed. This tree has renown for the strength of its wood and the longevity of its life-span, causing it to be held as a life-symbol of tenacity and endurance. Yew yields the best arrows, and arrow tips were sometimes spread with the considered poisonous yew berry. Yew staves and shepherd crooks are considered fortunate and protective against beasts of prey, vampires and lightning bolts, if waved in the air.

Birds eat yew berries and take no ill from them. This tree is a good companion close to dairies, as it gives excellent weather protection against hot sun and gales both of which are inimical to the delicate process of butter- and cheese-making. Also yew makes strong, weatherproof fences and gates, and famed bows. This tree is a chosen nesting place of hawks, a bird beneficial to farmlands.

Use   External only. The leaves made into a strong brew and applied cold to nervous twitchings, soothe them. The leaves dampened and ignited, smoke away gnats and mosquitoes.

The Principal Minerals and Medicinal Plants rich in Them: Their Action

CALCIUM   Chamomile, chicory, cleavers, coltsfoot, dandelion, horsetail, meadowsweet, mistletoe, mustard, pimpernel, plantain, rest-harrow, shepherd's purse, silverweed, sorrel, toadflax, watercress, willow.
This mineral builds and maintains bones, teeth and nails, gives vitality, promotes healing of wounds, reduces acidity, prevents faulty food assimilation, safeguards health of the embryo.

CHLORINE   All herbs contain chlorine in the form of sodium chloride, all the grasses and nettles and comfrey are especially rich; also blackberries and raspberries.
This mineral maintains suppleness of joints and tendons, removes toxic elements from the organism, prevents over-formation of fatty tissue, promotes health of teeth and hair.

COPPER   Burdock, chickweed, chicory, cleavers (goose-grass), dandelion, fennel, garlic, hedge garlic (sauce-alone), horseradish, house leek, sea-holly, sorrel, yarrow.

This mineral aids the organs of digestion, tones the nerves, clears septic conditions of the tissues, strengthens and brightens the hair.

FLUORINE   Beet leaves, garlic, watercress.

This mineral is anti-infective, maintaining health of the entire body structure and tissues, keeps the bones disease-free, teeth, nails, ears. Strengthens the eyes.

IODINE   Asparagus, cleavers, garlic, Iceland moss, Irish moss, pimpernel, speedwell, sphagnum moss, sea-holly, and all the seaweeds.

This mineral is the supreme gland builder and conditioner, reducer of excess fatty tissue, safeguards the brain from toxins, removes toxic elements, promotes strong hair.

IRON   Artichoke, asparagus, bilberry, blackberry, brooklime, burdock, chicory, comfrey, cornflower, dandelion, dock, gentian, groundsel, ground-ivy, hawthorn, hops, nettle, parsley, periwinkle, raspberry, rest-harrow, rose, salep, scabious, scullcap, strawberry, toadflax, vervain, water-cress, wood-sage, wormwood.

This mineral is of premier importance to the blood, promotes oxygen absorption, builds red corpuscles, gives good pigment. Maintains disease resistance in the body, feeds nerve tissues, aids hair growth.

MAGNESIUM   Alder, artichoke, birch, broom, carrot leaves, cowslip, dandelion, hop, marshmallow, meadowsweet, mistletoe, mullein, oak, poppy, primrose, orchid, scabious, slippery elm, rest-harrow, rose, toadflax, walnut leaves.

This mineral promotes cleansing and restoration of the

organism, reducing excess acidity, calming the nerves. Promotes health of the skin and fine texture.

PHOSPHORUS   Anise, asparagus, calamus, chickweed, cornflower, dill, fenugreek, golden rod, linseed, liquorice, marigold, meadowsweet, sea-holly, sunflower, sweet flag, sorrel, watercress.

This mineral builds and maintains the brain, teeth and hair, all bony structure. Promotes keen eyesight and good nerve coordination.

POTASSIUM   Birch, borage, calamus, carrot leaves, chamomile, coltsfoot, comfrey, couch grass, cowslip, dandelion, elder, eyebright, fennel, honeysuckle, lady's mantle, meadowsweet, mistletoe, mullein, nettle, oak, peony, peppermint, plantain, primrose, rhubarb, scullcap, toadflax, walnut leaves, wormwood.

This mineral promotes general healing of the tissues, tones the bowels, gall bladder and liver. Encourages healing of diseased tissues, relieves pain.

SILICON   Asparagus, bed-straw, cleavers, dandelion, flax, holly, horsetail, sea-holly, strawberry, thistle, stalks of all grasses and cereals – including wheat and oat straw.

This mineral promotes and maintains strength of hair, hardens teeth and nails, strengthens the eyes. Maintains suppleness of limbs, ligaments and skin.

SODIUM   Alder, cleavers, clover, comfrey, dill, fennel, garlic, marsh-mallow, marguerite, meadowsweet, mistletoe, nettle, rest-harrow, shepherd's purse, violet, woodruff.

This mineral is the premier alkalizer of the body, strengthener of the digestive juices. Aids iron assimilation of the body, reduces premature hardening of the tissues, prevents catarrh and disease of mucous membranes. Maintains health of the urinary system and kidneys.

SULPHUR Brooklime, broom, cabbage, calamus, cowslip, coltsfoot, daisy, eyebright, fennel, garlic, Irish moss, marigold, meadowsweet, mullein, nettle, pimpernel, plantain, poppy, primrose, rest-harrow, scabious, seaweeds, shepherd's purse, toadflax , watercress.

This mineral acts as purifier and tonic for the entire system, especially the blood. Maintains health of skin and hair, strengthens the glandular system and promotes flow of bile. Keeps the liver healthy.

WOOD ASH The ashes of wood – charcoal – are a well-known cleanser of the human and animal body. Charcoal is highly absorbent and will take into itself many impurities. Then being also laxative, it will pass these impurities out of the system. Likewise worms and worm ova are also removed to some extent by charcoal.

Wild animals know the benefits of eating charcoal and when they scent wood-smoke will come in herds to eat the resultant charcoal. I observed this in the New Forest of England, where there are often forest fires. Herds of wild deer and ponies come to eat the charcoal. Bees also use charcoal quite extensively.

Preparation of Charcoal Charcoal is made very simply merely by burning dry (clean) tree branches slowly, in deep pits. Slow burning is essential for charcoal making, and therefore to check fast burning damp down with water-soaked embers. Wood ash (or charcoal – if the burning is slow enough), is then scooped up and mixed into bran. Or for smaller animals, such as dogs, sheep, goats, if they will not take charcoal in its natural state, give mixed with milk. Average dose: One dessertspoon of charcoal twice daily (wood ash and charcoal are of equal value).

Charcoal Poultice   One pound grated raw carrots mixed well into a half-pound of powdered charcoal, then heated and applied quite hot. Or mashed turnip can be used instead of the carrot.

This gives an excellent drawing poultice for swellings, abscess, boils, and all types of inflammations. Do not bind too tightly, especially not the feet.

Hay

Gramineae   Species and wild flowers. What bread is to man so is hay to the animals which man has domesticated. And hay is not merely food, it is also medicine. Because of the importance of hay to the farmer – for the sheer survival of his animals – hay is loved, and there are many rites and rituals associated with its cultivation and making. Hay, of course, is not a herb. It is composed of dried grasses and wild flowers.

The beautiful scents over the hayfields at cutting time alone give belief to its mystical powers. The scent of new-mown hay (when it is true hay, filled with fragrant field flowers, and not merely plain cut grass), is something beautiful and memorable in the farmer's every year, and a comforting smell also for the animals for whom it is gathered and stored.

In the lunar calendar for the farmer, hay should be cut, weather permitting, when the moon is waxing near its fill, then the goodness is in the leaf and blade and in the field flowers, and not down in the root, which anyway is not required nor used in hay. Since men first domesticated wild animals, hay has had associations with the Church, and newly mown hay is strewn in the aisles as a fragrant tread for the worshippers, and plaited, and wild flowers garlanded, hay bales are stood around the altar, and there is hay incense in the churches.

Before the hay is cut, when on windless days sudden ripples are seen passing through the fields, the wiser farmers know that it is the benevolent spirit of the hay passing by – and country people still watch for the hay spirit.

Preparation   Hay should never be kiln-dried. It needs to be stood in airy mounds, shaped like the old-time bee skeps, and daily turned and tossed until fully and naturally weathered and dried by weather and touched by sun, moon and starlight. This is true hay possessing juice and body; whereas machine cut and compressed hay possesses only half the body and vitality of carefully seasoned hay. The bales of machined hay are frequently mouldy in the centre layers.

Use   As a nutritious and minerals-rich and medicinal fodder, and to maintain animals during times when inclement weather makes grazing impossible (land under snow or frost), and to line animal stomachs with bulk food to prevent 'blow' or colic when animals are to feed on pastures which are dew wet or very lush. No peasant farmer would ever consider letting his animals out to graze under such conditions without first giving each animal an armful of hay to eat.

Medicinal use   This is in the form of steamed hay: that is, hay is slowly cooked by steaming in very little water, the old-fashioned way was between two tin plates over a bucket of boiling water, the hay itself merely sprinkled with a little water to assist the softening process. When the hay is sufficiently soft, cool it off to tepid, and then smear well with honey. (Do not spoil the hay by letting it get over hot, nor the delicate health properties of honey by pouring it on hot hay.)

This steamed hay is fed to sick animals which, in such cases as fever, scouring, severe colic, need to be confined in stable or byre and fasted from all food, and given only water for several days, the fast then being broken on steamed hay with honey.

An old-fashioned but effective sheep tonic, also for other animals, is made from cooked hay two parts, and one part nettle greens. Fill an average size bucket one-third deep with this vegetable mixture, cover with hot water almost to the top, heat gently but do not allow to boil. After ten minutes on the heat, stand to brew. When tepid, strain, sweeten with two tablespoons of honey or molasses, and use in the drinking troughs.

A final use for hay is to pack it around newly born animals to keep them warm. (Note. A loud ticking alarm-clock wrapped in a warmed, fleecy cloth comforts orphaned animals who believe that their mother is with them.) Wean young animals from the milk and gruel, on to steamed hay.

A postscript on hay Since the earlier editions of this book, hay is being replaced in modern farming by silage and the fields given over to arable crops. Thus, a further blow at natural health.

Cleansing of Pastures

It is unnatural and unhealthy for many animals to graze on a small area of land for a long time. In the wild, the herds are always changing their grazing grounds, moving onwards to clean places. Constant change of pasture is difficult to provide in farming, especially in modern farming. The only way then left to prevent animal-sick land is to cleanse pastures by several methods: by firing, by liming, by spreading soot or salt, or by growing an antiseptic crop, and the best one is *mustard*, and ploughing this into the ground. Radish and turnip also cleanse the ground.

The veterinary doctor, Dr John Rhorbach, now also a specialist in veterinary herbal matters, wrote to me deploring modern farming. Not only did he lament the passing of the healthful meadow hay harvest, drying naturally on tripods, he also commented on the loss of knowledge of worms control of farm animals by careful and skilled planning and manipulation of pastures.

Management of Cereal Supplies

The protection of large supplies of cereals is a worldwide farming problem. The enemy is always there: rodents, and the insect pests – moths, weevils and ants.

For rodents, the farm cat is the best solution. I met a farmer in Austria who keeps a large snake in his barn to keep out the rats. The big brown common species of snake are known as vermin eaters and are harmless to man and cattle. Use of poison to kill vermin leads to a vicious circle (see Rats below). Traps are a better and more useful solution.

The damage from insect pests is as severe as from rodents and, again, there is no sure solution. Fortunately insects mostly attack cereals when they have softened in age, so the best plan is to avoid over-stocking and to keep supplies moving.

On the Greek mainland wheat, oats and barley are sometimes given some preservation help by immersing sacks of grain in the sea. Weighted down by rocks, they are kept in the water for half an hour or so until the grains are well salted, which repels insects. The grains are then sun and wind dried on special grain mats woven of natural fibres.

Some Greek farmers also sea-plunge their supplies of dried garlic, keeping the garlic submerged for an all-over dip only. They sea-salt the garlic to prevent it from sprouting during annual storage.

When one has electricity a good machine to instal in the granaries is what I saw in use in Garboldisham Windmill, Diss, Norfolk, England, from which I have obtained supplies of flaked cereals in large amounts for many years. Those cereals have always been in prime condition with no insect damage and when I visited the mill I was impressed by the absence of insects, though the large supplies of cereals in flaked or flour form were a great attraction for such pests.

In the main part of the mill there was in use a machine called an Insect-o-cutor, the foremost use of which is to catch the small white-headed blow moths, which love to invade grain mills and are mostly active between April and October (I visited in September). The machine has an ultra-violet light which, because it uses only about 20 watts of electricity an hour, can be left on continuously. The insects are attracted to the flickering blue light behind which are series of wires. When an insect hits one of these, a 400-volt charge of electricity in the wire kills the insect which then falls into a tray below. The Insect-o-cutor obviously does not catch every insect, but it is very effective, especially in the dark when the moths are worst and it is, of course, much better than the use of far-carrying insecticides.

Cleansing of Farm Buildings

Farm buildings such as cow-houses, stables and poultry houses, need cleansing against parasites (skin vermin and worms), and rodents, cockroaches, scorpions, snakes, any and all of which like to make such places also their dwelling places to prey on the inhabitants, or to live off the food on which they feed, and all of which vermin endanger the health of the housed animals.

The best fumigation which I came across on all my travels, and which since I have used many times and recommended to other farmers (who have likewise been very pleased with the results) I learnt in Spain on the Sierra mountain range beyond Granada. This is a herbal fumigation, and entirely non-poisonous. The herb used is cayenne pepper (in powder form). This can be used alone, but it is further improved by the addition of garlic hulms (the dried skins and stems), and dried cow or horse dung.

Firstly seal up the building completely (using dampened cloths to close up any cracks or spaces amid doors. A quarter pound of cayenne pepper (powdered) to an average size building of about twenty feet square, two ounces are also effective for milder fumigation. The cayenne pepper requires to burn slowly. For heating, an oil stove can be used. Upon the stove place a tin lid, or a square of cut tin. On this spread the pepper (along or with the other ingredients), sprinkle with a little petrol or paraffin to facilitate the ignition. The pepper gives out pungent fumes which kill by suffocation, *not* by poisoning and is therefore, unlike chemical poison sprays.

Juniper berries and foliage are also effective as a fumigant. I learnt their use in the Balearic Islands. Seal the area, as for cayenne fumigation, place leafy branches of juniper in a tin, apply a little petrol and ignite; or put a quantity of the dried berries on to hot charcoal ashes. Another very useful form of fumigation is the burning of southernwood herb, fresh or dried.

Soon after fumigation, when the building has been aired by the opening of windows and doors, the animals and poultry can return.

Hedgerows

Hedgerows, not fencing, are the best investment for the farmer, for controlling movements of farm stock. Hedgerows pay high dividends in both health and efficiency. They provide shelter for the animals, as natural wind-breaks, and also shelter for the wild birds which clean up the insect pests on farms and in the orchards and vegetable gardens. Fencing declines in strength and usefulness throughout the year, whereas, in contrast, hedgerows improve with age, growing stronger and denser.

Healthful and good barrier hedgerow bushes and trees to plant are hawthorns, sloe, blackthorn, crab-apple, gorse, with honeysuckle and bryony to intertwine and increase the denseness of the hedgerow and also provide natural medicines. The same applies to all the hedge bushes and trees listed above, they give shelter, food and medicine for man, beast and bird.

The Moon

The moon exerts much influence on all plant and animal life. The females of both animal and bird are particularly affected by the moon, the menstruation cycle being moon orientated; the growth of the embryo is much under moon influence, the embryo being held in a bag of fluids. The Greek goddess Artemisia is the moon goddess and the plant family named after her, the Artemisias, are important for all female creatures, notably in the saving of life in difficult births.

The mental faculties of all creatures are also strongly moon-influenced: the very word lunatic comes from *luna*, the moon.

The moon is the queen of all waters, strongly influencing their flowing: queen of the spring tides and of the spring streams and rivers, of the sap within trees and plants, and of the body fluids of all living creatures, primarily the brain.

The planting of crops, tree grafting, and the harvesting of fruits and crops (especially cereals) were all in former times organized carefully according to the lunar calendar. But the harvest moon has now lost its meaning. The harvesting of crops (which fatten when the moon is waxing full) is seldom done by moon timing, but more usually at the convenience of the visiting grain cutting and drying machines, all done in haste with no attention paid to the essential slow maturing of the cut blades of grains or of fruits gathered for drying.

It is known to herbalists that certain plants are more influenced by the moon than are others. Artemis (Diana), the Greek moon goddess, was patron of wild deer as well as a famed huntress, but above all she was the protector of womankind, of all female creatures, human and animal, and of new-born infants. Therefore female animals seek out the moon herbs of the Artemisia group and, despite their bitterness, eat them regularly. The herb southernwood (*Artemisia aboratum*) gives great help in difficult births.

For complete health, all living things need contact with the moon, with its light and with its special plants, several species of which are condemned by modern scientists as being 'harmful'!

The importance of sunlight is recognized but the moon, equally important, is shut out from mankind (except the nomads and some primitive tribes) and also from most domestic animals, particularly the stabled ones in their unhealthy modern cattle barns and stables built from cement blocks and given cement floors – which insulate from vital earth contact, and often asbestos roofing.

How much better were the former cattle byres, now mostly standing roofless and forlorn, built from healthful natural stone, true examples of ancient building skills. Those old cattle shelters had permanently open doors allowing the animals to be out in moonlight, sunlight, rain, whenever and whichever they chose. Disease of farm stock was rare under such natural conditions, whereas today ill health is rampant and new diseases are being registered all the time.

The Moon shines in my body, but
my blind eyes cannot see it:
The Moon is within me, and so is
the Sun.

Kabir, famed teacher of ancient India

Rats!

Farmers and horse-raisers can do all the right, natural things for animal health yet never reach the maximum peak of good health because they harbour rats on their premises. The presence of rats causes disquiet and apprehension among all animals other than their enemies, the farm dogs and cats. The other animals fear the danger to their well-being which rats evoke. They have reason for those fears for the creature, the rat, is evil indeed!

First, it is a carrier of diseases, the most typical rat-borne ailments being foot-and-mouth, hepatitis, and rabies. Rats bring with them skin vermin, principally fleas but also lice and ticks, and are carriers of worms, particularly tape-worms.

Another danger is the skill of rats in attacking sleeping creatures: they seem to possess some mesmeric power so that the victim they attack does not waken speedily. It is known that a mouse can kill an elephant. (It gnaws the marrow from its feet until lameness sets in and the victim can no longer walk around to get its daily grazing.)

Recently, when I was in Norfolk, England, I saw goats which had hoof damage from rats. Subsequently, the goat-keeper shut cats in with the goats every night. That ended the rats problem.

On my travels I have seen many animals which have been attacked in sleep by rats. In fact, a favourite hawk of mine was killed in his sleep by a rat. When treating paralysed sheep in the Pennines of England in 1947, the winter of the great snow, I saw many sheep blinded by rats, which had gnawed out the eyes by night. I insisted that guards were kept over the sheep by man and dogs until I had cured them of their paralysis (which I was able to achieve). I have also, on travels, seen humans damaged when asleep at night, by rats – noses and ears eaten. Those are the human parts typically attacked by rats – by mice too.

I believe very much in the teaching of a wise Bedouin Arab concerning rats. He declared simply: 'Make the existence of rats so uncomfortable in your area that they will gladly remove themselves elsewhere.'

Poison is useless against rats because the clever ones do not eat it and, thus, survive. Poison also kills, at second hand, the natural prey of rats – foxes, owls and hawks – which are the best way to keep down the rodent population. Rat- and mice-eating snakes are also very helpful, as are dogs and cats. Fortunately my Afghan hounds are skilled ratters and mousers. One bitch of mine killed a near dozen of the highly dangerous Syrian rat, which used to devour my crops of grapes and olives. She tossed the rat with her big feet and then bit it. Recently, another Afghan bitch, in Greece, has killed a near dozen rats.

Traps are also useful, but do kill the enemy humanely when captured! I have a strong theory that if mankind occupied themselves with destroying the rat population of the world they would be kept too busy to fight their fellow men and, further there would be twice as much food available as a result.

Rodent damage of crops and stored food is vast indeed. For example, when a big agricultural project was launched recently in the Sudan, the rats came along and ate 70 per cent of the harvest. Never before has the population of rats and mice achieved such huge proportions. They are far more numerous than the human race; they are the biggest animal population of the modern world. Use of agricultural poisons, which rats cleverly avoid, is a basic cause of their increase because it has killed off large numbers of the natural enemies of rodents. Modern intensive farming also creates ideal conditions for the spread of rats.

Spanish folklore tells that God created neither the rat nor the mouse, the devil created both! The rats and mice are said to have sneaked into the Ark of Noah, sent there by the devil, to eat the food supplies and, most wicked of all, to gnaw a big hole in the Ark to kill all God's creatures by drowning. The rats made their hole, below the water-line, but the dogs and cats came along to protect the Ark. The dogs took turns in blocking the holes with their long muzzles until human help came. Then, further helped by the cats and owls, they attacked the rats whenever they tried to make more holes, and thus the Ark was saved!

3

Herbal Treatments for Sheep

The sheep is closely allied to the goat and the deer, especially in temperament and habit. It is naturally an animal of hill country and is a wide ranger, and does best on mixed grazing where the turf is rough and there is an abundance of herbs. However, as the sheep is primarily a 'nibbler', it is very helpful to fire heather and gorse tracts to encourage the young shoots and growth of tender grasses. It is well able to make use of, and to enjoy, woody vegetation, such as heather, whinberries, gorse, and tough foods such as reeds, sea grasses and seaweeds. It can survive in bleak pasture where other animals would starve, and is only surpassed in this respect by the thistle-eating donkey. It will thrive well on sedges, rushes, heaths, mosses and wiry grasses. In olden times the good grazing on typical island farms was reserved for the cattle. The sheep were often fenced off along the coastline where their only grazing, other than seaweeds, was on sparse sea-plants. That common seashore plant sea-samphire (of the Umbelliferae family) was always considered very helpful to and beneficial for sheep. It also makes an excellent pickle, in straight vinegar, for human use and will last well for years once pickled, using the preservative seeds of anise. Sheep were known to wade far out to sea, and even to swim, to obtain seaweeds from far rocks. The salt in their wool acted as a deterrent to body parasites, including the various sheep-attacking flies. The seashore flocks of the Scottish isles and of the coasts of Wales and Ireland were famed for their rugged health. Sheep require shade in very hot weather. To a hill animal by nature, damp, ill-drained pasture is especially harmful and is the common cause of many sheep ailments, including fluke. Salt air is very helpful to sheep, and unless they are in the proximity of sea air, they would benefit from organic iodine, in the form of seaweed, as frequent addition to their diet. The seaweed will also help to supply the crude salt that the sheep require to maintain health, and especially to remain worm free. Seaweed meal and foods can now be obtained from several firms in England and America. The animals like and flourish on them. The Spaniards say that salt given to sheep makes the wool fine and soft, strengthens the animals, and prevents foot-rot. Sea plants are most remarkably rich in vitamins; many varieties contain 1,000 times as much vitamin A and D as an equal weight of cod-liver oil. In addition there is the very high iodine content. In most of the old farming books the provision of salt is advised in all sheep pastures as a preventative against worms and fluke. The spreading of the pastures with salt is recommended, and it is observed how all the salt areas are grazed to a maximum by the sheep; one hundred weight or less of salt to the acre. But the crude natural variety only must be used – nothing synthetic. Molasses is the best tonic food for sheep; linseed oil the best general medicine, being a gentle purge as well as a good conditioner. It is mistaken economy to let ewes breed in their first year. Their strength is needed for maximum growth, not for producing lambs. Wait until their second year, then there will not be lambing problems nor birth of unthrifty lambs.

Putting ewes on to good green feed, especially the tonic herb mustard, several weeks before the breeding season begins, is a valuable practice. Overstocking, especially in lowland pastures, is one of the chief ills of modern sheep farming. In the last century it was ruled that two acres should be reckoned to every ewe per year; nowadays ewes are fortunate if they get two yards! And yet sheep, especially the ewe with her rich dung, with their gentle, non-destructive manner of grazing, are among the most important agents for soil fertility. They are rightly called 'the golden-hooved' animals.

Having lived for years on primitive Greek islands where there are no vets to doctor their livestock, I found their animals well cared for, and basically I learnt much in natural medicine from the farmers. Sheep were their principal animal and they have many excellent herbal remedies for them, which I was pleased to learn and use.

First, there is what they call 'horta'; everyone uses this great, green tonic, for man as well as animal. Horta is simply every variety of the dandelion family (including soft thistles) gathered in the early spring months when greenest, piled into a big pot, some salt added, and left to simmer with lid on for many hours. (The dandelion plants are dug up by the roots using a sharp, pronged tool.) The herbs are cut small before putting into the water and the liquid turns a bright green and has a rather bitter, but palatable taste. Some fresh lemon juice is added before drinking. This liquid is mixed into the water supply of any animal which requires a tonic or is ailing. Its medicinal property is highly tonic, also very blood-cleansing.

For a pick-me-up for sick sheep, the following mixture is much used and excellent results are observed. To every teaspoon of common tea, add one teaspoon marjoram (the pot variety, *onites*) and a half teaspoon powdered cinnamon. Then pour on a quantity of water and heat to make a strong brew. When tepid, add one teaspoon of honey to every cup of the brew. When cold, shake well, then pour into a plastics bottle ready for dosing the sheep. Now add a tablespoon of cognac (grape brandy) to every cup of the tea mixture. Shake well and give the mixture morning and night.

In fevers, follow the exact remedy above but add to the tea brew before heating several fresh or dried, finely cut, carnation flowers and six spice cloves. Some people add a couple of aspirins too; I prefer the alternative of a teaspoon of finely cut yarrow flowers or leaves.

In all internal treatments for sheep ailments, other than the very trivial complaints, the cure should begin with a short cleansing treatment in order to stimulate the organism to speedy removal of the causes of disease, which stimulation is never so effectively achieved by other methods as the natural one of fasting.

Internal Cleansing　Begin with a total fast of one day on water only; a purge to be given in the evening. For the purge soak seven large size senna pods in one small cupful of cold water, to which has been added a pinch of powdered ginger; soak for a minimum of six hours.

An alternative laxative to produce a quick purge (but which should not be used habitually) is Epsom salts or Glauber's salts. Five full teaspoonfuls of salt dissolved in hot water to which been added half a teaspoonful of ground ginger, and one teaspoonful of grated gentian root. Give when tepid. On the second day of the internal cleansing treatment give three laxative meals, or half a pint of milk and half a pint of water per feed, with the addition to each meal of two teaspoonfuls of molasses and linseed oil, or plain molasses if linseed oil is not available. Oil should always be given after salts to counteract their costive effect. In the evening purge as on the first day. On the third day feed bran mashes with molasses, merely one pound bran, two ounces molasses, the first meal in the morning; midday, feed two pounds; in the evening add a little steamed hay to the bran-molasses mash.

On the fourth day return to the usual diet. For the first two days of the treatment, which are purely fasting, the sheep should be kept from general grazing if possible and brought into a yard or kept in folds; this, of course, is difficult when large numbers of animals are being treated. A supply of fresh water should be kept available, preferably spring, well or brook water. Corporation water supply from taps is of low vitality. Garlic in tablet form, combined with other herbs or alone, or as a brew, should be given each morning. This greatly aids the cleansing work of the fast. Average dose is three four-grain herbal tablets daily, or one garlic root, or two whole plants brewed, in one pint water, one cupful of brew being given morning and night.

Sheep should always be dosed with much care as they are nervous animals and can easily be choked. Give charcoal throughout the internal cleansing treatment, either in small pieces or in tablet form, six three-grain tablets daily, or equivalent in wood charcoal.

Charcoal can easily be made by the slow burning of tree branches. Pine, oak, olive, eucalyptus, all make excellent charcoal. Whenever charcoal is purchased in pieces or tablet form, make sure that it is *vegetable* and not animal charcoal made from bones. The latter is valueless as a medicine, and in any case it is a health hazard to give herbiverous animals dead animal substances of any kind, though dried blood, fish products and other animal things are often forced on the herbivores to add cheap bulk to their dried commercial meals, dairy 'nuts', etc.

LAMBING If ewes were prepared for lambing throughout their pregnancy, lambing losses would be reduced to a minimum. Despite the so-called advances of science, losses remain very heavy.

Treatment   In-lamb ewes should always have access to plenty of fresh running water, as this is one of the most vital requisites of their daily diet. They should be allowed free and wide range grazing in order to prevent harmful fatness. Wide range gives them the advantage of taking a wide variety of herbs, especially cresses and twigs and leaves of the wild raspberry bushes. Raspberry leaf is the most important known herbal aid to speedy and easy parturition. It will grow on moorland, especially when there are rills or brooks there. Animals which were known as slow and difficult breeders have had easy and speedy lambings merely by the one addition of raspberry foliage to their diet. This applies to all female creatures, including the human being. When raspberry is not available, then briar-rose or blackberry can be used, only they are not nearly so powerful as raspberry. Linseed is another important aid to successful parturition.

Attention should be given to diet. In-lamb ewes should be kept on a light diet, the heavy feeding should follow *after* lambing, for high milk yield. The embryo should be kept small and muscular, not big and fat. Kale is a most important sheep feed, especially for in-lamb ewes, and is far better for them than root crops. The root crops should follow on after the ewes have lambed down, carrots and turnips being especially good; also oats for heavy milk yield which are rich in fat content. All the lucerne family increase fat content of milk, and are of general benefit to health. Most of the aromatic group of herbs, such as marjoram, sage, etc., increase milk yield. So also does milkwort and speedwell. (See Milk Production, Cows.)

Root crops must never be given frosted; fed thus they can cause abortion. They should not be fed alone without roughage. At least a portion of them should be sliced and mixed with wheaten straw. Hay can also be given for roughage, and some grain foods. Dry feeds fed with roots safeguard against scour, pulpy kidney and other ailments. This is accepted by most shepherds who study the dietary of their flocks. All ewes should be given a drink of tepid water immediately after lambing. As much water as they will drink. This is important, but is often neglected.

Difficult lambing and retention of afterbirth   The ewe should be kept fasting. She should then be drenched with a strong brew of raspberry leaf and linseed, strengthened with honey or molasses. All these substances are stimulating and tonic to the womb. Also feverfew herb can be added to the brew with much advantage. One handful of feverfew to one of raspberry. Further ivy leaves added, six to every half pint of liquid, are very helpful. The other birth-aid herb is *Artemisia*, the southernwood variety.

An old peasant remedy, used very successfully in the Pyrenean mountains and on the Spanish mainland, to bring down retained placenta after the birth, in all animals, is to horn down a quantity of the animal's own milk (the first milk when it is rich in colostrum). Ground ivy herb (a species of the mint family) can be added to this drench with advantage. Pennyroyal is also a well-proven remedy. Whenever available true ivy should be fed to ewes immediately after lambing, two handfuls of leaves per ewe. There should be plentiful grass kept for ewes after lambing, as it is the spring grasses, above all foods, which charge the milk flow with the vitality which will have such powerful effect upon the suckling lambs and which will help them into strong adulthood. Young grass is also a natural vermifuge, especially when the leys are planted with seed rich in herbs, including the clovers, mustard and the deep-rooting chicory and comfrey.

MILK FEVER   This is not common among ewes unless they are being milked for sale of their milk. Sheep milk is a popular commercial product in Mediterranean and Balkan lands, where it is highly valued. (For milk fever treatment – see Goats.)

WORMS   The many species of worms which attack sheep are among the most common sources of sheep ailments and the cause of the greatest losses. For worms, if they themselves are not the cause of death, can create such general debility of their host animals that other ailments, such as the common streptococcal and other bacterial infections, get a hold and destroy the animal. It is useless to dose for worms and to continue to keep the flocks on worm-infested pasture. When worms are proved in the flock, the animals must be dosed on the old ground and then moved immediately to clean land. The old worm-sick land should be cleansed by natural methods, such as heavily liming; growing a thick crop of mustard and ploughing in; heavily planting with garlic; or the old-fashioned method of spreading with soot.

When visiting farms I have over-often smelt the sour odour of sheep-sick ground, and invariably have found the symptoms of worm infestation in the flock.

Symptoms   Presence of worms is indicated by unthrifty appearance of the flock, including the lambs; discharging eyes, and often a husky cough which is given the name of 'husk' or 'hoose' in various parts of England; the cough is especially common in the lambs, who also often acquire the habit of eating quantities of earth.

Treatment   Garlic is the great specific, aided by molasses, for this herb possesses great powers of pulmonary penetration and the lungs of sheep are a common area for worm infestation and are difficult to reach with general worm drenches (such as the powerful – and highly dangerous – chemicals, which destroy the health of the animal along with the worms). Garlic is also an important worm preventative, and was formerly in regular use with sheep farmers in the Pennine mountain areas and in Ireland. The garlic referred to is the wild variety which grows abundantly in most parts of the world in many forms of broad and narrow leaf. When the plant is in leaf, which is generally in the early spring until midsummer, at a time when it is most needed by the flocks, the whole plant can be utilized. I noted on the hills of Galilee, in Israel, where wild garlic is a quite common herb, how keenly the goats and sheep graze every reachable leaf.

Feed finely chopped and mixed with bran and molasses, or make into medicine balls for those animals which will not eat it in any other form. One large, or two small plants, finely chopped, and mixed well with flour and black treacle into balls, the size of a walnut. Or flaked garlic root can be used throughout the year to make the medicine balls, or tablets of compressed garlic can be given, the average dosage for a sheep being two to three four-grain tablets once daily during treatment. Tapeworm and liver-fluke should be treated by the same method. In severe and deep-seated worm infestation, when immediate treatment is needed to save life, then a more potent treatment is needed, and the old and famed linseed-turpentine drench should be utilized, but given with all due caution on account of the potent properties of turpentine. For lambs: ten to fifty drops of turpentine, mixed with half an ounce to one and a half ounces of linseed oil, plus a pinch of ground ginger per dose. Adults: eighty drops of turpentine given in two ounces of linseed oil. The maximum turpentine dose for sheep is quarter to half an ounce per dose. If turpentine is given carelessly it enters the windpipe and can cause spasmodic closing of the mouth. To ensure safety from this, turpentine should be well soaked into a little dry oatmeal and the meal further mixed with a little cold oat gruel and linseed oil. Also treatment with N.R. Herbal Compound tablets (five antiseptic herbs, including garlic, rue, blue sage.)

All worm treatments should be given fasting, the lambs, however, being allowed to continue to feed from their mothers. Mustard seed (black or white variety), two ounces per lamb, given in milk also provide a safe vermifuge. Further, plant areas of mustard for the flock and let them graze it. Food additions of – raw grated carrot, raw desiccated coconut, and seeds of pumpkins, nasturtium, papaya, grapes, melon, are all worm removing. Likewise raw grated radish (common and horse), and turnip: also charcoal.

LIVER-FLUKE This parasite infests damp pastures for it must have damp, ill-drained places for its existence and completion of its life-cycle, the final stage of which takes place in a small snail shell. Garlic is a preventative. Centaury herb is an ancient peasant remedy. One ounce of herb being given daily; made into small balls with fat and flour. Lumps of rock salt should be available on the pastures.

Symptoms Jaundiced look of the eyes, rapid wasting and loss of wool. The back is roached and the abdomen drops.

Treatment Treat as for worms. Also give much chopped raw dandelion and centaury and flaked gentian root in the diet, also wormwood and southernwood. Capsules of oil of male fern are proved effective. In very advanced cases destruction of the animal is the best policy.

GID or STURDY This is caused by the cyst of a species of tapeworm. Dogs are the chief cause of the worm on the sheep pastures, though rabbits are also thought to be carriers. The worm segments dry up into egg form, and are eaten by the grazing sheep. They are then hatched out in the stomach and via the blood-stream enter the brain, where they form cysts.

Symptoms The infected animal shows a giddy gait, frequently falls, and is often unable to regain its feet.

Treatment Get the sheep on to clean pasture. Liming destroys the dried tapeworm segments deposited in the fields by dogs, and which are taken up by the sheep during grazing; also plough in heavy crops of mustard. Dosing with garlic is a deterrent to the development of the segments into the fatal bladder cysts. Likewise all sheepdogs should regularly be given garlic treatment as a worm preventative and cure; and in severe cases they should be dosed with male fern root or oil of male fern in capsule form. Once the cysts have formed in the brain, a surgical operation is the only effective cure. Aim always at prevention by keeping the sheepdogs free of tapeworm and thus safeguard the sheep themselves from infection from that source.

SCOUR (DIARRHOEA) This is a common ailment with sheep, especially during prolonged very cold or wet weather. The diarrhoea may also be the symptom of more severe diseases, such as black scour, which kills so many hill sheep; or caused by over-eating of rank or very sodden or over-rich green food, poisonous plants, etc. If treated immediately it is not difficult to cure, but if neglected death may result, especially in young lambs.

Symptoms Droppings become very moist and over-frequent. The wool on the hind quarters becomes very soiled and evil smelling from the loose excrement. The sheep show a failing appetite and look weak and emaciated; they bleat over-frequently. In black scour the excrement pours from the anus like black tar; and if not checked death rapidly develops, sometimes preceded by paralysis.

Treatment This should begin with a laxative drench to sweep out the putrid matter from the intestines. A quick and effective drench is one to two full ounces of Epsom salts dissolved in half a pint brew of dill seed water or give senna pods. (See Senna.) One small handful of dill seed boiled for five minutes in one pint of water, and brewed for two hours. Fast the sheep for twenty-four hours following the drench, give garlic brew or tablets, for internal disinfecting, in the evening. (See Internal Cleansing at the beginning of this chapter.) Then continue the treatment as instructed in Internal Cleansing – but do not purge further – introduce solid food as stated in the treatment. Highly recommended in all forms of diarrhoea, to thicken the milk-molasses feed, is powdered slippery elm (red elm) bark. This herbal substance acts as an internal poultice. It does not falsely cure the diarrhoea by blocking the bowels as with the chalky chemical powder products: it cures in the true sense of the word by its soothing and healing powers. Larkhall Natural Health (for address see p. 448) make a blend of slippery elm and other intestinal healing herbs, known as N. R. Gruel. This gruel has saved the lives of many animals of all kinds, including wild animals (young ones). It is my own formula, and I used this gruel when successfully treating many cases of the considered incurable black scour, among pedigree Swaledale sheep, in Swaledale, Yorkshire. In all cases of scour, keep the affected animals penned in a dry, warm place. Flaked barley should be the only cereal given for some time following the treatment. Boiled beets are good, also parsnips (which contain soothing bromine).

COCCIDIOSIS   (see Goats)

TETANUS   (see Goats)

METRITIS (Septic)   This generally occurs immediately after lambing, within twenty-four hours.

Symptoms Pinkish or brown discharge from the vagina, high fever, abdominal pains, coma.

Treatment This must be immediate. Removal of the lamb, fasting of the ewe for two days, followed by milk-molasses mono-diet. Dosing with garlic, flaked root, or two four-grain tablets, night and morning. Give one-inch sticks of liquorice juice in milk, twice daily. Keep the ewe warm. Internal douche with lavender brew. As soon as the discharge has ceased for several days at least, return the lamb to the mother.

MASTITIS (Garget) This is a general name for inflammation of the udder. The lambs should be allowed to suckle, the milk meanwhile being kept healthy by feeding large garlic balls or garlic tablets once or twice daily to the ewe, garlic possessing a potent power of entering the milk-stream; this power is not shared in like degree by any other known herb. In many countries sheep are kept mainly for their milk. This often means that they are deprived too soon of their lambs, and garget results.

Symptoms The ewe refuses to allow the lamb to feed. The udder becomes inflamed and very hard, also lumpy to the touch. The ewe often develops a fever.

Treatment Internally give garlic and a drench made from the scalding and brewing of wood sage: all parts of the plant are beneficial. A short fast should be given. Externally use a hot herbal application to reduce congestion. Apply to the udder flannel cloths dipped in hot brew of dock leaves. If sores are present elder should be added to the dock brew; or marsh-mallow ointment can be applied. To make such an ointment, the leaves and/or flowers or roots of marsh-mallow should be finely chopped and then made into pulp in boiling water; this is then stirred into melted vegetable fat, which should be allowed to solidify again before use. The wood sage possesses great power of removing pus accumulations in the udder and other parts of the organism. Failing a supply of wood sage use pulped cabbage leaves.

Some Yorkshire and Welsh hill farmers treat mastitis very drastically because they have not the time to give individual treatments to their large flocks. With a sharp knife they cut off the infected teat, and merely force out by hand-pressure the accumulated pus and the clotted milk. Certainly a very drastic method. Yorkshire farmers also apply warm packs of cow dung with good success.

SORE TEATS The delicate tissues of the teat sometimes become chapped, and develop deep fissures. The ewe then cannot tolerate the lamb feeding from her.

Treatment The teats should be alternately treated with warm almond oil as a salve, and bathed with a brew of equal parts of elder blossom or leaves and marsh-mallow leaves. (Dock leaves can be substituted for mallow if the former are not available.) Also proved very effective: raw cucumber juice applied.

FOOT ROT This is a difficult ailment to eradicate as the necessary treatment in order to effect a true cure requires much time and long application.

Symptoms The animal limps painfully and develops an unthrifty appearance due to the great pain, the disease developing rapidly and depriving it of its appetite and normal power of movement necessary for grazing. The feet are inflamed and internally ulcerated and foul smelling.

Treatment Change the pasture. The presence of foot rot indicates that all is not well with the land. Well purge the animals and then build up with good foods, such as oats, wheat, given crushed and mixed with molasses and pulped carrots; this last food is a very valuable tonic for sheep. Give plenty of green kale, rich in healing sulphur.

For external dressing of the feet: wash out all dirt from the clefts, cutting away sufficient horn to allow the inner sensitive parts of the foot to be reached. For dressing use pinewood tar or Stockholm tar mixed with powdered barley and molasses, which should be rubbed well into the feet and lower area of the legs. Or equal parts of Stockholm tar and castor oil make a good salve. To effect a speedy cure the sheep should be folded on to clean dry straw, or kept in a deep, straw-covered yard. Afterwards they must be pastured on dry ground. An effective treatment used by Welsh hill farmers is tar and salt: two or four ounces of salt to every half-pound of tar.

It must be remembered that the natural home of sheep is on stony hillsides, where vegetation is sparse. The exercise over hard ground and the leanness of body due to low diet, all keep the feet firm and in good condition. Damp, lowland pastures and rich feeding encourage foot rot.

STREPTOCOCCAL INFECTION This is a very wide term as there are so many forms of streptococci. However, at times of extreme debility, such as follows long starvation from green food following weeks of snowfall, or at times of very prolonged drought, streptococci, become over-predominant in the body and there is general emaciation, mucus discharge from the membranes of the eyes, nose, organs of reproduction, and sometimes from the ears. Paralysis of the back legs frequently develops, followed by rapid death.

Treatment Drench the animal three times daily with a mixture of powdered slippery elm, mixed with milk and molasses. Average dosage is one tablespoonful of molasses to one pint of milk. When strength returns to the animal, feed bran mashes with molasses, good non-dusty hay, pulped carrots, dry crushed oats. Peasestraw is also excellent for sheep, yellow turnips and lucerne.

Carrots are one of the finest natural tonics for all farm animals, from the cow to the hen. The stringy ends should be cut off before feeding, as they can bind together and form balls in the stomach or intestines, when many pounds of weight are being fed at one meal, and this can cause serious disorder. Garlic should be given as balls or tablets, to combat the streptococcal bacteria. And for a short period compressed chlorophyll in tablet form is important, as this green 'blood' of plants has an instant revitalizing effect on the chlorophyll-starved sheep. Sphagnum moss should be put into the water-troughs, and changed every three days. I have seen spectacular results from this combined treatment. After three days of treatment severely paralysed animals, condemned as incurable, were running and wall-jumping. Indeed, in all of my veterinary work the sheep cures have proved the most spectacular; the sheep farmers the most grateful, and also the most intelligent and unsparing in the carrying-out of the herbal treatments.

COLIC   (see Horses)

PARALYSIS   Paralysis can be caused by many things, from tumour on the brain or in the uterus, to poison or deficient diet, especially during heavy snowfalls or frosts, or even from a blow when crossing walls or going over or under gates.

Treatment   This can be internal or external. Internally: give concentrated iron-rich foods such as cresses, cleavers, comfrey, nettle, nasturtium – leaves, flowers, seeds; also molasses and raw, pulped carrots and beets. Other good, but expensive, remedies are pure honey, handful of raisins, red wine, all given in a bran mash. Remedial herbs are rosemary, sage, marjoram, finely minced and made into balls with honey and wheaten flour. Likewise give garlic leaves and roots, and mustard, whole herb or powder of the seeds; several tablespoons of each daily. Externally: massage with a strong, hot brew of mustard powder into which some drops of spirits of camphor and eucalyptus have been added; arnica added is also a great help. Apply on hot cloths, then follow with strong hand massage. On this treatment I cured a valuable breeding ewe of an Arkengarthdale, Yorkshire, England, herd which had been paralysed in both hind limbs for six weeks. The local farmers call her the 'miracle ewe'; she has since bred many lambs.

SCAB   This word covers many disorders of the skin in sheep. The condition may be purely mange, or a form of ringworm, or caused by lice infestation; but in all cases treatment is similar.

Treatment   Except in very cold weather, immediate clipping of the wool. Dipping in a solution of soapy water, drying, and then rubbing into all areas of the body the following wash. Brew tobacco powder, flaked garlic, and leaves of the wild geranium, as follows: into one gallon of cold water pour one pound of tobacco powder, four handfuls of cut garlic leaves or two shredded roots, two handfuls cut geranium leaves, bring to the boil and simmer for two minutes. Allow to brew for at least six hours; do not strain, rub well into the body. A more diluted solution can be used for lice and ringworm, using four handfuls of elder leaves in place of the tobacco, quassia wood chips can also be added, with much advantage when the skin is verminous. One handful boiled in with the mixture. N. R. (five herbs) Insect-repellent powder is proved effective made into a lotion, or as a powder for dusting. The treatment is absolutely harmless to the animal and is actually tonic to the skin and hair. All D.D.T. preparations (now, praise be, all banned) did great harm, more harm than can ever be analysed scientifically, the nerves and the eyes being the most damaged. It was proved that the milk supply could be poisoned by D.D.T. applied to the skin. Pure derris powder, which is a purely herbal product, can be used for mild cases of scab, with good results, either dry or as a dip, and was once a universally popular sheep dip before the modern drastic chemicals came into fashion. The tobacco-garlic application should be applied every few days until the skin is quite clean. Thereafter the sheep should be brought in the pens quite frequently and dry tobacco-derris dust applied. Doubtless if demand for this was sufficiently large, supplies would become more easily available, as tobacco dust is considered as a waste product.

There should always be internal treatment also, in skin diseases, even though they be of external parasitical form. For a healthy blood-stream and tough cell tissue and clean sweat-free body hair discourage the propagation of parasites. An abundance of garlic should be used, insects finding its pungent penetrative odour obnoxious.

All arsenical treatments should be avoided internally, also all other dangerous chemicals. Raw lemon juice (not bottled or canned) is applied for ringworm. As ringworm is a fungus-type skin parasite, in addition to cleansing with herbal lotion as described for scab, all air must be excluded from the fungus ring and then it will wither. Make an air-excluding glaze by covering over and beyond the fungus ring with raw, fresh lemon juice, or a glaze made by nail lacquer, or a light paste of egg white and liquid lime as used for whitewash (not the plastics type) can be used.

BROKEN LIMBS Sheep, being great wall and crag climbers, frequently suffer from broken limbs, especially forelegs. They can be repaired readily. I still consider splint and bandage to be the best method; especially the gypsy splint made from hollowed elder bough, and placed around the limb; lined internally with sphagnum moss, and kept in position by bandaging. Stand the limb in a bucketful of cold water thrice daily. Internally to aid the joining of the broken bone-parts, give daily a brew of chopped holly leaves and/or comfrey leaves fresh or a handful of herb or herbs to 1½ pints of water. In breakages, to allow for the usual early swelling of the limb, splinting should not be used for twenty-four hours, only light bandaging. Fast for one or two days to promote speedy healing.

RHEUMATISM AND ARTHRITIS These are ailments mainly caused by unsuitable pasture, damp, ill-drained, unhealthy land. The damp of the hill mists, however, is different, being natural to the sheep group of animals, and is beneficial, promoting dense and heavy wool. Lack of mineral in the diet due to insufficient variety in the grazing is another cause.

Symptoms Stiff gait, lameness without any sign of foot disease. Other parts of the body can also be affected, especially the neck, shoulder and back.

Treatment Look to the question of proper pasture. Internally give daily per sheep, a tablespoonful of paprika, which is a form of mild pepper, and is potently anti-rheumatic, and also rich in vitamins. Diet sheep for prevention and cure, using molasses daily; approximately two dessertspoonfuls. Parsley and comfrey are excellent, and so are ash, burdock, chickweed, celery – all when possible, including leaves and seed, and many lesser herbs given in Chapter 2. Cider vinegar or wine vinegar – one tablespoon to 1½ pints of water

– added to the drinking-troughs several times weekly, is a deterrent and a curative aid for rheumatism and arthritis. Spanish peasants give a compound of boiled rosemary herb and salt as a supreme cure for rheumatism. Two handfuls of rosemary heated gently in a pint of water to which half a tablespoonful of salt has been added. Give a drench, in two parts, daily. Also massage externally the affected joints, with the herb residue after the brew has been made. Further external lotions are: hot elder brew, a brew of shredded seaweed to which has been added one part of vinegar to three parts of cold seaweed brew or santolina herb infused in vinegar, applied hot. Also applications of warm cow dung bound with whitening are good.

FLY GALLS and SORE HEADS May and June are the most troublesome months of the year for the fly pests, when the eggs are deposited as forerunners of the maggots.

Symptoms Great uneasiness of the animal. Lumps and large festering sores appear.

Treatment Preventative dipping in N.R. Insect-repellent solution, see p. 447, or derris solution, or spraying with a solution of eucalyptus oil (in countries where there are eucalyptus trees, a strong brew of the leaves makes a very effective insect deterrent). It is notable that the koala bear which feeds on the foliage of the eucalyptus tree has a coat remarkably free from parasites (and the unblemished state of their skins is the reason for their being highly prized by furriers for their cruel trade). A strong elder leaves and garlic roots brew is also effective. If sores are present the places should be bathed with a brew of leaves or blossoms of elder or bramble. The old farming books, stressing the importance of using non-poisonous dips (long before this modern age of rampant poisons) all give tobacco as the best dip.

LICE and TICKS   Dip in a strong solution of derris, preferably powdered. A little eucalyptus oil can be added to the dip with great benefit. Camphorated oil is also effective.

Into the sores caused by the parasites there should be applied a strong solution of garlic leaves or roots. Give also garlic internally to disinfect the blood-stream and repel the skin parasites. Eucalyptus externally and garlic given internally have proved a very effective cure of tick fever in dogs and other animals.

Dusting with powdered N.R. Insect-repellent powder, or derris root and quassia chips is also effective. In severe infestation try and obtain tobacco dust, and use as a strong wash. One pound of tobacco to two parts of elder leaves brew; add one teaspoon eucalyptus oil.

MAGGOTS   An anti-maggot tip is given by Mr W. H. Humphreys. This is simply the application of a light smear of linseed oil, put on with a stiff brush. Mr Humphreys states: 'In May I dressed two hundred odd lambs (unshorn) with a light smear of linseed oil. These lambs were bushy.'

BRAXY   This is a blood disorder, producing clotting of the blood, and can cause speedy death. Sudden chilling is a common cause, also sudden change of diet from mean to over-rich.

Symptoms   Fever, hot mouth and nose; congested eyes, staggering gait.

Treatment   Fasting and quick drenching with strong Epsom salts and ground ginger. Followed by drenching with a solution of warm milk, molasses and oil of camphor (an average dose is from twelve to fifteen drops of camphor to one pint of milk). Give pure chlorophyll in tablet form. Apply hot flannels to the area of the bowels (dipped in hot brew of sage or thyme it is especially effective); and if the animal continues to be in great distress, then a warm-water enema containing a little ginger should be given. An old Highland remedy for prevention of braxy is the dosing of sheep with pigs' dung. This is a much-used peasant treatment and has received a lot of praise, although it is not one that I would want to use. The dung is mixed with fifteen times its volume of milk: 1½ pounds of dung given among a dozen sheep. Make sure that the pigs are worm free.

POISON Sheep, unless they come into contact with chemicals, sprayed grasses or other vegetation, are not common poison cases. They are slow and careful eaters, not greedy like goats. (See poison, Goats.)

RED WATER (see Cows)

HOVEN or DEW-BLOW (see Cows) This is caused by over-eating of rich, dew or rain-wet fodder in the spring or late summer following scanty rations. Clover or vetches are especially liable to cause hoven, also frosty vegetation.

BLINDNESS Cold and damp sometimes cause sudden blindness in sheep; usually a form of keratitis or 'blue-eye', and of a temporary nature.

Symptoms The animal appears very uneasy and hangs its head. On examination the eyes are found to be either covered with a fine white film, or to be of a light blue, solid appearance which looks very distressing. One or both eyes may be affected. The animal does not lose all of its appetite and will continue to graze unless totally deprived of sight. If the eyes are not treated promptly there is much wasting of the body.

Treatment Internally a short fast. Drenching with barley

gruel and molasses. A diet of bran and pulped carrots. Molasses and carrots are very beneficial in eye disorders, having a quick internal tonic effect on the eyes. The foliage of parsley should be fed with the roots. Parsley and fennel are further very potent remedial eye herbs, so are sunflower seeds. Externally: apply a brew of chickweed or balm or marshmallow leaves, bathing the eyes twice daily. Strain all brews for eye lotions. A brew of quince seeds is also an excellent remedy. The raw juice of cucumbers squeezed into the eyes is my own chosen remedy, learnt from the Arabs. Very diluted fresh lemon juice is another well-proven Arab remedy. Since I have also witnessed the great value of chamomile fortified with valerian root (finely sliced) and vervain: two teaspoons of chamomile to one of valerian – add a few sprigs of vervain, if available.

SHEEP DIPS   In former times, before the present widescale promotion of chemicals (backed by commercial interests), powdered herbs were used, choosing the most repellent bitter ones. There is no reason why they should not yet be used.

Chemical dips create further hazards because where the dip is dispersed there the poison lingers indefinitely: chemicals are there to stay on the earth – they never dissolve in the way of organic substances and they are always harmful to the animals on which they are used. In lands where natural animal care is still followed, sulphur springs are utilized for sheep dipping when available. Or a sea-water dam made by man and the flocks driven into that up to the head, and the head later washed down in a bucket of sea water.

In addition to the chemical dips, the Ministry of Agriculture advises dips of lime and sulphur, or tobacco dust and sulphur, all in solution. Such dips are far better than chemicals and can be used if desired. Double dipping is needed for the non-chemical dips: the flock has to be dipped on two different occasions at an interval of a few days, which is a disadvantage.

Additional useful and proved dip materials are derris powder, quassia wood chips, cinchona bark, wormseed herb, wormwood herb, all in powdered form in sulphur water solution. Bitter herbs, as detailed in this book, in fine powder form eked out by using a base of fine pine-bark dust or sifted wood ash, can be puff-sprayed on to the hairless parts of the bodies of animals to hinder lice and mosquitoes.

In the Greek islands, where the health standard of sheep is in the main very good, many farmers do not like to use chemicals on their sheep as dips or sprays; they consider their health is harmed thereby. When the sheep have been sheared, they merely bath them, first with hot water – no soap is used – then hose them down with cold water.

They use the ancient method of control of biting insects by keeping the sheep in the dark stone byres, roofed over, during the flies' season, and to protect against excessive sun heat. It is known that flies are around during certain months only and also that they bite only during daylight hours, so the flocks are put out to graze by night, free from torment. It is a pity and a mistake that the old-time stone sheep houses out in the fields have now largely disappeared. Those primitive buildings, easy to erect from local stone and mortared with mud and straw, served the sheep well and helped to maintain their general well-being. The sheep made much use of such places; they were a sort of sanctuary for them.

Lambs

If attention has been paid to the keep of the ewes throughout the in-lamb period, the lambs will be born active and sturdy, able to resist any amount of cold and damp.

One of the greatest causes of death in young lambs is

overcrowding in the pens. Young lambs develop very quickly and ample growing space must be provided for them. All young things from plants to animals require early 'thinning-out' so that limbs can have plenty of growing room, bodies ample food, and lungs the maximum of air. Sheep and lambs love the open air, and when in normal health will thrive in the hardest frosts. The lambing yards or pens must not be too sheltered or warm, for the animals will take chill later when sent out into open spring fields. The ewes from whom the lambs are feeding also require wide grazing range in order to make the best of milk which will ensure the future adult strength and health of their offspring. Also wide range is essential to ensure freedom from worms. The ewe's milk should be charged heavily with garlic, either by grazing the ewes where wild garlic is grown as part of the ley, or feeding garlic in a mash of bran and molasses.

Orphan lambs can be reared very well on a diet of N.R. gruel with honey (and if possible the milk of other ewes or goats).

WORMS The subject of worms in the adult ewe has already been fully dealt with, but I repeat here that lambs should be kept worm free in their early months, by the vitality, tonic and cleansing properties of the milk of a totally healthy ewe. They then but require dosing for worms in the autumn before they are turned out on to the moor or other rough grazing to make their adult growth. This autumn worming should be as sure a part of sheep care as the dusting of the wool with anti-vermin preparations. The best worming time each month is when the moon is waxing full or just on the wane.

Treatment The following medicine should be given to the lambs every morning for three successive days. The medicine is to be given fasting. One small teaspoonful oil of turpentine, mixed with two tablespoonfuls of oil of linseed, together with a half-teaspoonful of grated garlic, all blended into a sufficiency of milk, about three to four tablespoonfuls. One hour later give a feed of warm bran mash into which has been stirred one heaped tablespoonful of molasses.

CURDLED MILK and HAIR BALLS This ailment is said to be incurable, but I have cured many lambs. If, however, the cause is formation of balls of wool in the stomach, there is frequently death, for the wool balls block the opening from the stomach into the bowels, or sometimes it is the small intestine which is affected. Turkish peasants give big draughts of warm olive oil and powdered charcoal, and are sometimes successful in removing the obstruction. It is the shedding of much wool by sickly ewes which is a grave danger to suckling lambs. Keep the ewes healthy and this danger will be lessened. As part of the general care of lambing ewes, all loose hair should be taken from near their udders before lambing down. Also loose hair should be collected off the hedgerows, for lambs like to graze the young hedge shoots, especially hawthorn and bramble.

If the ewe has been kept on an over-mean diet until close to her time of lambing, and then suddenly is over-fed on large quantities of roots and indigestible and unnatural 'dairy' cakes and so forth, the milk becomes of a sticky consistency and is then highly indigestible and forms curd in the stomachs of the suckling lambs.

Symptoms Lambs affected with curd are seen to totter and are soon in a state of collapse; violent scouring generally develops. When wool balls have formed, the lambs exhibit spasms which resemble fits, and rapidly collapse.

Treatment The lambs should be taken immediately from the ewes, and promptly hand-fed on the following mixture, which will break up the curd and promote recovery. Make a strong tea of nettles. Any part of the nettle plant can be used including the roots if the plant be not yet in leaf when needed for treatment. After well brewing, re-heat the tea and pour over flaked barley. Allow to stand until the liquid thickens. Then squeeze out from the barley until this is left dry. Mix well into this one heaped tablespoonful of molasses to every half-pint of the brew.

Raw lemon juice in frequent doses of two tablespoonfuls is a much used Bedouin Arab remedy. Also a strong brew of sorrel, or feed the sorrel raw in handfuls.

Keep the lambs on this treatment for one day, giving drenches four hourly. On the second and third day add two parts of milk to one part of the herbal brew. It is understandable that milk other than the ewe's milk will have to be procured. The milk of goats is the best substitute; failing this, give cow's milk. Dried milks, pasteurized milks, must *never* be given.

If the condition of the lambs be very low with thready pulse, then give a stimulant of balls of honey (if possible fortified with two or three drops of oil of anise) pushed down the throat at intervals of several hours.

SCOUR (see Sheep) Lambs do not require the salts purge, and should not be fasted for longer than twenty-four hours. Through the fast they should be given balls of thick honey, the size of a walnut (six balls daily). A teaspoon each of finely minced sage and dill – or dill seed – can be added with advantage to every three honey balls.

COUGH This is most generally caused by worms or catarrh. Garlic with molasses or a strong draught of equal parts of sage and thyme, made into a strong tea and fortified with honey, is the specific for both. See also Worms, in adult sheep section.

RHEUMATISM or CROOK   Lambs sometimes develop a form of rheumatism which, if not treated properly, leaves the limbs permanently crooked. This is generally a cold weather ailment; exposure of unfit stock to east winds is a common cause.

Symptoms   The knees are generally first attacked. The joints swell and the swelling turns hard and stiff; the elbows are then the second seat of trouble. The semi-paralysed lambs should be carried at regular intervals to their mothers for suckling, in order to prevent their loss from starvation.

Treatment   Internally dose with garlic. Give paprika and molasses in bran mash. Externally apply hot flannels, also counter irritants, such as eucalyptus or turpentine. A north-country, and also a gypsy external treatment, is scourging with nettles. Powdered willow bark, very rich in calcium, is an excellent tonic for the limbs, as is finely cut comfrey.

NAVEL ILL   This ailment is peculiar to weakly stock with toxic blood-streams. It usually develops within two weeks after birth.

Symptoms   Staggering gait, congested eyes, sickly smell. The trouble generally begins with infected umbilicus, and spreads throughout the system, the joints being especially affected. Swellings in various parts of the body.

Treatment   Preventative treatment should be used on lambs from ewes who have previously had infected offspring. Dress navel area with a brew of garlic and sage, one handful of each with one tablespoon of witch hazel added, in 1½ pints of water. Or sprinkle the navel with dried, powdered rosemary.

Once the disease has developed the lambs should be dosed with garlic brew, four cloves flaked into half a pint mixture of milk and water, fasted for twelve hours, dosed with two dessertspoonfuls of linseed oil. Balls of honey should be fed as a stimulant. Return lambs to the ewe and watch carefully. Continue honey, garlic and linseed oil until the disease subsides. If the oil proves too laxative, reduce to two teaspoons daily.

From Marjorie, Lady Pryse, Ffynnon Caradog, Aberystwyth, Wales, who has her own historic pack of nature-reared foxhounds:

> I bless the day I discovered your books. I have had a small flock of Moorit (Shetland) sheep since 1932. They are always healthy and have *never* had injections or drugs of any kind. They drop their lambs with ease. The farmers around can't understand it. I've never had so many dead calves for the hounds as this year – from farms. All my animals have seaweed meal and bring forth their young unattended. Years of artificial fertilisers and drugs are taking their toll now with non-organic farms.

I could quote similar opinions in praise of natural (herbal) care of farm animals, for all the animals included in this book.

4

Herbal Treatments for Goats

Goats are a special love of mine, and my own two children grew up in their company and owe much of their excellent health to goat's milk and cheese. My goats – like my children – were Nature raised and I never had any health problems with them. Herbal medicine always gave me great results in restoring to health sick individual goats and herds belonging to others.

The goat is closely allied to the sheep being an animal of the hills and enjoying rough pasture. Goats are the most agile of the domestic animals, and above all they need abundant exercise for true health. The goat herds that I have seen in Mexico and Spain, and owned by the Bedouin Arabs in Israel, numbering many hundreds, leading the natural life of the mountains, are examples of animal rearing at its best. The food of those goat herds is largely the coarse mountain grasses, and the abundant aromatic herbs such as thyme, majoram, sage and a species of lavender. These goats never get concentrates. Unforgettable are the mohair goats of Turkey, native to the province of Angora. The Turks realize the importance of dry hill pastures for this animal, and that low, damp pastures cause lung weakness.

The milk of such animals is beyond description for its excellent flavour and the vitality that it imparts to the consumer; a great contrast to the flaccid, bitter-tasting milk of the tethered, stall-kept animals. The goat, like its cousin the deer, needs a portion of twigs, branches and bark of woodland trees for healthful diet and suffers in health if deprived of such fare. Goats are not really grazing animals; they, also like the deer, are more of a browsing nature. The ailments of the goat are closely allied to those of the sheep, with the difference that in many breeds the udder being unnaturally developed for its use as a commercial milk-producing animal, the goat has its major ailments in this area, and the organs of reproduction which in the female are so closely associated with the health of the udder.

As with sheep, the goat requires plenty of direct sunlight but also shelter from the sun in hot weather. On the Greek island of Rhodes I observed that, during the summer heat, the wise shepherds grazed their goats and sheep only in the cool hours. Grazing from late noon and all through the night, the animals went home to cool caves or byres early every morning before the sun was high. Abundant sweet water, iodine-rich foods and foods rich in aromatic oils. They also require access to rock salt in their diet, especially in hot climates. They also need much leafy and woody food other than grasses, indeed natural woodland grazing for total health. Crops to grow for goats are, oats planted along with vetches, for cutting whole, and barley (*the* goat cereal), daily and feeding both together, alfalfa, sunflower (the whole plant and seed heads), linseed, corn, including the inner cobs. Also flaked barley and rolled oats, wheat bran and dried beet pulp. In old farming manuals no other foods are listed. There is no mention of modern processed dairy foods which often contain dried blood and fish wastes.

In the winter diet of domestic goats, silage makes an excellent and nutritious change from dry hay, especially when prepared with molasses.

A health rule for goat care is to walk the herd every noon through woodland. When trained, they will not stray from their keeper and that herbal and twiggy-eating walk will ensure them great health.

For Worms, Scour, Foot rot, Scab, Ringworm, Lice, Rheumatism, see Sheep, Chapter 3.

MILK PRODUCTION (see this under Cows) Do not fail to massage the udder and gently bump it up and down in the way of suckling kids, after each milking. Goats are apt to hold back some milk. It is surprising how much extra milk this will give, and also will empty the udder completely.

Goats' milk makes delicious and healthful curd: the Arabs use a herb to curdle milk speedily and thickly: it is a type of hedge mustard, *hwere*, Arab name, Botanical name *Sisymbrium officinale*, Cruciferae. Merely place three or four pieces of herb into one pint fresh milk. The herb fed to kids helps them to digest milk very well. Thistle flowerets, fumitory plant and nettle juice also curdle milk for cheese. (See also Dairy Produce, p. 286.)

ABORTION This is not common in the goat. The best preventative measure is the giving of plenty of bone-forming foods immediately before and throughout pregnancy; also during the last months curtailing all foods which are known to have an exciting effect upon the uterus (this precaution being confined to animals which are known to have a tendency to abort). Cereals and nitrogenous foods come into this category.

Symptoms The animal develops lassitude and disinclination to eat. There are symptoms of general unease and the head is frequently turned towards the tail, and this is accompanied by much bleating.

Treatment Throughout the time of pregnancy all over-prepared foods should be avoided, this especially applies to

216

dairy nuts and cakes. Plenty of natural bone-forming, vitamin-rich and nerve-building foods should be given daily, the best foods for the female goat in this category being raw pulped carrots, crushed cabbage stalks, linseed, molasses, and all forms of green vegetables either wild produce or cultivated without the use of harmful artificial fertilizers. Leaves stripped from winter canes are excellent, as are sunflower seeds and carrot. Kale and mangolds in the late winter and early spring: mangolds need not be kept to ripen, but must not be fed frosted. In animals known to possess a tendency to abort, all cereals, with the exception of small quantities of rolled barley and chaff, should be avoided, or fed very sparingly, as they often cause over-excitement of the uterus in pregnant animals. Barley in any case is the best cereal for goats, being blood-cooling, an important quality in a species of milch whose blood easily overheats.

Berries and other fruits are a very important diet item for the goat, as it must be remembered that they are woodland- and mountain-grazing animals by ancestry. The fruit of the wild rose and the hawthorn are especially beneficial in keeping the reproductive system healthy. Raspberry leaves are a proved birth aid and have already been referred to in the section on the lambing down of sheep (see Chapter 3). Raspberry leaves are in habitual use with peasant goat-keepers in most of the Mediterranean lands. Also tansy leaves are proved to be excellent, and hollyhock root. When raspberry foliage is not available, the blackberry or wild rose can be used, but they are weaker. Give minerals-rich seaweed daily.

Above all avoid damp mouldy hay, and damp cereals, such food breeding fungi which are able to cause immediate abortion. The ergot fungus which is used in medicine as a powerful stimulant for the uterus, grows on rye heads and other cereals. Avoid also frosted roots, especially frosted turnips.

Also, as with the cow and the horse, the goat can be

nervously sympathetic to other aborting animals, and an aborting nanny must be isolated immediately from other members of the herd, and kept in isolation for several weeks so that she does not convey her scent to the others. The scent of the placenta has an exciting effect on other near-by animals. This fact has long been recognized by gypsies and other peoples knowledgeable about the minds of animals.

KIDDING The properly reared goat provides the perfect example of natural birth. No shepherd is required in attendance upon her. She bears her single or twin kids as easily as and naturally as defecation. And yet the modern goat-keeping books invariably contain a long chapter on the many ills of kidding. Understandably if the goat is shut in without sufficient exercise to keep her body strong and supple, and fed wrongly on over-rich concentrated foods, rendering her blood-stream sluggish and the kids over-heavy and inactive, breeding difficulties will result. There will either be inability to conceive, or to bear easily the offspring if conception should be achieved. The healthy goat will even kid misplaced offspring without assistance (as will the dog) because her uterus is so active and powerful.

Treatment The dietary remarks given for lambing in sheep are applicable in every respect to goats. Raspberry leaves and crushed linseed are the only special herbal items required other than daily attention to natural diet and exercise. The beneficial properties of raspberry can be increased by the addition of other sympathetic herbs. Two tablespoonfuls of finely chopped raspberry foliage should be fed daily, fortified with a further tablespoon of herbs made up of equal parts of peppermint, thyme and chamomile. If available feed fresh ivy, a handful per goat immediately after kidding. Also give water to drink. I used the ivy treatment very successfully when in charge of Prof. Edmond Bordeaux Szekely's herd, at Rancho La Puerta, Tecate, Mexico, during 1960. Formerly there had been losses of mothers and kids. On N.R. rearing and use of ivy after kidding, all losses ceased; writing to me, years after, Prof. Szekely informed me that the good results on my method continue. (See also Sheep.)

A life-saver in difficult births When something more potent than raspberry leaves or ergot of rye is needed (I have never used ergot, as it is commonly given by injection, but I've witnessed its use and seen it fail totally, mostly), I use my own special herbal brew which has saved numerous lives. Take eight medium size ivy leaves, one tablespoon southernwood (*Artemisia* species), a teaspoon of chopped sage, a few sprigs of rosemary to make a teaspoon, and six cloves. Placed in half a pint of cold water, using a lidded pan. Heat slowly to near boiling point, remove from heat. Keep covered, do not strain. When still warm add a dessertspoon of honey. Press the brew well with a wooden spoon, pour off the top clear liquid and give two tablespoons in a plastic bottle, slowly, into the side of the mouth. Repeat every two hours until the birth has been achieved. Then give a final dose as a pick-me-up.

MILK FEVER This is not so general as with cows, as the growth of the embryo does not put such a strain upon the organs of reproduction as with the cow. But eclampsia does occur, and death can result. The attack is notable for its severity, the animal falling to the ground in a form of coma and losing consciousness.

Symptoms This is not so rapid of development as with the cow. Generally there is no sudden collapse. The animal first develops a fever and lies down and ceases to eat. Soon a coma develops. The goat differs from other animals in milk fever by generally being affected some months after kidding, whereas with other animals it is usually in the early period after parturition.

Treatment This should be immediate. A strong drench of powdered seaweed should be given, plus molasses. A good average dose would be half a pound of powdered seaweed, one pound of molasses, well stirred into a small quantity of hot water, and then milk added to make a liquid drench. If green leaf extract tablets are available, give a handful as well. If the animal is not recovered in one hour, the drench should be repeated plus half a teaspoonful of powdered camphor. External treatment: this should consist of hot water packs, a sheet being soaked in hot water (hot but not sufficiently so to scald the skin), and the animal is then enveloped in this sheet. The sheet should be kept steaming.

Once the animal has been allowed to fall into a state of coma or near coma, it becomes dangerous to attempt any drenching, for the animal loses its power of swallowing. If the goat has not rallied within several hours following the herbal calcium drenching, then immediate treatment is a strong injection of chemical calcium into the blood, together with external hot pack treatment with a sheet. This is the only time I advise treatment by injection, and have never used it myself. In many cases of milk fever, air inflation of the udder is needed; this has to be done by an experienced person. Give also the herbal drench of seaweed powder and molasses, then also ensure the total emptying of the udder by milking and then use the air inflation treatment. Old farming books often tell of this treatment which apparently has been known for a hundred years. Cure by air inflation is often so rapid that it appears unnatural! The process is fully described in farming books old and new. I have never had to use the method myself, and therefore do not give it now.

MASTITIS or GARGET   The causes of this ailment are so complex and wide that the subject of mastitis in the milk-yielding animals requires literally a full-length book. Here it can be said but briefly, that a natural vegetable diet, with strict limitation of milk stimulating cake and artificial meals, abundance of exercise when in-kid, and regular use of garlic as a disinfectant both of the blood-stream and the milk, will do much to prevent mastitis.

Heavy yields should not be forced by concentrates only; selective breeding for good milkers should be carefully maintained in every herd.

The goat is an animal possessing good powers of recovery from most ailments, doubtless due to its inheritance of great vitality from its natural-living mountain-dwelling ancestors, and thus recovery from mastitis, treated by herbal methods, is speedy and complete: it is a great rarity for there to be loss of a quarter. The best cereals for goats, to promote udder health, are oats and millet; bran is important too. Peas and beans (well soaked in cold water) are a valuable food during the winter months. And an abundance of green foods; the sulphur-rich cabbage family and cresses are especially beneficial. Hedge cuttings are useful. Barley is the basic cereal.

Symptoms   Early symptoms are: failing appetite, a 'slotting' of the eyes, and also lameness of the limb against the inflamed quarter of the udder. The udder then becomes very inflamed and hard, and generally there is fever.

Treatment   This is similar to that given for Sheep (see Chapter 3), but the goat can take a longer fast at the start of the internal cleansing treatment, and should have two days on water only, or water and solution of molasses, with a purge given in the evening. An effective purge for goats is two ounces of Epsom salts, one ounce of linseed oil, half a teaspoonful of ground ginger, one teaspoonful of grated gentian root and two ounces of warm water, given mixed in oatmeal gruel to make 1½ pints. Kids can be given a quarter part of this laxative.

Sometimes in goats the internal complex structure of the udder causes one small hard area to remain in the area cured of the mastitis. This should be treated externally by hot applications instead of cold. A few drops of oil of eucalyptus should be added to the hot brew of dock leaves and there should be deep massage of the area, and gentle pressure applied by the fingers to expel the matter causing the hardness. Sometimes a small form of wart is left in the teat, preventing proper flow of the milk beyond a few drops at each pressing. This should be similarly treated with the hot herbal brew.

Sores on the teats should be treated similarly to those of Sheep. (See Chapter 3).

BLOOD IN MILK   This is generally caused by rough milking, or exposure to damp and cold; although if unattended by other abnormal symptoms, it may be present in the milk from natural causes immediately following kidding.

Symptoms   The udder generally feels hot to the touch. The milk is either stained with streaks of blood, or in an advanced form, comes from the udder a deep orange colour, almost like egg yolk.

Treatment   Give a short fast utilizing plenty of garlic. An average garlic dosage of four plants daily, or two four-grain tablets twice daily. Give a daily drench of wood sage. Follow the fast with a very laxative diet of green foods, bran mashes with molasses and pulped raw carrots. As part of the green food give daily two handfuls of wood sage. Apply warm cloths to the udder three times daily for one week or longer, during treatment and after the cure is completed. Recom-

mended, N.R. Herbal compound tablets for their antiseptic
properties.

POX   (see Cows)

TUMOURS   (see Cows)

WARTS   Goats, similar to cows often develop severe outbreaks of warts, especially in old age. The udder and teats are
often affected, and the warts may break and bleed during
milking.

Warts are usually caused by deficiencies in diet. In all my
experience of wild animals I have never seen a warty one!

Treatment   Increase iodine content of diet by much seaweed,
also cleavers. Try and provide further, sulphur-rich watercress and other cresses, and cabbage.

External: there are many herbal wart cures and they are far
better and more lasting than surgical treatment which often
spreads the trouble.

Amongst the best are – the applied white juice from stems
of dandelion, greater celandine, and from stalks of fig leaves,
also unripe green figs. Or apply raw lemon juice, or rub with
the downy insides of broad bean pods, or with the fruits, still
green, of rue herb.

STERILITY   Unbalanced diet is the general cause, with consequent ill functioning of the glandular metabolism. The
natural wild or mountain-pastured goats are very fertile, sterility being a great rarity.

Treatment   An abundance of aromatic herbs should be
included in the diet: thyme, mint, marjoram, sage, fennel,
etc. Abundant vitamin E should be provided, and to ensure
this, all cereals fed must be whole-grain and therefore contain

the all-vital germ. Linseed and liquorice, sunflower seeds and raw, finely minced seaweeds, also raspberry leaves, red clover, hops, roots of orchids (early purple), cyclamen flowers, angelica (whole plant), garlic and cayenne pepper, bryony roots, all are tonic and strengthening to the organs of reproduction, male and female. Mint, wild or garden, is especially beneficial for the male goat. Honey is a producer of fertility. Plenty of sunlight and exercise. All these listed fertility aids have brought many condemned barren goats into kid.

A practical aid for a nanny with a very acid system, is douching the vagina with a mild solution of soda or magnesia water daily while in season, and also a quarter of an hour before mating. This renders alkaline an over-acid condition of the vaginal membranes, which condition is destructive to the sperm of the male, and thereby prevents conception.

Females which fail to come into season should be dieted as above. They should get further a daily supply of wheat germ and sunflower seeds, plenty of mint, especially wild water mint, and rose hips, also liquorice.

They should be kept in close proximity with the male goat so that they get his glandular scent. They should run with him in the fields where the scent of his urine will impregnate the grass.

LEUCORRHOEA or the WHITES This is a white slimy discharge from the vagina which generally develops after a bad kidding. The discharge also occurs as a catarrhal infection and following a chill.

Symptoms White vaginal discharge. General debility accompanied by failing milk yield. Staring and falling coat.

Treatment A short internal cleansing fast. A tonic diet such as suggested for sterility owing to its beneficial action on the reproductive system. Give garlic daily either as diet or medicine; also raspberry leaves.

External treatment   Douche the vagina daily until discharge ceases. Two proved effective douches are: a weak solution of garlic brew, used at tepid heat, or a brew of dill seeds and lavender. The dill-lavender is made as follows: two tablespoonfuls of dill seeds, two tablespoonfuls of lavender, covered with a quart of cold water and brought to the boil for three minutes, keeping covered. Remove from the heat and brew for a minimum of six hours. Strain well before use and use at a tepid heat.

PNEUMONIA   Goats by nature being creatures of dry, rocky areas, and of high hillsides, are subject to pneumonia when kept in damp, draughty quarters, or exposed to sudden chills on journeys (when being transported to shows, matings, etc.). Goats bleat bitterly when tethered out in the rain, whereas most milch animals enjoy rain showers.

Symptoms   Chilly look with shivering bouts, followed by high fever. All food is refused and the goat looks miserable. There may be bouts of coughing.

Treatment   Remove the goat to dry quarters, but keep a window open for fresh air. Bed the goat on deep straw litter, and place pine boughs and rosemary foliage available. Leave a bucket of weak sage tea, sweetened with honey near the goat. The fever heat promotes great thirst and therefore the goat will accept medicinal drinks. Morning and night dose with pulped garlic cloves, four cloves per dose, or give N.R. garlic-rue tablets. Nightly give a dose of senna (see Senna). While high fever is present withhold all food, at most give a little steamed hay spread with molasses. If the lungs become very painful, apply a mustard pack as follows: spread over

the area and round to the backbone, a thick paste of powdered mustard with a little wine vinegar added in the mixing.
Press the paste well down through the hair to reach the skin.
Cover the mustard pack with sheets of brown paper, then
draw over all a woollen sweater, putting the forelegs of the
goat through the sleeves. As mustard packs are strong,
sponge off after forty minutes, using warm sage water, dry
well. Re-cover, but without inner paper sheets. When the
fever lessens, give thin oatmeal gruel sweetened with honey,
and a dessertspoon of sweet red wine added to every half
pint of gruel. When temperature has been normal for several
days, solid food can be given again.

BLADDER DISORDERS These are usually resultant from a
difficult kidding, or from the quite different cause of dietary
fault: an overconcentration of starches being given, and the
irritation of the kidneys, and thence the bladder, resulting;
especially likely if the cereals fed are unbalanced, i.e. not
whole-grain.

Symptoms Frequent passing of urine, generally with much
straining at time of voiding. Abnormal thirst. Stiff hind movement. Eyes are often congested.

Treatment Fasting. Laxative diet with plenty of linseed tea.
Feeding of handfuls of such vegetable things as parsley
leaves and roots, couch-grass leaves and roots, cherry stalks
and twigs, parsnips, horestail grass, comfrey, asparagus,
shepherd's purse, heather, chicory (whole plant), also raw
peas. All these listed things are highly beneficial to the urinary system. Give charcoal.

Diet should be laxative with only barley for cereal food.
Feed also pulped raw carrots and parsnips, seaweeds, also
fennel and dill.

COCCIDIOSIS In recent years, especially in America, this ailment (generally to rabbits!) is becoming increasingly diagnosed in goats, but in former goat books and old farming manuals relating to all types of livestock, this disease was never mentioned for goats. This new problem seems to me to stem from the increasing use of vaccines for a growing number of goat ailments which are all readily curable by simple fasting and herbal medicines. I *never* vaccinate, never use a syringe for anything, considering it an outrage to a body not made for quick medications. I view with horror the advice of orthodox medicine for vaccination of whole herds – and repeat vaccinations.

My advice is to avoid all unnatural treatments and to use the treatment advised for sheep (see Scour). Then immunize naturally with remedies proved over the ages of antiseptic herbs such as garlic, sage, thyme, rue, rosemary, wormwood and southernwood.

I was interested to note that on the old farms of the Balearic Islands all of these herbs were grown and no others (with the exception of an occasional santolina plant) for health protection of man and animal. They should also be grown on modern farms.

DIARRHOEA (SCOUR) (see Sheep)

FEET: OVER-GROWN The feet of goats need constant supervision. If the herd grazes on natural rocky terrain, the feet are kept in normal shape by the daily friction they encounter. But if the goat is on soft land – or worse, confined in paddocks or pens, then the outer horny layer of the hooves grows rapidly, and this will collect grit, small stones, dirt, etc. This foreign matter will soon cause soreness and inflammation, and eventually rot and lameness. Therefore feet must be given regular examination, and any excess growth pared down with a small hoof clipper. Oiling hooves is good for them, use pure lin-seed oil in which some rosemary has been infused for several weeks.

BAD LEGS AND FEET   Caused by over-rich diet, especially overuse of concentrates to increase milk yield. Also stabling on concrete flooring without sufficient cover litter is another cause.

Symptoms   Lameness, much heat and pain in legs and/or feet. If hooves are affected there is redness and inflammation. The goat crouches continually on its knees.

Treatment   Fast the goat, give daily garlic dosage. Place on a very green and laxative diet. Include one dessertspoonful of powdered wormwood in a bran and molasses mash, daily. Externally: poultice the legs, and/or feet, with a soothing and healing poultice of slippery elm and wormwood. Boil four ounces of powdered wormwood in 1½ quarts of water. Then stir the brew into one pound of powdered slippery elm, using sufficient of the brew to make a soft mass. Paste this mass around the areas to be treated and keep in place by use of an old stocking (preferably of cotton). The stocking should first be drawn over the leg, then tied around the hoof, and then turned down to receive the poultice in the hollow of the leg. Keep very moist. If stabled on concrete, make a thick layering with straw and bracken to keep the goat's feet off the stone flooring. A good foot dressing for general use is Stockholm tar.

ARTHRITIS   (see Sheep)

RHEUMATISM   (see Sheep)

BLOW or HOVEN   (see Cows)

POISONING   The goat falls ill from many sorts of poisoning, plant and mineral. Basically the treatment is the same: first speedy and thorough removal of the poison, and second, restorative treatment for the damaged internal organs, especially the intestinal tract which is generally left burnt and ulcerated; also for the injured nerves.

It is an important and interesting fact that goats which are allowed to graze freely in pasture and woodland are far less likely to get poisoned than goats which break out from confinement and whose only green fodder is that which is cut and fed to them. When such animals do break out of captivity, they fall ready victims to poison because their natural instinct in selective eating of the surrounding wild plants is entirely lacking. And if they are fed one of the poisonous plants, in error, in cut fodder they are sure cases of poison.

Here is an international list of plants poisonous to the grazing of animals of all kinds; birds and poultry seem able to eat poisonous leaves and berries and take no harm from them.

Of the plants: buttercup, greater celandine, foxglove, ragwort, larkspur, deadly nightshade, henbane, wild arum, good King Henry (in quantity), honeysuckle (in quantity: yet goats so love this plant it is called goats' foliage), morning glory, bryony (white), bindweed (in quantity), bracken and most ferns (in much quantity), winter heliotrope, monkshood, belladonna, greater fennel, castor-oil leaves and fruits (in quantity).

Of the small trees: yew, laburnum, rhododendrum, berries of laurel (in quantity), elder (in large quantity), alder.

Symptoms   These differ with the poison which the animal has taken. General symptoms are violent vomiting and diarrhoea, abnormal thirst, much discomfort accompanied by incessant bleating, striking of the ground with the feet, extremities very cold, body swelling. In strychnine, there are violent nervous spasms which contort the body and give the animal much pain. Phosphorus and strychnine poisoning, from rat extermination on farms, is the commonest poisoning among goats, for they are intelligent and wary feeders and not likely to partake of any of the poisonous plants. Safer to trap rats: not poison them.

Treatment Give the animal immediately a piece of washing soda, which produces instant vomiting. A goat would require a piece of soda about the size to fill a teaspoon (break into two pieces before pushing the soda dose down the throat). CAUTION: make sure you are using pure washing soda, *not* dangerous *caustic* soda, which is a poison. Follow this immediately with an enema of weak soda water.

Then give the animal a drench three times daily of the following mixture: two tablespoonfuls of pure powdered slippery (red elm) elm bark, plus one tablespoonful of honey, mixed into a half-pint drink with skimmed raw milk. In a case of phosphorus poisoning it is especially important that the milk should be skimmed, as no fat must be allowed to enter the animal's system for a minimum of two weeks. In between the elm bark and milk feeds the animal should be allowed as much water as it desires, although this is very contrary to orthodox treatment of poison cases. If the spasms of strychnine poisoning are very severe the animal should be kept under a narcotic injection for a half day to one day to lessen strain on the heart.

Night and morning give a medicinal dose of two tablespoonfuls of witch hazel extract; this heals burnt areas. This complete treatment must be followed for at least one week and continued until all vomiting and dysentery has ceased. Cold Indian or China tea, without milk or sugar, can also be given as a drink. To improve tea as a medicine, make it with strained barley water. Give charcoal in powder or tablet form, about two ounces daily. Rue and vervain are herbal aids against poison. Give a teaspoon of either, morning and night.

Then, when the first violent symptoms are over, a mash of flaked barley soaked in milk, plus molasses, can be given, retaining, however, as the first meal of the day, the elm-milk drench. The first barley, etc., meal should be small after the week of fluid diet, not more than two cupfuls for the first meal, so as not to overstrain the long-empty stomach; increasing daily to an average-sized feed. On the third day a little scythed grass can also be given. When recovery becomes noticeable, the animal can be put out to grass again, and its body built up with such tonic foods as linseed, sunflower seeds, kale, chicory and carrots.

During phosphorus poisoning treatment, there are often several relapses after the animal has been restored to solid foods, before complete recovery, for remember that phosphorus attacks that vital organ, the liver. Relapses are indicated by fresh outbreaks of violent diarrhoea, vomiting, cold extremities and subnormal temperature. Do not repeat the soda dosage, but return to several days on the fluid diet plus witch hazel. The elm bark and the witch hazel act as internal poultices, soothing the injured internal tissues; this is especially so when combined with honey.

In poison cases the animal must be kept warm, rugged if necessary, and surrounded by hot (blanket-covered) bricks in a hay bed. For, following poisoning, the body warmth becomes exhausted in the strenuous efforts made by the blood-stream to expel as quickly as possible the violent and dangerous irritants in the system, and thus the extremities often become dangerously cold. Give a course of N.R. Herbal Compound tablets, approximately four tablets per goat, morning and night. Mrs Lesley Harrison, Foxley British Saanens, has found these tablets excellent for her goats suffering from poisoning due to sprays on weeds. So have many other goat breeders.

Modern goat keepers have to contend with a new type of poisoning which is becoming quite common: it is a form of intestinal blockage as well as blood poisoning. The cause is the eating of pieces of plastic, nylon and insulating material (polystyrene), that white, foamy-looking thin board which seems an attractive food for goats when they find it and which is of petrol origin. Such debris can be wind-blown on to areas where goats are grazing or can endanger goats when the herds graze along the seashore. This synthetic material, when eaten, is apt to swell and block the intestinal tract so that faeces cannot be passed. There is then double poisoning, from putrid faecal matter and from the synthetic material. This type of poisoning causes the goat to swell in the stomach area, to cease to graze and to show acute pain symptoms similar to colic.

Treat as for colic, only continue fasting until the goat passes excreta again. Give drenches of linseed, and of powdered charcoal in milk. Give a strong laxative daily, castor oil or senna – castor oil for no more than two days. Charcoal is important because of its power to absorb and expel all impurities including poison, three 3 gr. tablets three times daily, or two teaspoons in milk.

CONSTIPATION   This is not very general in goats, occurring mostly among stall-kept animals not getting a sufficiency of herbage and hedge browsings.

Symptoms   Hard, dry faeces. Foul breath, inflamed eyes.

Treatment   Very green laxative diet, and use for several days of any one of the following reliable purges, much used by the old-fashioned herbalist. Two tablespoonfuls powdered liquorice, one dessertspoonful powdered ginger, made into a paste in two ounces of castor oil. Give in balls. Or, two tablespoonfuls powdered liquorice, one ounce grated soap, given in black treacle. Or, half-pound pulped figs, two ounces castor oil stirred in, given in two parts morning and night. Rhubarb root is helpful.

Silage is an excellent fodder. Also pulped carrots, parsnips, and all the berry fruits with the exception of bilberries, which are binding.

COLIC   In all forms this is a product of indigestion caused by faulty diet or over-exposure to dampness or chill winds. In kids the condition can be particularly severe, causing death.

Symptoms   Congested eyes, distended belly, roached back, an appearance of blow (see Hoven in Cows), striking of the ground with the feet. The kids will sometimes fling themselves about as though epileptic.

Treatment   Immediate fasting. Dosing with laxative, castor oil if necessary; warm water enemas. Fluid diet for several days, of barley meal gruel with milk and honey and slippery elm bark. Give chlorophyll (leaf extract) tablets. If the pains become very bad give a brew of liquorice, a walnut-size lump of the solidified juice dissolved in half a pint of hot strong dill water, four ounces dill seed well boiled in three-quarter pint of water, simmered for thirty minutes, brewed for a further thirty minutes, then strained. The draught to be given warm. A half-teaspoonful of grated gentian root, stirred in, will increase its efficacy. Other proven herbal treatments given as drenches are, a strong brew of mint and thyme, or an average brew of ground ivy or orchid roots (salep). As an after-cure once the colic pains have subsided, a strong dose of powdered charcoal in milk is excellent, also parsley peart.

External treatment. Keep the goat warm. Apply to the belly cloths dipped in warm mustard seed or mustard powder brew. Or rub with warm olive or salad oil, to which a few drops of oil of eucalyptus have been added.

JAUNDICE Treat as for colic, fasting, giving liquorice and dill, and charcoal (see also sheep-dogs for the special jaundice herbs).

EYE BLIGHT A form of eye blight or keratitis is the most general form of eye disorder in goats. The eyes become covered with a blue film and the animal appears to be in great pain, always seeking dark places in which to lie, and refusing food. The condition appears to be infectious. (For treatment see Blindness in Sheep, treatment of which has never failed to restore to health the many keratitis cases that I have treated.)

PARALYSIS This is not uncommon in the goat and there are many causes, a typical one being the eating of poison-sprayed vegetation. Eating belladonna herb is also a cause. Paralysis of hindquarters can be caused by a blow or fall, or severe constipation or even worms infestation. In the female there may also be a uterine tumour of size pressing on the nerves.

Symptoms The animal loses the use of its limbs, usually very quickly. Remedial treatment must be equally speedy to effect a cure.

Treatment Fast the animal, allowing only pure water and old hay. Some honeysuckle foliage and sage leaves and nettle (dried) can also be given as fodder. Make a strong brew of sage leaves, and add a teaspoon of powdered ginger to every half pint of brew. Give balls of wheaten flour and honey. Nightly for one week give a laxative of senna pods: ten pods, soaked all day in ten teaspoons of cold water, a half teaspoon of powdered ginger added. After four to six days on a diet of hay and sage brew, allow normal food, but also give much nettle (and nettle seed when available), molasses, garlic (leaves and bulbs), finely-cut rosemary mixed in bran. Externally: massage the limbs with a strong brew of mustard seed or powder. Hot vinegar can be used for the brew.

SUNSTROKE It must be stated once more that the goat is essentially a hill animal and should always have access to shelter from the sun (also from drenching rains). The goat being commonly a tethered animal when not being pastured in a herd, is too frequently subjected to punishment from sun and rain. I have seen many cases of sunstroke in goats. Tree shading is best, but stone shelters with open doors are also useful.

Symptoms Panting lungs; appearance of dizziness, with hanging head and unsteady legs, much bleating. A very high temperature or a sub-normal one. Rapid death may occur.

Treatment Place the animal immediately in the shade. Give a drench of a brew of mint leaves and sorrel, plus honey (which is a quick shock restorative). Give cold common tea (see TEA PLANT, Chapter 2). Sponge down the entire body with cold water and bind cold cloths of water fortified with a little vinegar around the head, horns and neck. Keep on a mono-diet of milk and honey for two days, but allow grass grazing in a place entirely in the shade. Handfuls of sorrel, given in a bran-molasses mash, is refrigerant and helpful. Keep the animal in tree shade, by tethering, for at least one week.

SKIN AILMENTS (see Sheep) In cases of lice the goat should be clipped all over and washed with soap, a little soda being added to the bath. The skin should then be dusted with derris or tobacco. Also recommended, N.R. (Five Herbs)

Insecticide powder for dusting and bathing. It is 100 per cent herbal.

In case of eczema, give a short internal cleansing fast (again see Sheep) using plenty of garlic internally, also buckthorn, burdock and sorrel. Externally, bathe with a brew of blackberry foliage. Elder can also be used, blossom and/or leaves, but blackberry is best.

TETANUS What I have written about coccidiosis in goats applies also to tetanus. This is a modern problem. The goat, by nature being an adventurous animal, liking to climb and leap, suffers many skin abrasions and wounds. Yet one never hears of tetanus among wild goats (nor among their close relation, wild deer) yet both are often injured by rock falls, tree spikes, etc. Because injuries are so common in goats – and so natural – I consider it extremely unwise to vaccinate against tetanus each time there is a wound, when it is extremely unlikely that the goat will develop tetanus and which, if developed, can be treated successfully in the natural way with fasting and the many antiseptic herbs. Wild goats and deer, when badly injured by biting dogs or when the males fight, wade out into the sea (if it is reachable) and cure themselves that way. They will also roll in sphagnum moss. (See also Cows, Wounds.)

WORMS (see Sheep) Remember to provide boxes of clean earth for the kids to eat. Important.

WOUNDS (see Cows) Goats are adventurous animals. In the wild their active character does not create problems, but in farm environment when there are artificial walls, barbed wire and spiked fencing, accidents are quite frequent. A basic prevention of accidents for all farm animals should be the provision of natural hedgerow fencing, planting the shrubs and trees suitable for the climate.

CAPRINE ARTHRITIC ENCEPHALITIS New viruses come along all the time in this modern era when the promised wonders of advanced medical science should have eliminated all disease. The viruses, which kill off valuable stock in quantity, are a direct result of unnatural rearing policies. Merely consider the orthodox advice that is given to combat the ailment. First, there is a total ban on imported goat semen. But the very use of this frozen semen, and of artificial insemination itself, are direct blows at the natural happiness and vitality of the female goat being so treated. Then a major piece of orthodox advice is that kids should be deprived of their mothers' colostrum and milk, and that the kids should be removed from their mothers at birth and then raised on cow products – probably dried milk is indicated and permitted. Even if such unnatural treatment did prevent the spread of the virus – and I do not credit that it does so – kids so raised will inherit poor health, which is likely to make them victims of other virus ailments, instead of building up their vitality and protecting them by feeding them herbs that have long been proved effective deterrents to disease. Of these the foremost is garlic (but whole garlic and not merely the extracted oil, which is an internal irritant and not a remedy); rue, wormwood or southernwood, sage, rosemary and cloves are also effective.

You can use the herbs either fresh or dried. If fresh, they must be cut very small; if dried, they should be powdered, or you can have them made up into an exact formula, as in my N.R. Herbal Compound tablets (H.C. tablets have been extremely helpful in preventing and curing all virus ailments, including rabies in dogs and foot-and-mouth in cattle.)

Kids should be allowed to benefit from their mothers' colostrum and milk and from the herbs in the milk flow. In order to prevent the herbs from contaminating the milk with their strong smells and tastes, the herbs should be fed to the mothers at milking time; they will have left the udder by the time of the next milking.

In conclusion, I should mention Mrs. Ann Petty, formerly of Quebec, Canada, and now of California, USA, who practised Natural Rearing for a number of years. She states that when she commenced her goat herd, the goats had every known (and unknown) disease, but year after year their health improved, and people came from 'far and wide' to admire their size, beauty and general strength.

Kids

Kids are mainly prone to the same ills as lambs. (See Sheep.) Unfortunately, as their mothers are commercial milk-producers, most kids are bottle-fed from an early age (sometimes from birth) instead of being allowed to feed naturally from their mothers' udders and, as with calves, never enjoy maximum health, which is the natural heritage of the udder-fed.

Naturally bred and reared kids are the healthiest of all the domestic animals, being very active from birth, precocious and highly intelligent. They are grazing strongly at the age of four weeks.

If the female goats have been carefully bred for milk production, as well as fed for it, they should be able to suckle one kid and also yield sufficient milk for the bucket to give a profit much above the cost of their keep. The kid will then obtain the benefit of total health, which will make it (if a female) an important and vital member of the herd when its own time comes to produce milk. Udder-reared kids will far surpass bottle-fed stock in general development and resistance to disease.

Kids to be bottle-fed must, if possible, stay with their mothers for at least one week. And those reared by hand from birth, must unfailingly be fed on the laxative 'first milk' (colostrum) of the mother.

In Spain and Mexico where I have met very hardy and healthy goats, the bottle is never used. The kids are taken from their mothers after the first week and kept apart on the farms or ranches. They are fed three times only, morning, midday and evening, being put then to suckle an old nurse goat, who will take as many as six kids. All day they have to seek food from young grass blades and fallen leaves: they get nothing else. That way they learn to graze very early. Some may get evening milk only from their true mother.

In bottle feeding six small feeds per day of warm milk should be given, the milk to be diluted with a tablespoonful of barley water to every half pint. A wine bottle is preferable, owing to its long neck. N.R. Products make a nutritious and soothing rearing gruel of tree barks and cereals for kids and lambs. If necessary kids can be given half goats' milk and half cows' milk in the feeding bottle, but of course full goats' milk is best.

Ground whole barley gradually should be introduced into the milk, also a little molasses (one teaspoonful to a pint of milk). Powdered slippery elm is a wonderful bone and muscle producer, and the calcium-rich powdered willow bark is also good. Then flaked oats and mashed raw carrot. A little powdered seaweed for full glandular development. Kids do well on a porridge of oatmeal, enriched with molasses.

Kids in the natural state, similar to the foal, are weaned very late, and will continue to feed from the mothers into early adulthood. The Arabs, who are rearers of such magnificent horses, highly prized milk as a food for herbivorous animals (realizing that it is vital vegetable matter in suspension) and they continue to feed milk to the best of their adult horses, and also to their racing camels. Also they feed honey to their best animals.

A kid should be getting milk from the udder or bottle until as late as six months of age. Early weaning retards growth, and no amount of rich feeding in adulthood can then bring the goat up to full size and total health. Suckling stimulates the mother's udder to full milk yield.

One of the best tonics for backward goat kids, is blackberry fruit. Handfuls of herb Robert (wild geranium) are also an excellent tonic, so is fumitory and all the aromatic seeds, such as dill, fennel, anise, celery, fenugreek.

Kids should be encouraged to take plenty of exercise in order to develop their limbs fully. Piles of thick tree branches, or sawn logs, should be placed in the pasture, to encourage the young ones to leap and climb, as they would do when living in the wild state. They will also enjoy nibbling at the bark.

From Diana Downes, Rt. 2, Box 108A, Dallas, Oregon, USA:

We raise Nubian goats and hope to show that natural care and rearing produces a superior animal. We bought the original stock from a man who was a Roumanian and who believed entirely in herbs and natural foods for people and goats. He said when we bought these goats: 'Let them out in all weathers if they wish, so they can go nibble on the wild herbs to cure themselves and preserve their health. You will never have a sick goat.' Certainly they were in beautiful condition then, and have remained beautiful and very healthy.

As I was working on the revision of this Goats chapter living in a remote part of southern Greece, I had an interesting experience. Down on to the beach near Leonidion came a magnificent herd of black goats, shining with health, rugged creatures. They came with a purpose! A recent storm had littered the shore with quantities of seaweed. The goats feasted on this, fighting each other with their long horns as each animal sought to get the most seaweed. They ate up all, then went away up the mountainside.

Ann Petty also wrote:

From March 1 through to March 20, my goats dropped me forty-four kids, whew! all the births either triplets or quadruplets, and that brings my herd to eighty! I have never had so many kids, but I've been feeding much natural iodine in kelp powder and your seaweed minerals blend food. The kids are on their feet and have had their first drink within fifteen minutes after their birth, amazing!

We are now many generations into N.R. and the herd undoubtedly improves all the time. Now people come from far and wide to see my goats, recommended by others, for I do no advertising, and join no societies. Nobody can believe their eyes, and they say in wonder, 'I've never seen goats like that before so big and such huge udders', etc.

I don't try and explain any more, people aren't able to understand – they say, 'It's wrong to raise kids on their dams' and 'wrong to let them go into the forest', and 'You don't give any chemical treatments?!' I find most of my goat interested visitors to be fixed believers in veterinary orthodoxy. And then they think they can raise much better animals than mine since they know the 'modern' methods, and they take away my kids convinced that they can beat me in a competition that does not even interest me! BUT IT IS THE GOATS PURCHASED HERE THAT WIN FOR THEM IN THE SHOWS (and that makes me laugh). Finally how nice to hear from you and have your thoughts on cows, that are so close to mine.

I had written to her about the pain that I feel whenever I think about the ending of a cow's life. That those ultra-sensitive animals, so gentle and kindly in their own ways, they must suffer deeply when butchered, should have to go to a public slaughter-house, those places of no escape and atmosphere of all-engulfing terror!

I know two cases of stampeding cattle escaping from the butcher, one a steer in Chicago, USA, the other a cow on the Sierra Nevada Mountains of Spain. In both cases a child was in their stampeding path. In Chicago, children were leaving a school and a child fell down in the panic caused by the onrushing animal; the steer amazingly stopped its onrush, stepped gently over the child, and then ran onwards. In Spain a small boy was in the middle of a narrow path by a mill, throwing stones into the mill stream. There was no hope for the two people near by to get to the child before an onrushing cow and to pull him out of danger, for sure he would be crushed to death. But, again, the cow curbed its onrush, sniffed at the child, then, walking carefully past the small human, continued its fear-maddened race down the mountainside. The two observers knew they had seen a miracle. One was myself – and the child was my son.

In a recent BBC programme – 'New Ideas' (a weekly series) – an individual farm slaughter-house was described (serves No. 10). I wish that such could be installed worldwide and thus remove much of the terror from animal slaughter – cattle, goats, sheep, horses, all.

5

Herbal Treatments for Cows

'Hast thou cattle? Have a care for them.'
The Bible

With the exception of poultry, cows are the most unhealthy of the domestic farm animals, doubtless because they, together with poultry, are the most commercialized. Ill health in both these classes of animals begins with the rearing of the young. Poultry chicks are deprived in the egg, and afterwards, of the natural healthful radiations from the body of their mother. The young of the cow are deprived of their mothers' milk, and when bucket-fed develop weak jaws, inferior digestive tracts and weakly legs, as compared to those reared on their mother as nature intended all calves to be raised.

It is well understandable that animals given such a bad and unnatural beginning to their lives develop into tubercular and infertile adults. The amount of disease present in modern cattle herds, despite all of the so-called advantages of scientific rearing, is tremendous. The following observation is taken from an old farming journal, published in the year 1885, and is most applicable to present-day wholesale depriving of calves of their mothers' milk, with substitution of all manner of milk imitations.

'Husk in calves is brought about by the absence, for the sake of economy, of the natural food of a calf. We are told by unsuccessful dairymen that milk makes no money, yet we find the calves are not allowed any!

'Stop the milk supply early in the life of a calf, leave the poor bellowing baby animal to the unsympathetic care of a careless and ignorant calf-herd, and if that calf does not become the victim of all the ills of calfdom, husk included, then the writer's long farming experience has all been in vain. Keep a healthy calf from the day of its birth, in the same pen as the calf suffering from husk, and give the healthy strong calf access to its mother's milk, and I defy you to convey to him the throat derangement from which his bed-fellow is suffering unnecessary martyrdom. Mercenary motives and mismanagement cause most of the ailments in animals of the farm.' (From *Farm and Home*, May 1885.) This quotation in every respect agrees with my own beliefs on the root cause of cattle ills; especially important in the quotation is the reported disease immunity of the naturally reared animal. Furthermore, not only is the deprivation of suckling bad for the calf, it is injurious to the health of the mother cow. Failure to suckle her calf is a frequent cause of glandular and udder ailments, also it may be the cause of uterine complications, because shrinkage of the uterus after parturition is much dependent on the nerve stimulus provided by the sucking calf.

Another cause of the general poor health of the commercial cow is the interference with the very important breeding rhythm of nature.

It is natural for most animals – and plants – to be born in the spring. The deer calves down in the spring and so do most other of the grazing, milk-producing mammals. It is the high prices obtained for winter dairy produce which induces the farmer to arrange for unnatural winter calvings. In spring calvings the cow experiences the most difficult months of her forty weeks' gestation during the winter months, when the weather is cool and there are few flies to torment her. In early spring the fresh juicy grasses will cleanse her bloodstream and develop her milking capacity, and likewise immediately after calving she is able to feed herself upon the young green food best suited for vital milk yield, and for the health of the calf. The calf will get milk charged with the vitality from sun-rich grasses, and will know the benefits of warm sun and tonic spring air on which to grow to healthy adulthood.

Equally important for disease prevention and cure in cattle is the provision of herbal leys, natural water supply (never from the corporation water works), and home-grown, whole-grain cereals, kept free from harmful chemical fertilizing and poison spraying. Without the provision of all the above given essentials of cattle rearing, whole health becomes an impossibility.

Lack of exercise is one of the great faults of the rearing of modern dairy cattle. Cows are provided with insufficient space for the roaming natural to the herd life of herbivorous animals. A healthy cow should be able to run without difficulty: the present day development of the heavy pendulous udder makes such exercise almost impossible. Less than fifty years ago dairy cows were regularly 'walked' by a cow-boy, to keep them in good fettle, for both milk production and breeding. Breeding animals – female and male – must get daily ample exercise to keep them in sound health. Otherwise the bloodstream, lungs and digestive tract all become unhealthy. Exercise is said by farmers to lessen milk production. That is only so in the unhealthy. There is also the quality of the milk to be considered as well as the quantity.

Unnaturally reared cattle exist, breed and yield milk, but they never show the wonderful vitality nor the disease resistance of the naturally reared, and this applies to all animals when the health of the natural is contrasted with the unnatural. Furthermore, the milk of wrongly and artificially fed cattle is bitter tasting, and turns sour so quickly that preserving by pasteurization becomes an essential of the marketing of such milk.

For Eye Disease, Skin Parasites, Rheumatism, see Sheep: for Leucorrhoea, see Goats. *Note*. Increase the dosage to treble or over of that prescribed for the two above-mentioned animals. During fasting treatment the prescribed should again be trebled or more, according to breed of cow. Average laxative dose is twenty to twenty-four large senna pods to one and a half cups of water, with a half (small) teaspoon of powdered ginger added. Garlic dose is two whole roots or entire plants, grated, raw, or brewed in one pint water – half pint mornings, half at night – or ten N.R. Herbal compound tablets.

Calving

If the in-calf cows, from time of service until calving, have had sufficient daily exercise, ample diet of natural foods, including those of a bulky and laxative nature, also plenty of fresh air, sunlight, and have been housed in dry and airy places, calving should be easy and straightforward. Even in complicated presentations easy births can be achieved if the above requisites have been supplied.

Two weeks before calving is due, feed a laxative diet, such as pulped carrots, bran mashes, ground oats and linseed meal. For several days before the actual calving, feed cut fresh grass and a warm bran mash sweetened with half a pint of molasses. Feed no other grain foods. Continue this diet for two days after calving. Then if all is normal, as it should be, put the cow back on to usual diet. For difficulties of birth, see Sheep.

ABORTION (see Goat section for treatments)   When abortion is epidemic in the herds, individual in-calf cows should be carefully watched. As soon as there are observed any symptoms of untoward uneasiness or any excessive vaginal discharge, the cow should be brought in from the fields and confined in paddock or yard for one week. She should during that time be strictly dieted, commencing with a one-day fast. The fast should be on water only, a laxative senna drench being given in the evening. All cereal feeding should cease, and diet should consist of clean, sweet hay, scythed grass, bran mashes with molasses, ground linseed, kale, pulped carrots, and sunflower seeds. The raspberry leaf daily dosage should be replaced by a concentration of vitamin C; one of the blackcurrant concentrates, or rose hip syrup. My personal choice is blackcurrant purée, an average daily dose is two tablespoonfuls once daily. This is expensive medicine, but is of little cost when compared with the loss of a calf through abortion, and the subsequent failure of the milk supply as an after-effect of abortion. Many of the Rosaceae family are valuable as an abortion preventative. Also give honey.

Blackcurrant leaves, strawberry leaves (wild and cultivated, if cultivated take care that chemical sprays have not been used), sweet briar leaves, rose hips, hawthorn haws, can all be fed with much advantage. A famed Somerset gypsy remedy for prevention of miscarriage in humans is the powdered dried root of garden hollyhocks; this remedy has been used with successful results in animals. A cow would require a daily dose of two dessertspoonfuls of powdered hollyhock roots, or rather more of the finely flaked fresh root stirred into half a pint of milk, one dessertspoonful of honey to be added.

Garlic to cleanse and disinfect the bloodstream should be given regularly to all in-calf animals.

It must be remembered also that the cow, similar to the goat and the mare, is highly influenced by nerves in relation to abortion; and neglect to consider this fact is one main reason for widespread abortion passing through the herd and being classified as an epidemic.

Mouldy hay and flowering grasses which may carry the fungus ergot – especially prevalent on rye, wild or cultivated – and in winter frosted roots, must all be kept from cows when in-calf. All are dangerous. Silage is also best avoided for cows which have any tendency to abort.

Finally, regular exercise is essential for breeding animals, both bull and cow. This is too often neglected and weakly offspring are consequently produced.

RETENTION OF AFTERBIRTH This trouble is rare in the goat and the sheep, but it is becoming increasingly prevalent among cows. It is significant that a very high percentage of such cow cases are those animals which have been subjected to artificial insemination instead of enjoying normal service by the bull. Doubtless the reason for the failure to expel the placenta, in those cows which have been impregnated by AI, is the fact that during service the uterus has not been properly stimulated and none of the normal nervous excitement has been aroused with the corresponding stimulus and awakening of the whole sensitive and highly vital glandular system. The action of the glands at the time of sexual intercourse has a most important and beneficial action upon the whole reproductive system, which benefit remains with the animal throughout the long period of gestation: glandular stimulation is wholly lacking in AI. The far-reaching effect of a powerful discharge of sperm on a properly excited animal is such that the odour of the sperm can be smelt several hours later upon the skin of the body in areas remote from the sexual organs and also in the breath. This could never be found after AI.

The female's emotional condition at the time of conception

has a great influence upon the vigour of the resultant embryo, low vitality being a general thing among artificially conceived animals. Doubtless, further, the lack of vigour of the embryo has a negative effect upon the uterus, and thus the birth is not fulfilled in the normal way and the final effort required for the expulsion of the afterbirth is lacking.

Naturally there are many other causes for failure to expel the afterbirth, such failure being quite common long before AI came into use. A major cause is low vitality of the cow at the time of parturition, and general lack of nervous tone. Only careful prenatal attention to diet can give the necessary all-round good health.

Treatment   The cow should always be given her calf to suckle as soon as she will accept it, for the stimulation of the udder by the suckling calf has an immediate effect upon the nerves of the uterus. Likewise she should also be allowed to lick clean all over the body of her calf, the skin of which, following the birth, possesses substances which are both attractive to the mother and important for her health. Likewise the early fluid in the cow's udder before the milk comes in is of vital importance to the new-born calf, being highly cleansing and tonic, and nothing could compensate the calf for the deprivation of this early fluid, colostrum. The importance of the colostrum and also the cleansing of the calf by the mother's tongue, is accepted by most of the so very practical early period farming journals and books, where it is stressed how greatly the process affects beneficially the nerves of the cow and calf. To induce a backward heifer to lick clean her first calf, the calf can be sprinkled with bran. This is an old peasant method.

The forced removal of retained afterbirth is usually far too early, nature should be given a chance to complete her own work at least until the passing of several days. When artificial removal becomes necessary then the orthodox method of hand removal, the inducing of violent contractions of the womb by injections of chemicals or fungi preparations, should be avoided for as long as possible, and instead the safe herbal treatments should be used. The herbal remedies are as follows: big drenches of strong brew of raspberry leaves mixed with feverfew, three parts of raspberry to one of feverfew herb, a quart drench with one pound molasses added, given to the cow, fasting, who should not be allowed any heavy foods until the afterbirth has come away. French gypsies recommend a strong draught of beer and brown sugar with grated nutmeg, to induce the afterbirth to come down: an average draught of half a gallon of beer, one pound of brown sugar and two ounces of nutmeg.

Another popular draught is: two quarts of pennyroyal (hedeoma) tea, one pound Epsom salts, two ounces of ground ginger, one pint of the cow's own milk. Linseed oil should be given two days later to remedy the costive effect of the salts.

As an after treatment, even after a normal birth, the cow should be fed four handfuls of fresh ivy leaves. Cows themselves seek out ivy and eat it keenly after calving, especially in cases of retained afterbirth. I noted this in the New Forest of England where cows trampled my herb garden while reaching for the abundant ivy which grew there. At the time that calving is due keep the cow on a fluid diet or on green, very laxative, feeding. At time of birth and immediately after birth, the body is far too occupied with the vital processes related to parturition, to expend valuable energy on digestion of food which is not required at such times, either for the nourishment of the cow herself or her calf. Diet should be very green, of scythed grasses and also green vegetables, bran mash and molasses should also be given, but she should be fasted on water, or water-milk-molasses, for one day immediately following calving. This natural treatment greatly helps the normal processes immediately following birth, encourages a thorough cleansing of the uterus, and removes the causes of future uterine or udder trouble, which so generally have their beginnings in mismanaged or unhealthy births.

AFTER-CALVING HAEMORRHAGE This is caused generally by the bursting of a blood-vessel or vessels generally following a difficult calving.

Treatment Raise the hind limbs several feet above the level of the front ones. Give vaginal douches of cold salt water to every quart of which should be added two tablespoonfuls of the astringent witch hazel. Or a strong brew of herb Robert plant or ivy leaves can be used with the witch hazel. Externally: apply cold cloths to the vaginal area and to the belly; for the vaginal cloths apply some witch hazel. A good tonic for all run-down conditions in cows, mares, etc., is a brew of powdered oak bark plus a little powdered ginger, made with one handful of herb to one quart of water.

MILK FEVER This trouble is becoming increasingly common in cows, and must again be associated with forced unnatural modern feeding and herd management. There appears to be no record of milk fever among the wild herbivorous animals during lactation. For instance, I have never yet on all of my moorland wanderings found the dead body of a hind killed by milk fever, and yet large numbers of domestic animals die annually from this ailment. Therefore, before a cow calves down, much attention should be paid to her diet to ensure that it is not too immediately milk-stimulating, and thus likely to cause overstrain of the system, already strained to full capacity by the last stages of pregnancy. For the same reason the cow's diet should be watched very carefully immediately following parturition; it should for a week or more be preferably a meagre diet, rather than an over-rich one. Let the diet be very laxative and green. The green element provides the abundance of calcium, the sudden over-drain of which is a basic cause of milk fever. Molasses, being very calcium rich, and not at all overheating as some farmers state, should also be given freely. Steamed hay (hay heated gently over a bucket of water to soften it), handfuls of water-cress and water-mint, crushed nettles, are all beneficial in the early days after calving. Preventive treatment in a threatened case of milk fever, or in cows known to have a tendency to the ailment, is a small daily dose of Epsom salts, to discourage immediate over-rapid production of milk. Two table-spoonfuls of salt given in one cupful of the cow's own milk is sufficient.

Symptoms Development of milk fever in the cow is usually very rapid. It must also be stated that it is not always associated with calving, although it is generally a subsequent ailment. Milk fever can sometimes occur many months afterwards, although such an occurrence is rare in cows. The cow becomes feverish, lows almost incessantly, and appears very uneasy. She rapidly loses control of her legs, and lies down and is unable to rise. Her eyes become very congested and her breathing and pulse rapid. If immediate and effective treatment is not then given, coma rapidly sets in, and death may follow. The horns and extremities usually become very chill.

Treatment This must be immediate. The cow must be prevented from stretching herself out upon the ground and getting her head down, by supporting her with bales of straw or hay. She should thus be kept propped up in a sitting position. If coma has not already set in, she should be given an immediate calcium and iodine-rich drench of two big handfuls of powdered seaweed mixed into two pounds of molasses, the molasses being mixed with warm water or milk to make it of a running, drinkable consistency. The drench can be repeated at hourly intervals. This treatment alone in mild cases of milk fever, taken in its very early stages, has restored cows to normal. The more orthodox treatment, essential in all cases of complete collapse of the animal, is inflation of the udder with air. This treatment has been in use in cattle medicine for half a century or more and is very effective. All firms who sell cattle foods and medical instruments, supply an apparatus for udder inflation, with full instructions for its use. The main points to watch when giving such treatment are: the absolute sterile condition of the needle used, so as not to cause any infection of the udder; and care that the air is not injected too rapidly into the udder, so as to cause inflammation. Air injection should be given very gently. If necessary the operation can be repeated three or four times. The principle behind the udder inflation is to prevent immediate further flow of milk into the udder, and thus to stop further loss of calcium and hormones from the bloodstream.

An alternative treatment to udder inflation, and much used in orthodox practice, is the injection of a strong dose of calcium solution into the bloodstream. This treatment requires skill and is best administered by a veterinary surgeon.

MASTITIS   The basic cause of mastitis is much the same as that of milk fever: unnatural rearing, especially dietary. The cow in total health experiences no lactation difficulties. Many farmers blame the use of milking machines. Personally I think that a chief cause is the deprivation of the cow of the pleasure and stimulus of suckling her calf. American farmers have proved that the quickest way to cure a cow of all udder ailments is to let a vigorous calf suckle her, making sure that the calf feeds from the affected quarters.

When machine milking is used, the cows if possible should be finished by hand. Also always massage the udder after milking, and bump it up and down in the way that calves do when feeding.

Herbal treatment has proved particularly successful in cure of mastitis. It was this disease, cured speedily and completely by my herbal treatment, which first interested Sir Albert Howard in herbs for cattle, and caused him to urge me to develop the work as fully as possible. It is my opinion that animals with mastitis, treated by orthodox methods with chemical drugs, and neglect of all fasting and special dietary treatment, never again possess normal health of the udder, a quarter of the udder very frequently being lost. Also unnatural treatment of mastitis often leads to later development of tuberculosis of the udder. While use of the sulphonamide drugs in large quantities – and even the modern over-refined or concentrated or synthetic substance into which the chemist has turned the natural mould penicillin – will often produce disorders of the kidneys, also foot diseases, and even help to induce abortion. These remarks apply likewise to most of the modern antibiotics. But herbal treatment is a tonic to the whole organism and will leave the cow so treated in better health than she enjoyed before the onset of the disease.

I first used the mastitis herbal treatment as long ago as 1939, for goats, and in 1946 adapted the goat treatment for cows, with the same successful results. By 1947, Sir Albert Howard was sending me all cases of mastitis whose owners had applied to him for advice. Treatments were always successful and herbal medicine for veterinary use grew rapidly in prestige.

Symptoms   The disease begins with attacks of shivering, and general unease of the animal is manifest. Appetite fails, the horns feel chilled and fever develops. Sometimes the temperature rises rapidly to 107°, high fever being a typical symptom of the ailment. The entire udder rapidly hardens and becomes very hot to the touch. Curdled material is found to be present when expressing the milk. As the udder further swells and hardens, the cow develops a peculiar straddling stance to prevent her hind legs from pressing upon the enlarged udder. In neglected cases mortification of the udder may set in.

Treatment   This must be immediate and very thorough. The main drawback with herbal treatment, for the busy farmer, is that it requires time and care. It is not the mere injection of some violent drug to suppress the symptoms and the affair ended; constant attention to the cow is required for a week or more. But the resultant complete health of the udder and the cow herself, especially if she be an animal of much value as a milk producer, is surely worth the time required, were it not also sufficient to feel that the very best is being done for the animal herself, quite apart from her value.

The cow must be confined indoors in the cowhouse throughout the early stages of the treatment. This should be well ventilated, for a cow in fever requires fresh air. Begin with a cleansing fast of two days. Water only is allowed. All straw or other bedding must be enclosed in sacks to prevent the cow from eating during the fast, the litter-stuffed sacks being placed on the floor for bedding. Cows both in health and sickness should always have sufficient litter on which to lie, to prevent any kneeling on bare stone. Each evening of the fast a laxative drench of twenty large senna pods should be given, the senna pods to be soaked in half a pint of cold water for a minimum of six hours; one teaspoonful of ground

255

ginger to be added to the brew. The whole brew to be given at one dose. Break the fast on the third morning with a drench of two pints milk, half-pint tepid water, and ten heaped table-spoonfuls molasses added. At midday feed a meal of steamed hay, approximately one-third of a gallon bucket of sweet hay, softened by heating gently over hot water for one hour. Add to the hay two pounds of bran and ten tablespoonfuls of mol-asses. Repeat the meal in the evening. Do not give further senna laxative brew. Keep on this diet for three days, but increasing the quantity of the feed according to the size and appetite of the animal being treated. The medicinal herbs to be used throughout the treatment are garlic and wood sage, wood sage or common (blue flower) sage, sage and garlic being specific for the cure of udder ailments. The garlic dosage is two whole roots grated into one pint of water, half-pint given morning and night, or six to eight four-grain garlic tablets. The tablet dose can be given morning and night if necessary. N.R. Herbal Compound tablets contain blue sage in addition to wild garlic.

The blue sage is given as a brew during the fast, two handfuls of the herb, finely cut, brewed in 1½ pints of water, two tablespoonfuls honey added. Give as a single drench in the early morning. When the fast is ended the herb can be given finely cut, mixed with bran and molasses. Give also, when available, several handfuls twice daily of raspberry foliage and herb Robert, also southernwood.

When the body temperature returns to normal, the cow should be turned out to grass, except in severe weather (sunlight is always beneficial in udder disorders). To complete the efficiency of the treatment the cow should be allowed to suckle her calf for several weeks, when back in the field.

External treatment Some external aid must be given to relieve the udder. This should consist of cold packs to dispel the fever and encourage the expulsion of the pus accumulation from the teats. A brew of common dock leaves should be used for the cold pack. Two handfuls of dock leaves brewed in one pint of water. Soak flannel in the brew and well bathe the udder and teats, with cold brew, following very gentle milking. This should be done three times daily, or more often if necessary. In cases of very bad inflammation packs should be made by soaking thick swabs of cotton wool in the dock brew, covering with flannel, and then binding with an external sheet bandage to keep in place. If necessary the cow's head should be tied short, to prevent her from removing the udder pack.

If the udder is very congested, feeling very hard, then the brew should be used hot.

When the cow is back in the field continued attention should be paid to the daily diet. In addition to the green feed that she will get from the field grazing, the cow should be given twice-daily a feed of sweet hay, a normal ration for her breed, a supply of compost-grown oats, and a mash of bran and molasses. As a convalescent tonic, steamed beetroot is excellent, the leaves, raw, also being fed to utilize their high mineral content, especially fluorine. Feed also blood-cooling and minerals-rich comfrey foliage.

Final note to mastitis treatment. It sometimes happens that the general cure of the ailment is very speedy following the herbal treatment; all fever departs, and the udder returns to normal, with one exception. A small area of hardness sometimes persists in one quarter. If this persists for as long as three weeks, a short, intensive treatment is then indicated. A one-day fast, one-day fluid diet, milk-water-molasses, the garlic and sage dosage to be doubled. Repeat the external treatment of the udder, but apply the dock leaves brew hot instead of cold (cold to remove inflammation: hot to dispel disease bacteria in the tissues and to reduce congestion). A few drops of eucalyptus oil or peppermint oil can be added to the hot brew with advantage.

DRY MASTITIS   This ailment can attack the udder of a cow when she is dry. It is often caused by sudden chill during hot weather, or unsuitable overheating diet. Thus the ailment is more prevalent in late summer and early autumn than at other times. It is rare in winter. The condition is more stubborn to cure than common mastitis.

Symptoms   These are the same as for common mastitis, but there is generally less fever and less swelling of the udder. Sometimes the swelling is confined to only one quarter.

Treatment   The same as for common mastitis (see above). But replace the senna laxative dose with one of Epsom salt. Give three to four ounces of Epsom salt dissolved in three-quarter pint of warm milk, four dessertspoonfuls molasses added. Give the usual garlic treatment. The udder should be rubbed and fomented with hot dock brew, and the affected quarters drawn thrice daily. Continue the treatment until the udder is normal.

LEUCORRHOEA   (See Goats)

SORE TEATS   (See Sheep)

COW POX   This is a fairly common ailment, and is considered to be infectious, being carried by the milker's hands from one cow's udder to others. It is a mild ailment and readily curable.

Symptoms   Red marks appear on the teats and on the udder at the base of the teats, usually of oval shape; they speedily begin suppurating. The cow sometimes develops a slight fever.

Treatment   A short fast, followed by laxative diet, essentially of a green nature. Internal dosing with garlic. Feed plenty of elder foliage in the diet, and watercress when available, also brooklime and bramble foliage. Externally: bathe with a brew of elder leaves (and flowers when in season) and dock leaves, equal parts, two handfuls of each, finely cut, to one quart water. A brew of flaked garlic root is also very effective. The elder-dock brew has cured large open ulcers on the teats of a Devon shorthorn cow, in five days, when the cow had been troubled with the suppurating ulcers for two years, making milking difficult because of their bleeding into the milk.

GONORRHOEA   This is an ailment of the sexual organs of the bull and cow. Over-fatness, through prolonged lack of exercise, burdens the internal sexual organs with fatty tissue, and is an important cause of infertility in cattle, and predisposes the animals to venereal ailments.

Symptoms   The sexual organs of the infected animals become highly inflamed, and pus is generated. There is difficulty in voiding urine and much pain is indicated. The animal loses condition and develops fever symptoms. There is generally frequent bellowing and the animal grinds its teeth.

Treatment   Fasting. Much internal use of garlic and a daily strong drench of brewed dill seed and sage: one handful of each to one quart of water. Laxative diet. Give both bulls and cows a daily handful of raspberry leaves to tone up the reproductive organs. Give carrots and chopped onion in the diet, also water-mint and green hops.

If improvement is slow, give a one-week course of a daily strong laxative: twenty-four pods of senna, two ounces powdered ginger, four ounces chopped chamomile flowers, to 1½ pints of cold water. The chamomile flowers should be brought to the boil in the water, and well brewed, and when cold the brew should be poured over the senna and ginger and the pods left to soak in the liquid for a minimum of six hours. Give half-pint drenches three times daily. External: bathing or douching with a brew of dill seed and elder leaves, in equal parts, brewed in one quart of water. Or brew of marsh-mallow plant, or lavender plant, or quince leaves. Massage with witch hazel extract to allay irritation and inflammation of the tissues.

COLIC This is not an ailment general to cows. It is caused usually by some irritant acting upon the lining of the intestinal tract. Some foreign body may be the cause, when surgical treatment must be used, common bodies being pieces of wire, tin, also nails: with the increasing use of wire enclosures upon the farm, so proportionally increases the danger of pieces of wire intake to the cows; hedges are the natural enclosure for cattle, they provide food as well as fencing.

Symptoms The animal becomes very restless and bellows consistently. At short intervals it draws its back feet up to its belly and paws the ground. (See Indigestion.)

Treatment Short internal cleansing fasting. Laxative diet, giving barley meal (with molasses) as the only permissible cereal. Give also as part of the diet the following compound powder meal mixed with milk and honey, as both fortifier and healer: one cupful slippery elm powder, one cupful powdered dill seed, one half-cupful powdered arrowroot, half-cupful barley flour. (This can be supplied, ready blended, by N.R. products.)

If the condition does not yield to dietary treatment, then drench twice daily with the following: two pints warm water, half a pound molasses, half an ounce oil of peppermint, two teaspoonfuls powdered cinnamon. Externally: apply hot cloths to the belly area. During convalescence give twice daily tablespoonful doses of powdered charcoal in milk. Oatmeal gruel with molasses makes an excellent convalescent aid; one ounce of powdered gentian can be added to every quart of gruel.

INDIGESTION This is the result of a prolonged unnatural diet. The cow is habitually a creature of exceptional digestive powers; what strong legs are to the horse to give it its supreme equine qualities, so are a powerful stomach and intestines to the cow, to give the especial bovine qualities. The ideal diet for the cow is the product of green pastures rich in herbs and charged with the vitality of sunlight, together with sun-irradiated water of brooks or spring. The modern diet is far removed from this.

At the end of each day the cow should get some sweet unchopped hay, and the following mixture morning and evening. A gallon of bran made into a mash with boiled nettle tea, made by boiling five handfuls of nettles in one quart water; two pounds of ground linseed; two pounds crushed wheat and oats; a quart of sunflower seeds; sufficient pulped carrots to keep the bowels well open. Carrots are best given mixed with wheaten straw and a little chaff. Remove the stringy ends from carrots.

The cow should be in an open yard when not in the pasture. Cow cabbage, lucerne, Russian comfrey, swedes, wholegrain oats, are all good milk producers and keep a cow in good prime condition. Silage is also a good alternative to hay as a change.

The pasture should not be under two years old for wintering stock.

Access to watercress beds in the early spring and late autumn is a wonderful cow tonic. An important tonic also is ground ivy, a common woodland herb, but the cows should not be allowed to gorge themselves as they will do if not controlled, because an over-abundance of the herb renders the milk bitter-tasting. Herb Robert, or wild geranium as it is sometimes called, is a powerful cow medicine conditioner, so is cranesbill, of the same family.

Cows eat with great pleasure the shooting leaves of hedges and trees in the early spring months. That way they will partake of the highly beneficial leaves and twigs of such shrubs as elder, willow, hawthorn, wild rose, bramble, hazel, ash and so forth. Hop shoots are a fine tonic for all the digestive organs.

A herbal tonic for cows with poor appetite is made as follows: powdered gentian root four drachms, powdered ginger four drachms, and caraway and anise seeds one ounce, with two ounces of powdered charcoal, well mixed into a quart of warm ale, to be given nightly for one to two weeks.

Treatment Indigestion when not treated in its early stages can become as painful for the animal as colic. Treatment is the same as for colic (see above). It should be said here that molasses (treacle) with its special properties of nerve soothing and mild aperient, is an indispensable preventive of 'stomach staggers', caused through indigestion, the most frequent ailment of dairy cows under present-day forcing conditions. Honey is also valuable, as is plain vegetable charcoal, a heaped tablespoon twice daily, or same quantity in tablet form.

LOSS OF CUD This is indicated by the incapacity of the stomach to bring back into mouth for further chewing the half-masticated food.

Symptoms Sickly appearance, poor appetite, dropping of food, much dribbling of saliva.

Treatment A short fast. Completely green diet with the exception of bran and molasses. Give tonic balls of nearly similar ingredients to the herbal tonic for indigestion. One teaspoonful grated gentian root, one teaspoonful grated liquorice stick, one ounce allspice, one ounce aniseed, made into balls with flour and honey.

BLOW or DEW-BLOW or HOVEN The cause of blow is uncertain. I favour the theory that it is caused by over-engorgement due to the over-eating of spring grasses following the long winter period of scarcity of such fare; the over-eating being especially dangerous when the grass is heavily rain- or dew-wet, or frosted. When rich succulent spring grasses are bolted without proper mastication, and very cold from the spring dews or frosts, indigestion, with much fermentation, sets in, and carbonic gas is then generated, the abdominal area swelling in a remarkable way becoming almost twice its normal size. There is equal danger of this in late summer and early autumn, when again herbage becomes very chilled or frosted. Unless the blown condition is relieved promptly, death may result from a number of causes, heart failure, a burst blood-vessel, or literal rupture of the intestines due to internal pressure of the gas. So serious is this condition that it is quite a general – but very health-destructive – method, to puncture the body side with a sharp knife to permit immediate release of the gas. Peasants in Mexico, where there are heavy early morning spring frosts, and cattle are frequently dew-blown, drag their blown cattle up steep mountain crags, holding the animals on ropes in an almost perpendicular position to induce the gas to escape through the anus. I have seen a far better method, and each time it has been used it has given unfailing good results. The method was shown to me by a German herdsman with Mrs. E. M. Bellhouse's Jersey herd in Devonshire, with which herd

I shared so much interesting pioneer herbal work with the owner.

Symptoms The internal gas generated usually forms in the first stomach or rumen which becomes very distended with enormously blown sides, causing the animal to stand in great discomfort; breathing becomes laboured and the animal groans in deep distress. Eventually the animal collapses.

Treatment A good preventive treatment is always to feed some dry hay to the herd before letting them graze dew- or rain-wet green fodder. It is further helpful to sprinkle the hay with dry bran (quite a generous amount); this helps to lessen the fermentation which often results from wet green food.

A practical German cure of blow when it has developed, is here given.

Make a rope from twisted hay or straw – anything of the sort immediately available. Push this aid far back into the cow's mouth in order to prevent the animal from biting through it, keeping transverse like a gag, the use of the rope being to compel the mouth to open and thus to promote continual chewing. In order to accelerate the chewing, which in turn promotes the expulsion of a large amount of the gas, take some warm dung from the cow's anus and push this into the mouth. As the cow is a cleanly animal this will cause much disgust and will promote extra rapid and strong chewing in order to be rid of the dung in her mouth. Meanwhile, rubber tubing, such as a piece of hose piping or even a spare part of a milking machine, should be thrust up the anus and worked about in order to expel further gas from that outlet of the body. The cure is rapid, the swollen body deflating before the eyes of the attendant, in similar manner to a punctured motor tyre; and in under one hour the animal is transformed from a condition near to death to quite normal health.

A quart drench of strong linseed tea should be given to complete the cure; five handfuls of flax seed well boiled in a quart of water, then steeped; also powdered charcoal or crushed charcoal tablets given in milk, are good to further purify the intestines of all lingering gas. Also a drench of a brew of the herb parsley peart. A drench of Luisa herb proved effective too.

Preventive treatment   The following advice given by a farmer under the initials of J. W. R. (Warwickshire) in the 1886 issue of *Farm and Home* journal, is full of sound common sense, and is well worth quoting from:

'You can with little trouble prevent the occurrence (Dew-Blow in Cows), and that will be better than cure. During the spring change-over of diet, give one and a half pints of linseed oil on an empty stomach twice a week, and bring the cows in every night before the dew falls. In the cow shed give the animal some good hay, and a feed in the morning also. Give only a little hay at night, but let the cows have as much as they will take in the morning. Do not turn out the cows until the dew is off the grass, or when it is wet from rain. The herbage becomes more indigestible when wet, and particularly so when frosted. To cure the complaint nothing is better than linseed oil, given in one and a half pint doses, and such doses may be repeated without fear, for linseed oil is as harmless to the cow as is castor oil to the child. The taking of the cows from the pasture at night will not generally have to be kept up above ten days or a fortnight at most, only while the grass matures a little, and while the cow's stomach becomes accustomed to its work and ceases to feed so ravenously.'

MAWBOUND or GRAIN SICKNESS   This is produced through over-feeding of grain foods, especially concentrated cake and meals. If treatment is not careful and prompt the animal will die.

Symptoms The cow shows great unease and becomes very costive. The breathing becomes deranged with much panting, and the cow grunts continually, this being the most typical symptom of the complaint. Suffocation often results.

Treatment Immediate fasting. A stiff laxative drench of linseed oil, two pints. Follow this by a brew of sage leaves, three large handfuls of herb to one quart of water, making half a gallon drench, to which should be added one pound of molasses. Repeat the brew every three hours until the animal's condition improves. Give warm enemas containing one-half teaspoonful of oil of eucalyptus to every quart of plain water; approximately three to four quarts of liquid make an effective enema. Give home-made wood charcoal or charcoal tablets from pharmacy shops, three times more than the human dose. When the animal's breathing becomes normal again, utilize a general laxative diet. But the linseed oil drenches should be continued for three to five days, reducing the amount daily down to one-half pint. If the pulse is found to be very rapid, chop some rosemary very finely and make teaspoonful doses into medicine balls, by mixing with flour and honey. Give one ball every four hours. The laxative diet should be maintained for at least three weeks. Plenty of sweet hay, carrots and chicory should be fed. When grain foods are again introduced they should begin with barley, and should be given crushed or flaked. One part of linseed meal should be added to every three parts of grain.

JAUNDICE This complaint may follow from a sudden chill, but the general cause is unsuitable diet, especially over-prolonged use of concentrated unnatural cakes and meals. Also chemical vermifuges often damage the liver and produce a tendency to jaundice. The trouble can also be caused by blood infection carried by rats. It is the derangement of the bile flow which is the basic cause of the complaint and until this is normalized the yellow pigment will continue to be noticeable, especially in the eyes.

Symptoms Yellowness of the eyes and also below the anus, costiveness, foul-smelling mouth. The animal is very lethargic and shows disinclination to eat. Abnormal thirst is often present.

Treatment A short fast with strong (non-oily) purge. Senna pods are suitable (see Senna). All fatty foods should be avoided in the diet; therefore no linseed or sunflower products should be given. Also avoid giving pulse foods. Give an abundance of dandelion in the diet, roots (grated) can be included too, plus a twice-daily handful of toadflax plant. Also recommended are fumitory, goose-grass (cleavers), sea-holly, centaury, blue flag iris. Otherwise the diet should be mainly grass and other green leafy vegetables, bran, molasses, carrots and seaweed. Give charcoal tablets. External treatment: apply a pack of flannel soaked in a hot brew of gentian root, covering widely the area of the liver. (Also give some of the gentian brew internally. Give bitters: wormwood and southernwood.)

The following is an old farrier herbal remedy for jaundice which has given very good results: one teaspoonful powdered gentian, one teaspoonful powdered ginger, half an ounce of Barbados aloes, four ounces of common salt (not the artificial or over-purified table variety: Tidman's sea-salt is good), one quart home-brewed ale, made into a gruel with oatmeal. Gum of aloes is obtainable from most herbalists.

WORMS (see Horses) Worms are far more prevalent in horses than cattle, excepting those worm species which enter through the skin, borne by summer flies. The following is an excellent dressing for treatment of warble fly in cattle. The principle of the dressing is the killing of the larvae in the warbles by using a dressing which will close the breathing pores and thus stop development of the fly. Tobacco powder and limewash make the dressing, the following quantity being sufficient for twenty-four cattle. Eight pounds tobacco powder and four pounds of fresh lime are steeped for two days in one gallon of water. The liquid is strained through coarse sacking and is applied to the backs of the animals with a stiff brush. Treatment should begin at the first appearance of the warble swellings in January or February, and should be frequently repeated until after June.

RED WATER, or BLACK WATER, or MUIR ILL (also a disease of sheep) This is generally accepted as being a 'disease of poverty'. Particularly affected by the disease are cattle kept on undrained, waterlogged land, usually aggravated by provision only of stagnant water for drinking. A further source of the ill is orchard or copse-wood grazing, where the ground has become sour and the grass lifeless and rank through deprivation of sunlight and sufficient free air. The disease is most prevalent at the back end of the year, though winter outbreaks amongst stalled animals are not infrequent. Milking cows fed on the too general winter diet of musty, chlorophyll-drained hay, greasy, devitalized manufactured cattle foods, and frosted root vegetables, develop red water symptoms. Also tick ravages are a typical forerunner of the disease. Orthodox medicine upholds that ticks are the invariable cause. As I do not accept the Pasteur germ theory of disease, the orthodox opinion is likewise unacceptable. However, *one* form of the disease has a proven association with the bite of a tick species.

Symptoms There is an appearance of general wasting, with ears, horns and extremities feeling chill to the touch. The spine is roached. In the tick form of the ailment the tick bite introduces into the blood system an organism which attacks the red corpuscles. The corpuscular remains expelled by the kidneys turn the urine red.

Treatment Foremost the animal must be changed to dry pasture if on an ill-drained one. If the animals are stalled, then attention must be paid to damp buildings. The animals must be well dusted with derris powder, or derris-wormwood, equal parts. Internal treatment must commence with a short laxative fast. Also drench with a brew of herb Robert daily: this species of wild (or garden) geranium, common in the world's flora, is an accepted peasant remedy for 'murrain'. Follow by a dry, but nourishing diet, in which should feature sweet unchopped hay, bran, charcoal products, whites of eggs and a little molasses. The egg whites counteract the excretion of albumen in the urine, which is a feature of murrain disease. There is no more helpful diet for this condition than old beans or peas mixed with chopped hay, as such diet further restores albumen to the system in a cheap and beneficial form. Desiccated coconut also restores albumen. In mild cases the above given diet will generally prove sufficient to effect a cure, but in more severe cases there must be twice daily dosage of the following gruel: whites of two eggs, two ounces powdered marsh-mallow root, two ounces slippery elm bark, one ounce orris root, two dessertspoonfuls honey, mixed into one quart of milk-water (equal parts). Externally: warm packs to the bladder and kidney areas, also enemas of warm water and peppermint oil, twenty drops of peppermint to one quart of water.

BLADDER AND KIDNEY DISORDERS (see Goats)

COLD, COUGH, CATARRH   (see Horses)

PNEUMONIA   There are many causes for this serious complaint among cattle: damp, ill-ventilated, sun-deprived buildings, combined with the feeding of dusty hay and frosted roots are the commonest causes of the ill. Further, over-rich unnatural diets to force up the milk-yield, which clog the bloodstream and cause excessive formation of mucus, the lungs having so much traffic with the bloodstream being made unhealthy thereby.

The pus-forming bacteria pneumococci would not be present in large numbers unless there were sufficient mucus and other toxic accumulations to nourish them; the truly healthy animal does not succumb to pneumonia because there is nothing in the body to afford a sufficiency of breeding material for disease bacteria.

Symptoms   Very cold extremities despite the presence of high fever. The lungs are panting incessantly and also showing much straining, the ribs are very arched and the eyes much congested.

Treatment   Assist a general cleansing of the body, especially of the lungs, by fasting. Two days on a honey and water diet. Then follow with a fluid diet of milk, molasses, honey, slippery elm powder, two tablespoonfuls of each stirred into one quart of warm milk. No solid foods should be given while high fever is present. Give a strong dose of garlic: this is of tremendous importance in treatment of ailments of the respiratory organs. Garlic dose should be four roots shredded and brewed in one pint of water, a pint drench being given twice daily. Or six, four-grain garlic tablets given twice daily. Pine-tree shoots and spruce make a very good internal drench. If very high fever continues, a strong brew of yarrow herb should be given (see Yarrow): this promotes sweating.

Give a daily laxative while the cow is on fluids.

If the lungs are very congested, treat as follows: fill a nosebag with hot, wet bran and grated friar's balsam; or oil of eucalyptus can be used; two ounces of friar's balsam to the nosebag, or one dessertspoonful of eucalyptus oil stirred into the bran. Tie this round the nose and bind around the horns (for fuller instructions for making a steam bag see Horses, under Pneumonia). Well steam out the nostrils, and continue the treatment at frequent intervals until the breathing becomes easier.

Make balls of two teaspoonfuls grated camphor, three tablespoonfuls of molasses and a little barley flour to bind them. This should make approximately eight balls. Give two balls twice daily.

There should never be suppression of the symptoms with sulphonamide drugs. Such treatment suppresses but never wholly cures, and severe derangement of kidneys, liver and brain, also foot ailments, are common after-effects of such drugs, more harmful to the animal long-term than the pneumonia disease itself.

Keep the cow well rugged up and littered up to the belly for warmth, but allow plenty of fresh air no matter how cold the weather may be. The cow must be kept warm by rugging and bedding and the use of a heater if necessary: but the animal's head must have access to all possible fresh air in order to help the congested lungs. If the lungs are very painful and congested, a plaster of fresh cow dung can be used. Smear fresh cow dung over the chest areas, sides and back. Cover well, remove after several hours. Gypsies use the cow dung pack for pneumonia in humans and have great faith in this remedy.

When heaters (kerosene) are used, all parts must be kept absolutely clean, no kerosene to be spilt on the heater when filling. With absolute cleanliness there will be no harmful fumes. The best heating for stables of sick animals in winter months, is the common storm lantern. Storm lanterns should be hung on long nails to keep them away from the wall and hung well out of reach of the animals.

DYSENTERY This is a serious condition and should not be confused with diarrhoea which is generally of little consequence to the cow and is frequent when cattle are out at spring grass.

Symptoms The contrasting symptoms of diarrhoea and dysentery will be given in order to facilitate the distinguishing of the one from the other. Diarrhoea: general in spring, no fever or pain present, appetite remains keen. Dysentery: this is more general in older animals. There is much internal fever; much pain, faeces show blood, appetite is totally lost.

Treatment Apply the internal cleansing treatment as given (above) for pneumonia. For medicine give abundant honey and slippery elm, a moderate amount of garlic for disinfection, two garlic roots once daily, grated and brewed in one pint water, or six four-grain garlic tablets; chlorophyll tablets, six four-grain, and charcoal; a handful of powdered charcoal, or equal weight in tablets. As the intestines heal, milk should be added to the honey-slippery-elm gruel, and grated gentian root; two small teaspoonfuls of the latter to one and a half pints of the gruel. A drench of whortleberry or bilberry plant, or juice of the lightly boiled and crushed berries, is very effective in prolonged dysentery. So also is a strong brew of blackcurrant leaves.

When dysentery lessens, the gruel diet should be broken with the feeding, for several days, of a warm mash of flaked barley, to which a little powdered marsh-mallow root can be added with advantage. Raw whole eggs are often prescribed in orthodox medicine for scour and dysentery in cattle and calves; they are too fermentative and should not be given. Arrowroot and kaolin powders are other popular treatments in orthodox medicine, but are too clogging and artificially binding; they do not restore or heal the disordered intestines, and should not be given without addition of other herbs.

RHEUMATISM   (see Sheep)

WOUNDS   Wash the surface very clean with cold water, slightly salted, then bathe with a cleansing and healing herbal brew, possessing disinfectant properties. Use preferably comfrey plant or elder leaves and/or blossoms, or rosemary – whole herb. If knapweed herb is available, add some of this to the brew; it is an excellent astringent and tonic. The common daisy plant is also astringent and tonic. Approximate quantities for the brew would be two large handfuls of finely chopped comfrey and elder, or rosemary, to one quart of water. If knapweed or daisy are added, take half a handful, and mix with the other herbs. When bathing the wound, apply fairly hot for the first treatments; the subsequent treatments should receive cold applications. Bathe at least three times daily. Rub also into the wound some of the green leafage residue from the herbal brews, mixed with a small amount of vinegar, as there is generally also local bruising of tissues if the wounds be sizeable. One or two teaspoonfuls of vinegar to one cupful of green herb pulp. Plantain leaves yield a very soothing mucilage, valuable in treating inflamed surroundings of wounds, and adder's tongue ointment is highly curative in old wounds, so is the jelly from most cacti leaves.

A famed gypsy remedy for really severe wounds, especially the large areas of flesh which are frequently torn open by barbed wire, is the use of a brew of acorn cups first applied externally to stem the bleeding, then treatment of the inner wound areas with black pepper. The open surface is well sprinkled with black pepper, which acts as a powerful disinfectant and also stimulates healing. The wound is then sewn up and left to heal naturally. Dried and powdered rosemary is also an excellent sprinkling herb for wounds. For more shallow wounds from wire, sharp wood, etc. apply the healing herbal oil advised for bites and stings. (See Adder bites.)

When the udder is torn on wire and there is leakage of milk, cotton pads of the astringent witch hazel should be pasted into position with adhesive tape, the witch hazel being constantly renewed as the pads dry. Or a cloth bag can be fitted over the whole udder to help keep the witch hazel pads in place. The punctures can be plugged further with some cobwebs (spider). I very rarely sew wounds, and many have been large enough to insert one's hand into them, I merely wash them with a strong brew of rosemary plant, and then further sprinkle with that herb, dried and powdered. I do not use bandages, but keep the wound uncovered so that the animal itself may keep the injuries open (that is when the animal is able to reach the place with its healing saliva and tongue).

During all wound treatments there should be internal dosage with garlic or other antiseptic herbs, to keep the bloodstream healthy and thus avoid infection.

For soothing all types of wound and the promotion of healing, apply fresh leaves, with stalks removed. The best of the healing leaves are: vine, castor oil, geranium, mallow, hollyhock, cabbage. A handful of the leaves, washed in cold water, are placed on wounds and kept in place by cold-water-dampened cotton bandages. Apply fresh leaves every three hours.

NETTLE-RASH or URTICARIA This is an ailment more general to cattle in hot climates and is seldom to be met with in its acute form in temperate climate countries. It can cause death.

Symptoms Face, head and neck start to swell and become very hot to the touch. It is mostly a complaint of the lymphatic system. Respiration may become affected and death result.

Treatment Fasting. Brew of stringent herbs. Sorrel leaves and oak bark, one handful of each to one quart of water. Witch hazel bark can also be used and seaweed (bladderwrack variety). Knapweed is a general tonic for all glandular weakness, including that of the lymph glands. Give a laxative diet. External treatment: massage well with a strong brew of dock leaves. Elder flowers can be added to the dock brew with much advantage. Or the healing natural jelly obtained from many species of cacti, can be used.

WOODY-TONGUE This is becoming an infrequent ailment, perhaps owing to the increasing value of cows, and therefore the greater care being given to individual animals so that the woody-tongue malady is not allowed to reach the stage when the tongue hardens. The exact origin of the disease remains doubtful, although it is certainly a form of glandular disorder, especially of the lymphatic glands, probably caused by a parasitic bacterial attack. One cause may be a ray fungus taken in when the mouth or cheek tissues are pierced by awned vegetation. The condition is a sign of positive health degeneration; really healthy animals are not subject to such a disease.

Symptoms A hardening of the tissues around the tongue, inner cheeks and lower jaw. A typical case shows much distress, refusing food, and standing with the head kept lowered and tongue hanging out. The condition is often fatal.

Treatment This should begin with the usual short internal cleansing, fasting and dieting to tone up the entire system. For a glandular tonic an abundant use of seaweed is indicated, approximately one pound daily of the crude weed given in a mash of bran and molasses. Also knapweed, two handfuls of the flower heads fed once daily, and/or goose-grass. Garlic should be given plentifully to cleanse and tone the system, including the lymph flow. Externally the hardened areas of tissues should be well massaged with a seaweed-vinegar lotion. The tongue also must be massaged. The lotion is harmless if swallowed; it is indeed beneficial. The lotion is three parts of a strong brew of seaweed to one part of vinegar; and one dessertspoonful of paprika added to every pint of lotion.

The gypsies use fungi very successfully to cure woody-tongue. They use especially wild mushrooms and a variety of common toadstool with a blue stalk, which they call *Blueleg-gis*. Gloucestershire gypsies boil the big black woodland slugs (first killed), with the fungi; they consider the jelly-like mucus substance thus obtained to be beneficial both for internal and external treatment.

Penicillin, being of the fungi group, could also give useful assistance, providing it has not been rendered too over-refined; it is better to use penicillin fungus in its crude form, scraping the green mould off stale bread and making a solution in water. One teaspoonful mould to one small cupful water.

ANAEMIA This is a serious condition in the cow, for it is indicative of the whole digestive system being at fault, when the cow is unable to extract sufficient chlorophyll during its grazing to maintain the proper proportion of red blood corpuscles. (The anaemia cure for humans in which liver is utilized, has been found to rely upon a substance known as folic acid, for its curative effect, this substance being stored in liver, and deriving its name from *folia* – leaf.) A cow subsisting mainly on herbage – grass foliage – should be able to resist anaemia. The disease is uncommon. I have met with one case in England, in a Jersey cow, but in countries where there is often a lack of green food owing to sun scorching, such as Mexico and Spain, I have met the complaint more frequently.

Symptoms   General appearance of lassitude, poor appetite, cold extremities and horns. The gums, inner eyelids and anus area are all bloodless, being almost white.

Treatment   A short fast (two days) to cleanse and tone the system. Then a very green diet, also iron-rich foods such as molasses, oats, watercress, bramble (including fruits), rest-harrow, chicory, chickweed, burdock. Iodine-rich foods such as seaweed, Iceland moss, Irish moss, white cabbage, carrots and artichokes. Expose the animal to all possible sunlight; do not confine in cow-house.

WARTS   This is mainly a glandular condition. It is quite common to young bullocks. Warts spread quickly if the condition is not treated promptly.

Treatment   Diet must be made very mineral and vitamin rich. Seaweed should be given daily, also dried cleavers – both highly iodine rich. Garlic should also be given. Externally: the warts should be well rubbed with the downy insides of bean skins. The foliage of runner beans can also be used. The white juice pressed from unripe figs, poppy fruits when green, rue fruits when green, dandelion stems and roots, stems of the greater celandine, are all effective. Raw potato is fairly useful.

FELON   This is not a general disease and is found mostly among stall-fed animals.

Symptoms   The teeth appear loose, and the nose is dry; the coat is staring, and the animal avoids being touched; there is much lethargy.

Treatment   This should begin with fasting and powerful purging with Epsom or Glauber's salt, first: eight dessertspoonfuls of salts in three-quarters of a pint of warm water, plus one teaspoonful ground ginger. Follow this with half a pint of linseed oil for four days. Give a nourishing diet and include in it plenty of barley meal and sunflower seeds, both of which are good for tooth trouble. Give also molasses. External treatment: rub the strained skin with a brew of hop leaves and/or flowers. Bathe the gums with a brew of rosemary flowers or herb, mixed with salt; one teaspoonful of salt to a half-pint of the brew.

FOUL IN THE FOOT   This is to the cow what foot rot is to the sheep. Inflammation sets in between parts of the foot, producing a discharge of fetid matter, the condition causing great pain. The foot will often dry up, thus partly withering, and the animal becomes permanently lame.

Symptoms   Lameness; heated extremities; failing appetite. These symptoms are soon followed by foul discharge from the hooves.

Treatment   Place the animal on a short cleansing fast, followed by laxative diet which should include plenty of bran mashes and molasses, with pulped carrots and abundant green herbs, including dandelion leaves, chicory and elder tops. External treatment: well wash out the foot with hot soapy water, carefully cutting out all loose and decayed flesh. Then draw out the foul matter by poulticing very frequently for one night and day with linseed bags, cotton cloth bags filled with linseed meal. Tie the poultice bags of hot linseed meal firmly around the foot to ensure the bag remaining in position, and cover with an old sock. After the poulticing treatment is concluded, when all fetid matter seems to have been brought out of the foot, then cleanse again with soap and water and anoint with Stockholm tar. Final treatment is to confine the raw and open feet in stockings, preferably well lined with sphagnum moss or other absorbent material.

TUMOURS Tumours can form in almost any part of the body. They should be given both internal and external treatment. Little seems to be gained by surgical removal, such treatment often rapidly spreading the trouble and hastening death. It is the cause of the ailment which should be removed, the tumour may then be induced to wither. Remember also that blows on soft tissue, especially the udder, can cause tumours. Therefore, take care. A cleansing treatment is necessary: (follow that for Anaemia). Herbs and foods beneficial for treatment of tumours: Garlic, violet leaves and flowers, wild pansies, rose hips, comfrey, mustard flowers and leaves, radish, rock-rose, turnip, marsh-mallow leaves, thistle, eucalyptus leaves, red clover tops, watercress, vine leaves and tendrils. Turnip (root) and the three last items on the list, are the most famed of all. Eating daily an abundance of raw turnips and garlic is a sound old peasant treatment for cure of tumours. Twenty-one days is the prescribed duration of the cure.

External massage of the lumps with the following mixture is useful: garlic cloves in castor oil (six cloves to every ounce of castor oil). Cut up the cloves small, place in the oil, in a jar, cover the jar top with lid or paper top sealed with rubber band, stand jar in a pan of hot (not boiling) water, and heat gently for half an hour. Then thicken the mixture with powdered seaweed and rub into the lump morning and night.

A course of Herbal Compound tablets, being highly antiseptic, should be given.

SKIN AILMENTS, RINGWORM, ETC (see Sheep)

TUBERCULOSIS (see below)

JOHNE'S DISEASE (see below)

FOOT-AND-MOUTH DISEASE When cattle are found to be suffering from any of the three above-listed ailments, they are generally destroyed. In England foot-and-mouth disease destruction is compulsory by law.

All three ailments are curable by internal cleansing with fasting and laxative diet, and abundant use of that supreme disinfectant herb, garlic; also moving to fresh pasture rich in vitality of natural herbs and grass. The accepted best prevention of tuberculosis is the open-air life, sunlight and well ventilated cattle sheds, comparable with the requirements for tuberculosis prevention in the human species.

Professor Szekely teaches, concerning human beings, that all disease is curable; only the patients themselves are incurable sometimes, because they have not the will power or perhaps the intelligence to carry out the often lengthy and arduous natural treatments. In the case of animals, likewise all disease is curable, but sometimes the animal dies because the owner has not the perseverance or intelligence to follow the natural herbal treatments which are never lightning-quick cures as with the chemical drugs, but in the true manner of natural medicine are often as slow as the growth of the herbs from which the medicines themselves are made. Or sometimes the animal is so wholly degenerate in health through man's unnatural and commercial-minded rearing for many generations, that the body simply does not possess the general health recuperative powers that are natural to all substance that is in life.

In TUBERCULOSIS: garlic, oil of eucalyptus and powdered Iceland moss are the long-proved most powerful herbal remedies; in JOHNE'S DISEASE: garlic and all the aromatics, such as thyme, sage, anise, fennel; in FOOT-AND-MOUTH: garlic, rue, wormwood, eucalyptus, fenugreek and sage.

Within recent years, by telegram and air letters, I advised on herbal treatment for foot-and-mouth outbreak in the well-known dairy herd of the Prince of Venosa (Alberico Boncompagni Ludovisi), Rome, Italy. In his herd those cases treated did not develop any chronic symptoms, and the rest of the herd remained immune, dosed with herbs already listed under Foot-and-Mouth. We both agreed that successful treatment of this herd could not be considered conclusive. The cattle might have recovered without the herbs, as they are well cared for, and have been for a long time, by natural methods. But the herbs did help and this same treatment would certainly be used again if there should be a further outbreak.

DRYING OFF MILK Cows should not be milked too close to calving, for generally they never again prove to be such good milkers no matter how generously they are fed on natural and vital diet. Cows should be dried off six to eight weeks before calving; and this should be done through two treatments, astringent and sparse diet and external regulation of the milking times. The annual dry period for cows is one of the essentials of a high milk yield in each lactation.

In the diet all oily foods such as linseed and cotton cake should be stopped, and grain foods fed very sparingly, being confined mostly to bran. Also pulse foods to be given sparingly. An abundance of green foods to be given, pulped carrots and molasses. Curtail the usual twice or thrice daily milking to once daily for one week to ten days. After that period of decreased milkings, commence to draw the bag out twice or thrice per week only, until the milk taken turns to dregs. It is then recommended to milk out very occasionally, such as once a fortnight until only a little thin, colourless liquid can be expressed. The cow can then be considered as dry, only her udder should be examined once weekly, so that if one quarter appears larger than the other, the contents of the enlarged one can be drawn out again. A mild laxative such as fifteen senna pods daily, soaked in cold water of a half-pint quantity, for seven hours, and a quarter teaspoonful of powdered ginger added, helps to condition the cow during the drying-off-period. Mint, especially water-mint, lessens the milk flow; two handfuls should be fed twice daily. Two handfuls of periwinkle herb can be given every other day for two weeks. Epsom salt will also dry up milk, an ounce dose given on alternative days over a period. Give also cranesbill and asparagus.

MILK PRODUCTION: DIET AND MILK   Milk is the product of two main processes, the breaking down of the delicate, sensitive tissues of the milk glands, and intake of matter from the blood system. The output of milk is mainly influenced by two factors: hereditary ability to produce milk, i.e. heavy milk yields on both bull and cow lineage, and also, dietary. Both factors must be carefully supplied if constant and heavy milk yields are to be produced. The amount of water absorbed by the blood from the vegetable juices intaken in the animal's diet and from the water drunk is carefully controlled by the delicate chemistry of the blood, all surplus and all waste liquid being drawn off by the kidneys and passed into the urinary system for expelling in the form of urine, of which matter the cow passes copious amounts, non-acid and charged with vitality and beneficial to the earth. As milk is approximately 87 per cent water, the absolute importance of the provision of sweet water can be understood. Chlorine-treated corporation water can never produce really vital milk. Cows instinctively will avoid such water whenever possible, and seek natural supply from brooks, rivers, etc. The provision of abundant succulent food, which is the natural diet of the cow, such as juicy grasses and herbs, berries, fruits and vegetables, both root and leaf, does increase the milk flow but does not materially increase the ration of water therein. It is the relative quantities of butterfat and casein that are altered in a notable manner by a change in food.

The effect upon the milk of various substances which pass into it directly from the blood system has been well proved. Chemical drugs are especially rapid in their entry into the milk, becoming detectable in a very short time. One big firm of chemical manufacturers, lauding their chemical worm drench, felt compelled to warn its users that it would both colour and impart taste to the milk during its use on the cows. But the firm then suggests that only half the herd be drenched at one time, so that the coloured chemical-tasting milk of the treated cows, when mixed with the pure milk of the untreated ones, will dilute the milk for sale, which will not then prove distasteful to the consumer. How beneficial indeed for the consumers to be getting worm drench in their milk! And this applies to all chemicals; because of their penetrative powers into the milk glands they are a menace to the health of man. However, it is the herbivorous milk-yielding animals which alter the chemistry of their milk from their food intake more powerfully than other species. This power of the cow and the goat to flavour their milk readily from their food could be turned to much advantage, and delicious flavour and health giving properties imparted to milk, cream and butter and cheese by the feeding to the cow of the beneficial aromatic herbs, such as thyme, marjoram, sage, lavender and rosemary, just as any other fodder crop is regularly fed; also sweet briar rose foliage, sweet vernal grass, bean blossom and clover, and the good sharp tang and disinfecting powers of mustard, fenugreek, nettle and water-cresses. (The iron in watercresses and wild water-mint is so powerful that it gives very dark colour to, and affects the taste of the yolk of duck eggs, when those birds have fed greatly upon them.) Molasses imparts sweetness to the milk; as also do calamus leaves and root; linseed, sunflower seeds, oats, carrots, elder blossom, pine kernels, sweet (Indian) corn-cob leaves and foliage, buckwheat, buttercup and marigold, all increase the butterfat and give richness to colour. Seeds and leaves of fennel, borage, balm, marsh-mallow (leaves and root), milkwort, anise and blue melilot ('curd herb' – clover family), sow-thistle, all increase milk. Also fennel hearts and roots, and hearts of the dwarf palm, which are much used by Arab herdsmen, and milkwort, clover and sage. Buckwheat, buttercup and marigold, all increase the butterfat and give richness to colour. Seeds and leaves of fennel, borage, balm, anise and blue melilot ('curd-herb'), sow-thistle and carob pods (St John's Bread), all increase milk.

Protein and calcium must figure generously in the daily ration, especially during high lactation, for the cow gives out generously these substances in her milk, and will deplete her own body supplies if necessary. Lucerne, peas and beans, lentils, will all supply protein, wholegrain cereals, herbs, root crops, willow twigs and boughs, will yield calcium. Warm cloths applied to the udder, and massage with warm hands, all stimulate easy milk flow. As do also gentleness on the part of the milker and friendly speech to the cows being milked. Fear in the milking shed lessens the milk yield. Songs of the milk-maids at milking time, were once considered essential to give high milk yield.

When milk production stimulants are required for milking records and so forth, then at least let them be as natural as possible. Instead of prepared 'cooked' cattle cakes, dairy nuts, chemical mineral tonics and so on, let the concentrates be such as wholegrain organically grown cereals, especially oats, linseed, sweetcorn – all fed crushed. Crushed peas and beans, fenugreek, ground seaweed, and sunflower heads which should be fed whole. Cattle spice can contain powdered seed of fenugreek, with some powdered carob pods, whole dill and coriander seeds, a pinch of cut-up cloves and ginger, and in countries where this is cheap, sesame seeds.

Mangolds, hay, oat straw and kale, are usual winter food supplements. An average diet for a milking cow, apart from the additions of seeds, vegetable minerals, etc., is five pounds of crushed oats daily (some barley can be given instead as a change, plus, in winter, between 15 to 20 pounds of kale and 12 to 15 pounds of good hay.) See also Goats, for a natural diet which is equally applicable to cattle, only that the latter require more grassy and less shrubby substance in their diet.

Heifers can winter out and get as much as they require of mangolds, oat straw and good hay. The youngest ones get some crushed oats extra. In Arab countries where the nature-reared herds are usually very healthy and sturdy, milking cows get cut and carted mallow greens instead of hay. Mallow is a very common weed in the East and will reach man height. Cattle will also eat gorse when it has been pounded with a mallet into a bruised soft food. Gorse is typical fodder of England's New Forest for ponies and cattle.

In the Canary Islands much of water-reed leaves is fed to the animals, particularly dairy cows. The dried haulm of maize – the residue after removal of the grains – is crushed and well soaked and lightly sweetened, to make it more appetising, and fed to the cows.

Dairy Produce and Herbs

There are herbs used to curdle milk, they are: lady's bed-straw, butterwort, *hwere* the Arab curd-herb which is often used for the Arab staple food, *Leben*, thick, soured milk (often preserved for a half year and more without refrigeration by rolling into small balls and bottling in unsealed jars of olive oil). Also sorrel (common) and lemon and nettle together with bed-straw to aid in the making of Double Gloucester cheese. The macerated flowers and seeds of melilot (*officinalis*) are used for flavouring Gruyere cheese, dill seed and leaves (and sometimes thyme) for the Fetah (of Mediterranean lands) sheep and goat cheese, marjoram leaves and flowers for French Camargue sheep cheese, and the white sap from unripe figs for Italian Ricotta cheese. Fig sap is also used in Greece. Grape seeds (residue from wine presses) are roasted and pressed into the outsides of cheeses as a preservative, and more thyme and marjoram used with the grape seed to form an outer cover for the cheeses. Powdered charcoal made into a paste with olive oil is also used as an outer cover for hard-type cheeses.

In the Spanish Balearic Islands, I made a very useful discovery of thistle as an alternative to rennet for the making of cheese, using the flowerets of several species of the big purple thistle (see Thistle, Chapter 2, for details). The rich milk of ewe or goat is necessary, although some farmers mix half cow milk with goat or ewe milk. Excellent long-keeping cheeses are made with the thistle flowerets as curdling agent and the cheeses are superior in taste to rennet cheeses (rennet is produced from the stomachs of butchered young calves).

The thistle flowerets of the *Cynara* species of several varieties, but especially *Cynara lumilis*, are gathered before they seed and produce thistledown. The flowerets are air-dried and are then stored in glass jars or tins, to last for the whole of the cheese-making season, which is usually eight months of the year, but in their flowering time the flowerets can be used fresh from the thistle heads. Artichoke flowerets can also be used.

The flowerets are prepared for the cheese curdling by pounding then in a pestle and mortar. Then a little warm water is added (I prefer to use warmed cheese whey), enough water to cover lightly the pulped cheese herb. After five minutes soaking, the mixture is again pounded and left to soak further. This is repeated several times until a dark brown liquid is produced. The liquid is then strained and added to the milk, preferably used warm from the udder. Failing this, the milk should be warmed to normal udder milk heat. The general proportion is five heaped teaspoons of the dried thistle flowerets to every gallon of milk. If too much herb is used it will spoil the delicate flavour of the cheeses, and might cause some indigestion.

The curdling of the milk is dependent on temperature; it takes an hour or so in warm weather, longer in cold. Sheep or goat milks are preferred because they curdle better, or a mixture of milks. The curds are then poured into a large piece of cheesecloth and left to drain until they become quite hard. The curds are then lightly salted as a preserving measure and are put into cheese presses, which can be of metal or straw cheese baskets. In the Balearics, strips of tin are lined with cotton cloth and tied around the cheese, the strips being tightened by use of a strong thread through holes as the cheese shrinks. The drying cheeses are air-dried on hanging wooden boards out of reach of rodents and cats. They are sometimes stood on rosemary and/or bunched sage placed beneath them on the drying boards. This adds to the flavour and aids drainage. The cheeses are turned several times in the drying, which usually takes one week. The dried cheeses are then either eaten fresh or are secured by strings and hung from the farmhouse ceiling beams to mature there and to provide good cheese throughout the year. Sprinkling of the tops of cheese with flowers of thyme and seeds of anise acts as a preservative.

Recipes

CREAM CHEESE   Two methods are given.

Put one tablespoon of coarse salt and a sprig of each of those herbs of the *Scarborough Fair* folk song – 'parsley, sage, rosemary and thyme' – into a pint of hot water and infuse them until the water is well flavoured and has turned cold. Stir well and then dip a cotton cloth into the herb water and wring it. Next, pour a pint of creamy milk of twenty-four hours' standing into the cloth, tie it tightly and place on a deep, pot plate in a cool place. Change the salty-herbs cloth every three hours scraping off all the cheese and transferring to a fresh cloth prepared as above. Do this every three hours, beginning in the early morning. The cheese will be ready for the farm meal of the evening. (Recipe from Yorkshire, England, of the year 1885).

Tie some thick cream in a bag of muslin, prepared as above, wringing out in cold, salted brew. Hang it up so that the watery portion drains away. The muslin, after preparation in the herbal water should be changed twice daily. When the cheese ceases to drip, it is ready for eating and only requires pressing into shape and further flavouring with a little more sprinkled salt. Add also a sprinkle of finely-cut basil.

CHEESE WHEY CHEESE   The whey from pressed or dripped cheeses can be utilized. This is especially done in the Balearic Islands with the residue from the thistle-curdled cheese-making. The cheese water is heated (preferably over a wood fire as the wood smoke flavours the cheese tastefully. A thick white substance forms out from the whey and is called *Ricotta*. It is pressed into moulds and eaten fresh, usually flavoured with a little salt, dried rubbed thyme and basil. The thin liquid now left is used as a refreshing drink, flavoured with honey and lemon, or it is given as a blood-cleansing medicine to farm livestock.

LEMON JUICE CHEESE This is an instant cheese and can be eaten immediately. Add enough juice from freshly-cut lemons to curdle well a small quantity of milk. Then add a few lemon leaves, finely chopped, and some fresh mint leaves. Stir the curds well, press through muslin and eat as a soft cheese. (Island of Rhodes, Greece.)

HERB CHEESES Herbs have long been associated with the white cheeses made from the milk of sheep and goats. Externally, for sprinkling over the cheeses and forking into them there is in general use the leaves of such herbs as thyme, basil, marjoram, balm, dill, mint, parsley (leaves and seed), celery (leaves and seed), and chives and young onion tops.

Every spring I make 'green' cheeses – white cheese turned green and very aromatic tasting by fine cutting of any or all the above herbs and forking them into the cheese adding, for extra flavour, a little salt, pepper and herbal oil (oil in which the aromatic herbs, including those given above and with the addition of rosemary and sage, have been infused for several weeks).

Green sage cheese was a very popular delicacy in England in former times when herbs were in very wide use. White cheese was cut into layers, each layer sprinkled with crushed sage leaves and a little salt and then pressed heavily in a cheese press until the sage was entirely absorbed into the cheese. It was then tinted with the green juice from pressed, fresh parsley.

Other cheeses were tinted an attractive yellow colour from the use of lady's bed-straw (the whole herb), or the golden flowers of tansy or cowslip, mustard, corn marigold petals (a few only), honeysuckle flowers and yellow lucerne blossom.

HERBAL BUTTER A block of butter, preferably salted, is melted gently in semi-liquid form. Into this is well mixed with a fork any, or as many as can be obtained, of the following herbs – marjoram, thyme, basil, lemon balm, dill, chervil, coriander seeds, celery seed (very little). All herbs must be rubbed off the stems and then finely minced and seeds must be crushed. For extra flavour and colour the golden flowers, as given in the previous recipe, may be used.

For resetting the butter after adding the herbs, old-fashioned butter moulds give added attraction to the butter in such designs as swan, rose, thistle, fern frond, bell, crown, half moon, etc.

Natural Cleansing Material for the Dairy

Instead of using detergents for the cleansing of metal milk churns and wooden cheese presses, boards, etc., remember that, in times before detergents were available, use was made instead of such harmless things as wood ash, salt, sand, with bunched herbs such as rosemary, sage, couch-grass, thistle, gorse (all free, from the fields or garden) to scour metal new-coin bright and to make wood stain-free and good-textured. Detergents are apt to linger within the things in which they are used, and they sour the earth when drained away.

Another great herbal help is horsetail grass. Although called a grass, it is of a fern-type family. Being rich in silica, it is an excellent scourer for churns, pans, etc., also, being of a shape able to enter glass bottles of oil lamps, it is a very useful cleaner of such things.

Calves

The Masai tribe of Central Africa judge the health of their cows by their calves. A cow which produces a strong, forward calf, is the one to be prized above all. The speed with which a new-born calf gets on to its feet is the standard by which the Masai judge a cow's merits.

Preparation for the health of the calf should commence even before the cow is served by the bull. Indeed, there should be long health preparation of the breeding cows in order to ensure the maximum health for the calves to be born, and on which will depend the future success of the herd. The bulls, too, should be kept in the highest state of health and should not be allowed to serve too many cows. It is significant that in recent years bulls at artificial insemination centres have developed foot-and-mouth disease.

If the cow and the bull both be in total health, the health of the resultant calf bred from them cannot help but be excellent, and possess very powerful natural resistance to disease. The worms and skin ailments common to calves, will not be able to afflict the well-bred calf, unless its pre-natal good health inheritance be spoilt later by unnatural rearing.

Calves are best born out in the fields, unless the weather be too severe. If such a practice be followed habitually it would much lessen the risk of abortion in the herd, due to strong birth odours in airless stables.

REARING   If the calf is not allowed to feed from its mother, then rearing by a nurse cow is the only other really healthful method. In Mexico, Spain, Arabia and other countries where natural animal husbandry is habitually practised, the calves are allowed to run with their mothers on the hill pastures and feed from the parent. Indeed all the family pasture together, bull, cow and calf. The calves only partially use up their mother's heavy milk yield (unnaturally heavy, because cows have been line-bred through the centuries for milk production) and there is plenty of milk left for the owner of the herd.

If calves are not permitted to feed from their natural mothers, try to provide a nurse cow. A good nurse cow giving three gallons daily will be observed to share her milk quite evenly among six calves given to her to suckle.

If, however, calves must be bucket-fed, then, having of course first obtained sufficiency of the vital pre-milk fluid, colostrum, from the mother, they should get three to four quarts of sweet milk per day for the first week, increasing this gradually. It should be said here, concerning colostrum, that it possesses both important laxative properties and five times the amount of albumenoid present in ordinary milk. Some hay tea should be made by boiling for five minutes, and brewing for two to four hours, using six handfuls of hay to a quart of water, and adding two tablespoonfuls of the tea to every quart of milk given. A dessertspoonful of honey or molasses twice daily is very beneficial and generally tonic and preventive of indigestion, so also in N.R. Gruel.

The most general causes of death among young calves are sudden and extreme changes in temperature, over, under or irregular feeding, worm infestation, food poisoning. Calves should always be kept slightly hungry, digestive troubles due to the calves consuming more food than they can digest are thus avoided.

The benefit of the calf being allowed to suckle is not only the strong and natural jaw formation thereby obtained, but also the effect upon the whole digestive system; for when the calf sucks, the saliva is caused to flow freely, and the milk enters the stomach mixed with its natural and correct proportion of

saliva, whereas a calf bucket-fed feeds so quickly that salivation is almost entirely absent. For instance a half-gallon
measure of milk is a good average ration for a calf feeding at
the udder, a gallon per day is necessary for most calves
feeding from a bucket.

As soon as the calves can eat, their milk and grass diet
should be supplemented with sweet hay, alfalfa, pulped carrots, crushed or flaked oats, some rolled barley, and as a
tonic, sunflower seeds.

Brown sugar or treacle with a little powdered ginger can be
given in water or buttermilk, as a tonic, especially to backward calves. Malt flour is also excellent and certainly seaweed
is important.

Calf-meal Recipe   The following appeared in the journal *Farm
and Home*, in an 1886 issue, but it still remains an excellent
recipe for home-made meal: 'One bushel each of old beans,
wheat, and oats, and a quarter of a bushel of linseed, ground
together and mixed with fourteen pounds of any good cattle
spice.' Calves should be encouraged to take dried powder
meals by first sprinkling them on their noses.

A good grain mix for calves, to be fed when they are older,
is: twenty pounds yellow corn meal, ten pounds wheat bran,
twenty pounds whole milk, thirty pounds crushed (or flaked)
oats, and twenty pounds linseed meal (with full oil content)
plus 3 per cent seaweed minerals mixture, mixed in. *Note.*
Tests have shown that with the exception of Indian corn, no
other plant food fed alone can sustain life.

The most important rule of calf feeding is not to allow the
calf solid foods until after it has taken its milk. The milk,
which passes direct to the last stomach, would wash down
the solid food before it is fully digested, if fed after the intake
of solid food, and the semi-digested food is very likely to
cause irritation of the digestive tract, also scouring.

Milk fed to the calf should never be pasteurized, nor should it be fed cold, especially in winter, but it should be heated gently to natural heat of the cow's milk as taken from the udder.

A good basic feed of weaning is: ground whole barley, one part, flaked oats two parts, steamed flaked corn, one part, and ground linseed (full oil), one part, with two tablespoons of molasses.

There is an old-time motto which says, 'the eye of the master fattens the cattle'. That means simply that it is the care of the individual farmer or loyal herdsman who studies the special needs of every animal with regards to daily diet.

When a nurse cow is not available the calves can still be suckled without undue detriment to the milk selling. The calf should be allowed to suckle a different quarter daily, the other three-quarters being milked for sale. When the calf is suckled, its milk requirements are less than when bucket-fed. Approximately half a gallon of milk daily, increasing proportionally, is the general requirement of a calf. Feeding should be regular and should be thrice daily for the first three weeks. When solid food is taken, the milk feeds can be reduced to two. Allow the calf no more than it will take eagerly. Indeed, keep calves hungry and thus avoid digestive troubles caused by their eating of more food than they can fully digest, with consequent sour stomach, scouring and worm troubles.

scour (see Sheep) The treatment used for lambs has proved very successful for scouring calves. I first used the treatment on a calf in Mexico, found abandoned by its mother on the mountainside, and considered as dying. The cure was speedy and entirely successful and since then many valuable calves have been cured with the simple herbal treatment. The dosage given for lambs should be trebled for calves. It should also be said here that the speediest cure for scouring bucket-fed calves is to let them suck from a healthy cow.

HAIR BALLS   Calves sometimes sicken from the formation of hair balls in the stomach or intestines. Caused by licking and sucking themselves or other calves; more usual when being artificially reared on the bucket. This is not as serious as in lambs.

Symptoms   Cough, blown belly, and some inflammation can be ascertained, as the calf cries when light pressure is applied to belly.

Treatment   Strong dosage of warm castor oil and powdered charcoal. One cupful oil to four tablespoonfuls charcoal. Laxative diet, including bran mash with molasses.

WORMS (see Sheep)   It is generally the bucket-fed calves which are troubled with worms, the digestive systems of the bucket-feds never being as strong or as internally clean as the suckled calves', and hence worms are able to obtain anchorage and to multiply until they become an actual malady. When worm infestation develops, the animal must be fasted, internally cleansed, and dosed with one of the non-poisonous worm removers as given for sheep, merely increasing the sheep dosage according to size of animal being treated. Plenty of roughage should be given in the diet, wheat straw, chaff, hay, oily seeds and other like foods.

Calves will also suffer from the worm ailment in husk (or hoose), similar to that found in lambs. It is due to the presence of a nematoid worm in the throat area and bronchial tubes. (See Sheep.)

For weakly and very young calves a drench of a quart of buttermilk is a good mild worm expellant. Also a brew of wormwood herb or purging (mountain) flax, or nettle foliage boiled in whey.

SKIN AILMENTS (see Sheep) A successful gypsy remedy for ringworm in calves, is the smearing of the affected areas with a thin paste of powdered mustard, only watch out for blistering, and therefore remove and renew at frequent intervals. Raw lemon juice applied twice daily, is also curative. Lice may be destroyed by several dressings of buttermilk and vinegar in equal parts, well rubbed in. Some brew of quassia chips can be added to the dressing with advantage. Poisonous substances should not be used as the calf is prone to lick itself and other calves. Even tobacco lotion is risky for calves.

LUNG AILMENTS (see Adult Cow)

COMMON COLD The common cold in the calf can readily turn into pneumonia if the animal is not treated promptly. To cleanse the calf of mucus discharges there should be internal cleansing treatment, followed by a laxative diet.

Symptoms Emaciated appearance, mucus discharge from eye and nose; growth not normal, being over-slow due to the prolonged mucus-clogging of the body. Scour is often present.

Treatment Fast the calf for one day, and give strong garlic dosage for several days: approximately two to three four-grain tablets daily. Then follow with leaf-extract tablets. Give also N.R. Slippery Elm Gruel, on account of its internal soothing powers and its high bone and muscle-building properties.

Finally there is a tribute from Alberico Boncompagni Ludovisi, Prince of Venosa, Rome, Italy, who writes, 'What a bold crusader you are indeed for the wellbeing of the animals. You deserve success, for your work is highly to be praised.' The Prince of Venosa has a famous dairy herd in addition to his pointers who are now many generations N.R.

At the time this new edition was going to print, the Prince of Venosa, encouraging an Italian publisher to take on the dogs and cats herbal (which has been achieved), stated:

> I think that all of the de Baïracli Levy herbals deserve high marks by any standards. By now I have known her through our mutual correspondence and her books for nearly thirty years, and I must say that my dairy cattle and dog breeding on my farm near Rome was always successful because of my having followed her sound advice to the letter.

6

Herbal Treatments for Horses

Legend tells that the horse, stallion and mare were created from the sea waves and emerged pure and white as sea-foam. Certainly the horse flourishes when raised by the sea or within reach of sea winds. This animal also does well on sea herbs, especially on sea spinach, sea reeds, sea samphire, and certainly benefits greatly from the addition to the daily food of iodine and general minerals-rich seaweed (of most types, though deep-sea kelp is the preferred one).

Then further legend from Greece (where this section of the book is being written) tells of Chiron the centaur (half horse, half man) who, long ago, was so wise in knowledge of medicinal herbs that heroes and demi-gods went to him worshipfully to be his pupils.

The horse in general is a healthy animal. This statement is applicable especially to the early generations descended from wild or semi-wild stock – Exmoor, New Forest, Welsh, ponies, to name but three of the many of the natural living horses found in England. The native Arabian horse possesses superlative health.

A high percentage of farm horses, if kept out at pasture and not made prematurely aged through overwork, also have a high standard of health. Whereas race-horses, hunters and hacks, the majority of which spend many months of their lives confined in stables, and are further subjected to much physicking with chemicals, largely are of a poor standard of health and are commonly sufferers from numerous health aberrations of the legs and feet: this is especially true of race-horses when raced at two years old. The unnatural practice of hogging manes and docking tails has far-reaching harmful effects on the general health of horses; the more immediate effects make the horse fly-nervous with consequent loss of weight, and also remove from vital parts of the body natural protection against cold and damp and insect pests. Likewise a gelded horse, so common in England, can never know maximum health, because its body is no longer whole, and the natural rhythm of the body is thus disorganized. A factor which further predisposes the horse to diseases of the feet, is the shoeing of horses without due thought to the natural structure and purpose of the hoof. Stabling on concrete is the general modern rule for pedigree stock, both horses and cows. For short periods little harm is done, but for long periods, as in the case of racehorses, it is unhealthy because the animal is cut off from vital radiations of the earth. Barefoot walking is wise and beneficial for humans, for the reason of the earth radiations and it is notable how firmly the healthy nomad gypsies insist on remaining bare-foot people, and leave their horses unshod for long intervals: earth contact is essential for the whole health of the equine species. Kept on concrete it will be prone to the same troubles as the human foot constantly wearing rubber-soled boots.

On the credit side of general horse rearing is the all-important fact that foals are always kept with the mares, to be reared as nature intended, on the milk of the brood mares; thus, foals have a great advantage over the commonly reared calves, bucket-fed and dieted on milk substitutes.

It is also quite general for the foals to be reared out in the fields at their mothers' sides, not separated from all maternal care as with many calves. A further advantage is that foals are generally born in the spring, the natural time for grass-eating animals, as there are no winter milk-selling requirements to encourage winter births, as with cows.

Before describing the actual veterinary treatments to be listed in this section, the following advice must be given concerning the use of drenching in the various disease treatments. The horse is a very excitable animal to doctor, and should be carefully drenched by horning only small quantities of the liquid at a time, until the full drench is taken. It is wiser policy to take all necessary amount of time in patient horning of medicines, than having later to treat a sick horse for fluid in the lungs from hurried horning.

Finally, when fasting a horse, it will be necessary to confine in the stable and tie close up to prevent any form of eating: or apply a horse muzzle. Water should be available. For the senna purge a horse can take twenty or more large pods soaked in half a pint of water, a quarter of a teaspoonful of powdered ginger added. General garlic dosage is: two whole roots (or four whole plants) grated and brewed in one pint water: half a pint of the brew to be given morning and night. Or give six to eight four-grain garlic tablets. A horse will fast well for two to three days. Exercise should be given to fasting horses, a brisk ten-minutes' walk morning and evening, preferably over grassland: this will oxygenate the blood-stream and aid the fast. Do not permit any grazing. For further fasting details and the breaking of the fast see the Mastitis treatment for Cows.

MARES (for Abortion, Retention of Afterbirth and Mastitis, see Cows) Retention of afterbirth is rarer in mares than in cows, but is far more dangerous, and must be treated very thoroughly. Mastitis is rare and is usually of a mild form.

WORMS They are over-common in the domestic horse, and

are of four principal kinds: thread, round, tape and bot. Red threadworm is the commonest and the most troublesome to the horse. There is one small, round worm which affects the rectum, and a small sucking form of round worm which attacks the intestines, holding on to the intestinal walls by its head. Finally, there is the bot-worm and the common tapeworm. The general treatment for all worms is a short cleansing fast combined with internal dosing with garlic: followed by a laxative diet. It must be stressed that it is hopeless to expect to free, and keep free, a horse of worms when after treatment it is kept on horse-sick land impregnated with worm ova. Many stables have been in use for hundreds of years, their paddocks also in almost continuous use, never rested, never cleansed, and therefore infested with worms. Such sick pastures are quite commonly the sole grazing and exercising for the unfortunate domestic horse. Those paddocks have become entirely depleted of such common plants as mustard, wild turnip, couch grass, brambles, green fern and broom tops, ash twigs and elder, which are all worm expellent.

It is senseless to confine horses in stables and expect them to remain worm-free; wide-range grass grazing is essential for the health of the horse. Deprivation of grazing brings development of the numerous equine ailments common among the grain-fed van horses of the cities and racehorses.

Symptoms The general appearance is unthrifty, with tight coat and general emaciation despite greedy appetite. Eye discharge and cough are often present. However, some horses can harbour worms and keep in a fat condition.

Treatment For mild cases of worms in horses and foals, garlic treatment given morning and night is generally sufficient. Merely add three to four grated roots of garlic to a mash of bran and molasses, continuing the treatment for several weeks; or give nightly, for two weeks, six four-grain garlic tablets. All worm treatments are best given when the moon is waxing and near the full. The worms are then stirring, breeding and easier to dislodge. This is a French peasant belief which I have found to possess much truth. Also feed plenty of pulped carrots, first removing any stringy ends. Further, provide access to couch grass and brambles.

Guard against bot-worm by the practical measure of allowing the horse always to keep its full length of mane and tail, which is nature's main provision against fly attacks, as the horse-fly is the carrier of this worm; and also by rubbing with garlic brew or oil of camphor or eucalyptus or oil waste (sump oil from garages) the areas where the horse-fly likes to deposit its eggs, for these eggs when swallowed will develop into bot-worm. I learnt this oil waste treatment from a mule-driver in Tiberias, Israel, who in turn had learnt this from Spanish gypsies. I have since found that this anti-fly treatment is in popular use with Mexican horsemen. The waste oil is merely applied with a cloth or lightly sprayed (avoiding the eyes) on all areas of animals where flies especially trouble them. It is very effective and is harmless. A little oil of eucalyptus can be added to the sump oil with increased good effects. I have received thanks for this simple treatment from animal owners, world wide.

Early spring grass is one of the best and most natural vermifuges for horses and cows. The milk of mares when they are feeding on the spring grasses, and also on the shooting leaves of hedges and trees (they share the cow's liking for such spring food and eat with avidity all that they can reach), will have a vermifugal effect upon the suckling foal, which is highly beneficial, and essential to true well-being.

For a state of worm infestation fasting is necessary, general treatment being a preliminary two-days' cleansing fast, then night and morning dosage of balls made from three to four grated garlic roots bound with flour and honey or treacle, or three to four N.R. Herbal Compound tablets, followed one hour later by a drench of one pint of linseed oil (if procurable), otherwise substitute four pints of cane molasses stirred into a mixture of equal parts of warm water and milk – one pint, with eight tablespoonfuls castor oil added. Then feed a warm mash of bran with further molasses, and turn the horse out to grass. Feed also broom tops and all possible seedy things, such as pumpkin, mustard, seeded parsley, nasturtium, melons, etc.

The oldest and most famed equine worm ball, which is non-poisonous, is aloes, made from six to eight drams of aloes juice (1 dram = ⅛ oz). The animal has to be prepared previously for the aloes ball by feeding on cold bran mashes for twenty-four hours.

For persistent tapeworm: fast the horse for one day, a total fast, which means even withholding all water. In the evening of the same day give one wineglassful of turpentine (approximately two ounces) mixed into one pint of linseed oil (or molasses substitute). One hour later give a large warm mash of bran and molasses. Four days later give another pint of linseed, now without the turpentine; repeat the whole treatment in two weeks' time if necessary. (See Sheep, for safe method of giving turpentine.) Turpentine can also be given by lumps of sugar. Use up the prescribed turpentine dosage by lumps of sugar, soaking the turpentine into the sugar lumps, but not over-heavily so as to prevent the horse from eating the sugar.

I have found male fern very effective in deep-seated tapeworm. For the horse, male fern is best given as extract in capsules. Such are obtainable from herbalists, sold for human use. Treble the dose prescribed for humans. It is essential that tapeworm treatment should be given when the moon is waxing close to full and not when it is waning. However, unfortunately, with modern man's increasing reliance on chemicals for all the ills of animals in his care, male fern capsules are now difficult to obtain. Home-made pills from cayenne (red hot) pepper, in powder form, mixed with powdered wormwood, four teaspoonfuls pepper to two teaspoonfuls wormwood, made into balls with honey and flour. Coat them very well because of burning property. Human saliva or saliva from the horse will help to bond the pills. Roll well down the throat.

COUGH This is often present in wormy horses and in animals long confined in the dusty and vitality-impairing atmosphere of stables.

Treatment For local relief of the cough give a drench of brewed cherry tree twigs, one pint, with one tablespoonful of honey, and one tablespoonful black treacle added. An alternative and proved excellent drench is a brew of equal parts pine needles and elder twigs, blossom or leaves: approximately two handfuls of each of the herbs brewed in one quart of water. Give a drench of one pint. Or coltsfoot can replace the pine and elder. When mouths are sore or inflamed bathe with a brew of blackcurrant shoots or leaves, or sage. Feed also on a handful each of sage leaves and borage (whole plant), finely chopped and mixed into bran.

Give a good tonic. The following farrier recipe makes an excellent cordial ball for horses. Anise seeds, one pound; ground ginger, one pound; ground liquorice, one pound, and one handful of caraway seeds. Add sufficient treacle to form a mass. Give one ounce of this mixture every morning, fasting.

COMMON COLD, CATARRH In the horse and foal this is frequently inflammation of the *Rimma glottis*, or top of the windpipe, which is covered with a delicate membrane, more sensitive than the nerve itself. This is generally the root cause of catarrh and cough in the horse; dust is a very general irritant of this organ. The reason for the cartilages of the windpipe being so widely affected in the horse, is that they have been made extra-sensitive as a safeguard to the lungs, the most vital area of the horse's body, because the horse is, above all, a running creature, and the best and strongest of legs are of little use if the animal does not possess powerful lungs.

Apart from dusty atmosphere and the other unhealthy factors of long-time stable confinement, diet also plays an important part in the causation of the common cold and attendant catarrhal symptoms. Scalded and cooked foods, and over-use of all cereals whether prepared or raw, are all catarrhal producing, being highly mucus-forming. Then there is lack of the fibrous roughage obtainable from hedge-row herbs and bushes, both of which are natural and favoured foods of the horse.

Added to the above are the harmful influences of draughty, ill-ventilated stabling, concrete flooring which is always 'sweaty', and over-use of rugging which deprives the skin of its breathing powers and puts over-heavy work upon the lungs. It is significant that the common cold so frequent to the domestic horse is almost unknown among the many breeds of wild horse. I am opposed to concrete flooring, as it is cruel to the feet. But in damp climates it is considered an essential of animal rearing for the maintenance of hygiene. Concrete is in use in the stables of the leading studs. Concrete should always be covered with deep litter of straw, bracken, etc.

Coughs are common symptoms of many equine ailments and therefore should never be neglected.

Symptoms Distaste for all food, generally accompanied by

great thirst. Staring coat, drooping head, mane and tail. Eyes dull and inflamed, often exuding pus. Nostrils discharging.

Treatment Fast for one to two days. This should then be followed by a cleansing diet, which should include abundant carrots. Also some paprika, a teaspoonful daily on the food. Avoid for some weeks all of the nitrogenous foods, such as peas and beans, also avoid oats. Dusty hay must be rigidly excluded from the diet; all hay given during treatment should be well dampened with a solution of water and molasses. Silage is beneficial. Dose with garlic night and morning, and if the throat seems to be sore, then give a twice-daily drench of honey and elder-blossom brew, or honey and blackcurrant bush (any part), leaves, twigs, or fruit – fruit is the most beneficial for throat cure. Honey and lemon juice is also excellent. Press the juice of two large, ripe lemons into half a pint of warm water, stir in two tablespoonfuls honey. An alternate excellent treatment is the sage plant, as given under Cough. The discharging nostrils should be cleansed with a brew of elder blossom or meadowsweet, the nostrils being well cleaned out with cotton wool. Diluted lemon juice can also be used, one teaspoonful to one large cup tepid water.

SINUS INFECTION This infection can be found in all climates. A thick yellow and foul-smelling discharge pours from the nostrils and the horse breathes badly. In Tecate, Mexico, a good riding stallion belonging to Natcho Frederico was to be shot because of sinus disease considered incurable. It became impossible either to ride or work the horse. I cured the horse speedily with the following treatment.

Treatment Fasting and internal cleansing. (See Common Cold.) Heavy dosing with garlic, also feeding garlic. Rinsing out the nostrils with lemon juice: one teaspoonful fresh juice to half cup tepid water.

INFLUENZA   This ailment is common to the domestic horse, usually in damp climates. As with the common cold, diet is a contributory cause, especially over-feeding with rich mucus-forming foods; equally bad is lack of the abundance of green foods required by the horse at all times, including winter. Poor water, long stable confinement, especially when unlittered concrete floors are in use, lack of ventilation, all lower the health of the animal and prepare its organism for an attack of influenza.

Symptoms   Copious and incessant discharge from eyes and nostrils. Mouth sweaty and foul smelling, often showing inflamed gums and inner cheeks. The coat is staring, and breathing is laboured. There is weakness of the legs, and in advanced cases where treatment has been neglected or unnatural, the use of the legs may be lost with the resultant inability of the animal to stand. Fever is present, the temperature sometimes rising very severely.

Treatment   As for common cold. Garlic dosage should be increased. A wad of cotton wool should be dipped into warm water and a generous amount of eucalyptus oil applied, and with this the area of the lungs should be very well massaged. The body should then be covered with a light-weight blanket. The facial areas where there is congestion should also be massaged with the eucalyptus oil in solution, twenty drops of oil to one tablespoonful of hot water.

Finally a half-teaspoonful of eucalyptus oil can be mixed with a tablespoonful of stiff honey or treacle and this paste then smeared over the tongue, three times daily.

Following the two days' fast (or longer, if high fever continues), diet should be laxative, consisting mainly of bran mashes with molasses to which can be added chopped onion. Also an abundance of pulped carrots should be fed, plus green food and sweet hay. Give also a teaspoonful of paprika daily, and preferably made into pills with flour and thick honey, to check the burning properties until swallowed.

In cases of great debility, following influenza, a nightly drench of ale can be given, this to be fortified with brown sugar or molasses.

Allow plenty of cold drinking water throughout the treatment. A brew of blackcurrant leaves can be added to the drinking water with much advantage, or equally good are meadowsweet flowers, two handfuls of flowers brewed in one quart of water.

Gypsies give very successfully cold hay tea, fortified with honey or molasses. Sage plant mixed into the hay tea makes this drink yet more beneficial.

FLIES To protect against flies, first always let the horse keep its full and natural length of mane and tail, with which it swishes away flies. Then treat areas where flies gather by applying a light rub of waste motor oil (sump oil, obtainable free from most garages). Add a few drops oil of eucalyptus per pint for extra good effect. Avoid the eyes.

Rubbing strong wine vinegar morning and night into the hooves and up to the fetlocks penetrates the body and discourages flies and mosquitoes. Hang bunches of flowering elecampane (*Inula viscosa*, Compositae) in stables. This sticky plant catches flies which are then drowned by immersing the bunches. Also hang bunches of sage, rosemary and chamomile.

PNEUMONIA or BRONCHITIS These ailments are often aftermaths of the common cold or influenza.

In pneumonia the ailment is notable for the chilled extremities, a symptom which remains even when very high fever should develop, the temperature quite frequently approaching or passing the 105° mark.

The horse stands with forelegs wide apart, back roached, lungs straining and panting, ribs very arched and prominent. The eyes are highly congested. Cold extremities are a major symptom of this ailment: congested eyes also. There is commonly a discharge of watery fluid from eyes and nostrils. A distinguishing and notable symptom is the wheezing respiration. There is generally a great thirst.

Treatment This is similar for both lung ailments, and consists of the treatment as given for influenza. Preliminary fasting with daily use of laxatives is the premier treatment. There should be generous use of oil of eucalyptus throughout the treatment. A steam nosebag is often necessary to relieve the congested lungs.

To make a steam bag Half-fill a sack with bran or sawdust (pine sawdust is the best). Make a hole in one side of the sack halfway down, so that hot water can be poured on to the bran or sawdust, etc., and to allow a little air to mix with the steam. One tablespoonful of eucalyptus oil can be poured on to the bran-sawdust, or a tablespoonful of turpentine. Thoroughly soak the contents of the bag with boiling water, so that a fierce steam is caused to arise. Apply the bag thrice daily.

The legs should be kept warm with flannel wrappings. Diet as for influenza.

BROKEN WIND This is a form of asthma; the horse develops a wheezing form of breathing, especially accentuated when indoors. There is no accepted cure. Tubing can be used and horses so treated have won important races. Herbal treatment can give much relief. Shrewd horse-coper gypsies have many treatments for disguising broken-winded animals, but not for curing.

Horses with this trouble should never be brought indoors,

even in the most severe weather. The horse must be kept off all hay as a basic part of the treatment.

Symptoms Wheezing breath, congested eyes, staring coat, generally unthrifty appearance.

Treatment Use a modified form of the camphor-molasses treatment as prescribed for pneumonia in cows (see Chapter 5); this will give speedy relief. A steam nosebag with eucalyptus or friar's balsam is also very helpful in severe cases. Diet should be without hay, which should be replaced by clean wheat straw, fresh oats and pulped carrots and all possible green food. The straw and oats should be dampened with a solution of molasses in water, and one quart of bran added to every gallon of oats fed.

PINK EYE This complaint often follows after lung ailments, although it can also be found quite independently of any other disorder.

Symptoms Pink colour of the mucous membranes of the eyes. The general health of the animal is always found to be poor; a general cause of this complaint of the eyes is a toxic or debilitated state of the whole organism.

Treatment A short cleansing fast. Thorough resting. Keep the bowels open by a daily dose of two ounces Epsom salts. In strong physique a horse can take as much as fourteen ounces of Epsom salts at one dose. Laxative and almost wholly green diet. Include, however, molasses and above all, carrots and fennel herb, these three things having a direct and very beneficial effect upon the eyes. Use also a brew of fennel or chickweed herb externally to heal and strengthen the membranes of the eyes. A brew of chamomile is one of the most soothing of eye lotions; add a few drops of pure honey to every two dessertspoons of the chamomile brew.

A very excellent eye lotion is a brew of chickweed, fennel or marsh-mallow herb (all three can be combined if desired), mixed with warm raw milk, three parts of herb to one of milk, the eyes to be bathed twice daily, using cotton wool swabs. Clary herb, of the sage family, is a famed farrier's remedy for pink eye.

Raw cucumber juice is excellent for external and internal application; merely squeeze the juice of a freshly cut cucumber directly on to the eyelids and on to the eyes.

A good blood tonic for this condition is hay tea fortified with anise seed and brown sugar, a handful of anise seed to be brewed along with every quart of hay tea made, and two tablespoonfuls of brown sugar to be added to each quart after brewing.

FEVER   The general presence of fever in the horse is basically as a symptom of some other ailment, especially disorders of the lungs or intestines. Fever in both mild and severe form can be caused directly from poor stable management: overheated and unhygienic buildings, overcrowding, giving an overheating diet after being out at grass; failure to dry down sufficiently after long exercise in the rain. Another common cause is failure to unstrap the girths immediately on return from exercise or work – such being a basic rule of good horse care.

Symptoms   Temperature raised often as high as 103° to 105°. The pulse rate becomes much increased, also respiration becomes rapid. Urine is generally much decreased, highly coloured and very hot.

Treatment   Fasting and the giving of laxatives is most important while much fever is present. Promote sweating with a strong brew of yarrow or meadowsweet, or an equal mixture of both. A drench with a strong brew of sorrel is also helpful, or with a cordial of redcurrant fruits and honey, or brew of redcurrant leaves when the fruits are not in season.

The following recipe is an old Somerset fever drench to cleanse the system and promote sweating: one quart of warmed ale; half an ounce of ginger, half an ounce of anise seeds, one dessertspoonful of grated nutmeg, one table-spoonful of melted honey.

A cheap and effective strong physic to reduce a plethoric condition of the blood is a drench of eight pounds of hot black treacle.

Always allow plenty of fresh cold water for fever cases: cold hay tea is also excellent. Add some parsley when making the tea; parsley seed is especially good.

The bowels must be kept open with laxatives, such as senna, and if necessary warm water enemas should be given, a tablespoonful of garlic or elder brew to be added to every pint of warm water used. A gallon of water is a general quantity for a horse or cow enema.

COLIC   There are many causes of this common disorder of the horse. Some of the usual causes are: the eating of frost-encrusted grass, or frosted roots, and heavy feeding when the animal is exhausted after a hard day's work. It is under-standable that when the body is charged with the acid toxins of over-fatigue the digestive system, so complicated in the horse, will not be able to function properly; a hard-worked horse should always be rested for several hours before feed-ing. Watering the horse immediately when it comes into the stable hot is a cause of colic. So is feeding a fatigued horse and watering afterwards, instead of correctly watering it and allowing ample time *before* feeding. Over-surfeiting with water is also a common cause, this unnatural thirst being produced by the harmful deprivation of water for long periods, the horse being an abundant and frequent water drinker, and if kept without a ready supply of water it will develop the bad and harmful habit of over-drinking at such times as it is able to get any water. For this reason, one of the first provisions of horse-rearing should be ready access to clean flowing streams in fields or paddocks. Horses should not be kept dependent on bucket-fed water. This is especially important where brood mares are concerned as they need the vitality and earth salts obtainable from flowing brook or clean river water. Indeed this over-surfeiting with cold water can produce abortion in brood mares.

Indigestible food provides another cause; mouldy, damp, fermenting hay, very new hay, too much clover, overfeeding with peas and beans, insufficiently prepared linseed and hot foods – all indigestible.

Symptoms Much resemble those of inflammation of the bowels but are distinguishable by the fact that the pains are not consistent as in common inflammation, but are sudden and of a very sharp and severe nature. Intervals of ease follow the pains. Further distinguishing symptoms are that in colic the ears and legs remain warm and the strength is not very quickly affected. The pulse also is not at first affected, except when the animal is in the throes of the pain attacks. These attacks, which are of an extreme griping nature, are indicated by the sudden raising of the horse's head, the curling of the upper lip, the striking of the belly with the hind feet, attempt at voiding urine, and quick collapse on the ground where the animal rolls frantically upon its back. Pressure of the human hands applied to the area of the bowels gives temporary relief, but in ordinary inflammation the whole belly area is so tender no pressure can be tolerated.

Treatment If the pains of colic are not speedily and effectively relieved, death will result in many cases. Preventive treatment is all-important, because once a horse is attacked by gripes it will quite habitually have a return of the trouble a number of times during its lifetime.

For those horses with a tendency to the gripes, carted bucket-fed water should always be sun-warmed (or otherwise warmed) before being given. No new fodder should be allowed before the following March at the earliest date: by 'new' is meant the growth of the last year. Peas, beans, and potatoes, all being fermentative if the system is at all deranged, should be avoided. Always feed a quantity of dry hay before the horse is put out to graze, *if there have been heavy dews or rains*. An ample diet can replace the above fermentative foods provided that it is of a laxative nature.

Feed all hay long and uncut and give no roots other than carrots which should have their stringy ends removed. When the colic is cured and cereals – grains – are once more included in the diet, they should be fed mixed with cut hay. This mixture is recommended not for the giving of extra bulk in the feed, the horse not having need of a very bulky diet, but to make the food lighter and more porous in the stomach, thus enabling the digestive juices to work the food more easily. The high amount of chaff in oats is one of the reasons why it is such a suitable cereal for the horse. Give a handful of charcoal daily, or that amount in charcoal tablets, to complete the curative treatment. Give also fennel or dill (the latter as seed) when available or give dandelion leaves.

For relief of the actual pains give a drench as follows: into a quart of warm milk, stir one tablespoonful of grated gentian root, one tablespoonful of melted Spanish liquorice juice, half a teaspoonful of oil of peppermint, four tablespoonfuls of melted honey. If the drench does not give quick relief, then half a dessertspoonful of powdered ginger should be added to the mixture.

Apply warm cloths to the stomach area, preferably soaked in a brew, for giving of external warmth and stimulation:

such as a strong brew of hop tops or flowers, or thyme, or mustard (the whole herb or in its powdered form). Give the horse a very deep straw bed to prevent harm to its body when rolling and kicking during the colic attacks.

If the horse does not expel the accumulated gas through the rectum sufficiently quickly, enemas of warm water should be given, three to four quarts – as much as the horse will take comfortably.

For a laxative, linseed oil should be used, one and a half pints every other day until the horse is cured of the colic. Thereafter give the same quantity dosage once a week for several months, to ensure the bowels are kept open and as a preventive against the return of the disturbing agent or agents which caused the original sickness.

For milder cases of indigestion the horse can be physicked with Epsom salts or treacle, a fourteen-ounce drench of salts, or eight-pound drench of treacle. The salts should always be followed, one or two days later, by a pint of linseed oil to overcome costiveness caused by the salts.

Feed as much fennel as the horse will take: an old-fashioned but excellent colic remedy.

INFLAMMATION OF THE BOWELS   The onset of this ailment is usually very rapid, and the causes are similar to those of colic, although in this ailment external conditions are the more general cause: sudden chilling, long exposure to draughts, failure to dry down well after much sweating or after over-wetting in rain or snow.

Symptoms   Very rapid pulse, hurried and distressed breathing. The extremities are unnaturally cold or very hot. The nose is dry and hot. Cold sweat areas appear on the body. The condition is more severe than the colic and its treatment must be very prompt, unceasing and thorough, until the animal is relieved of the condition.

Treatment This is similar to that given for colic (see above). But more abundant use must be made of honey, both for relief of the inflammation and to restore promptly the greatly depleted nervous energy resultant from the complaint. Maintain strength also with oatmeal gruel, to every quart of which two ounces of grated gentian root should be added. Spanish gypsies use a brew of horsetail grass for soothing inflamed bowels.

DIARRHOEA (see Sheep) It should be noted, as with cows, that the horse being primarily a grass-eating animal, some loosening of the bowels is quite natural in the spring months.

RHEUMATISM (see Sheep) For diet, give good hay and a generous ration of oats and bran. Chopped celery plant, stems and leaves, also watercress, parsley – including the roots – and comfrey, should be included with the oats when available, plus a little molasses, and the horse should get at least two handfuls of nettles (lightly boiled, two minutes only) daily. Dock, juniper bark, burdock, willow bark, are all proved excellent, and handfuls of primrose flowers mixed in bran mashes. A gypsy name for rheumatism in horses is 'flying lameness', on account of the trouble frequently shifting from one area of the body to another. Local relief should not be considered cure. The whole body must be rendered pain-free for a period of months, before cure can be sure. A brew of rosemary and salt (see Sheep) is proved excellent.

JAUNDICE (see Cows) The horse responds especially well to a brew of hops for the relief of jaundice. Speedwell herb, three handfuls fed daily, is a popular remedy of the French gypsies.

INFLAMMATION OF THE KIDNEYS This is generally caused

by long exposure to cold and damp, or the carrying of over-heavy weights on long distances, also over-use of grain foods with their high content of calcium salts not readily assimilable, which place a heavy strain upon the kidneys and often prove directly irritating to the delicate internal kidney tissues.

Symptoms A peculiar stiff and unnatural hind gait. The affected horse cannot tolerate pressure applied to the kidney area. There is a constant attempt to void urine, and the little that is passed is both thick and dark hued. There is a great thirst.

Treatment As for colic. But the drenches advised for colic should be replaced with one of parsley roots or leaves, four handfuls of the herb boiled and brewed in one quart of water, with two tablespoonsfuls of honey added when the temperature of the brew decreases to tepid.

Chicory herb can be added to the parsley brew with advantage or can be used alone in place of the parsley. Cherry stalks or twigs are also a well-proved cure, as also is horsetail grass, and couch grass, all of which should be made according to the instructions given for the parsley brew.

Steamed nettles and pulped carrots should be added abundantly to the convalescent diet. Barley is the best cereal to be used for kidney cases. Feed also couch grass.

External treatment Hot cloths, soaked in a brew of hops or thyme or mustard, should be applied over the area of the loins.

GRAVEL The same treatment as for kidney disorders should be followed (see above). Couch grass should always be added to the parsley or any of the other herbs given for the cure of nephritis (inflamed kidneys). Warm milk and molasses is highly beneficial for this complaint, fortified with slippery elm (one heaped tablespoonful of the tree bark to the quart), and nutmeg, two teaspoonfuls.

In gravel, no grain foods should be fed for a period of one to three months. Diet should be hay, green feed and pulped roots, and hedgerow cuttings. Of the cereals only bran is permitted, and this should be fed daily, with molasses, in sufficient quantity to keep the bowels well open.

FISTULOUS WITHERS This ailment is generally listed as incurable, owing to the fact that any cure achieved is almost always temporary, the fistula reappearing after apparent cure. Indeed the only people whom I know who describe the treatment as curable, are the gypsies. A case of veterinary-diagnosed fistulous withers in a show mare, owned by Mrs. Gwendoline Slater of Ditchling, Sussex, was a test case for me in an English farming journal for which I was giving veterinary herbal advice.

The young riding mare had been condemned as incurable, by many persons, including veterinary experts. Temporary cures had been achieved previously but the treatments had been merely of a suppressive kind and the trouble had returned each time. The Sussex Agricultural Department took a personal interest in this case, and made available things, then in short supply, that I prescribed for the treatment. The herbal cure proved completely successful and the fistular trouble never returned to the mare, and very many years have passed since. I still correspond with Mrs. Slater about her other animals, and the fistulous withers case has remained in excellent health. Here is my treatment as printed in the journal.

Fistulous Withers:

I note what you say about your horse's condition being considered as incurable; in animals there are no incurable ailments. But some animals through long-term unnatural rearing of ancestors and offspring do not possess the natural recovery powers necessary for the cure of disease. It was a pity that the horse was ever subjected to vaccine (or injections) of any sort, for such unnatural practice is generally suppressive and harmful. I see no reason why herbal therapy should not obtain a cure; more severe ailments have responded to treatment, and permanent cure achieved.

There are two basic necessities for restoring horses to health. Natural grazing (free from all chemical treatment) with an abundance of hedgerow herbs and clean, natural, brook or spring drinking water: without these two conditions health recovery is doubtful and maintenance of whole health extremely difficult.

Treatment Commence with a twenty-four hours' fast, giving water only. The following day give two feeds of laxative diet – scythed green grass and bran mash with two desertspoonfuls molasses per feed. Third day repeat, giving three meals per day. This treatment should be followed while keeping the animal in stable.

Allow as much drinking water as the case desires. Then, fourth day, put out at grass again. Continue to give a daily morning feed of bran and molasses and add to this one handful each of chopped watercress and garlic leaves (wild garlic grows in nearly every county in England, if trouble is taken to find it). Give two teaspoonfuls of powdered seaweed with this meal. Repeat the fast, etc. treatment first days of every month. Externally make a brew of potato peelings, and bathe the infected area with this brew. A few handfuls of elder leaves can be brewed with the potato peelings with advantage.

SCAB TISSUE and PROUDFLESH   In the horse, following after wounds, there is often development of unsightly horny areas or proudflesh. Both these conditions can be alleviated by making a rub of two parts castor oil, one part of vinegar, and one teaspoonful spirits of camphor, stirred in every half pint of the mixture. Apply rather hot, morning and night, massage strongly into the areas.

MANGE (see Sheep Scab, also Sheep-dogs)   Especial attention should be given to the care of the mane and tail in horse grooming. A scurfy mane and tail can be cleansed by rubbing briskly with a warm, strong brew of rosemary herb, and then massaging well with a little castor oil which stimulates long and supple hair growth. Also maidenhair fern is an important hair tonic. One handful fed twice daily in bran and molasses mash. Finally, seaweed is proved excellent. For removal of scurf, rub with a cloth soaked in witch hazel.

A brew of burdock root is a well-known gypsy prescription for aiding growth of good hair on the horse. A horse with mange requires a preliminary all-over washing with warm, soapy water to which a little soda has been added, followed by thorough cleansing with a hose-pipe, before any curative treatment be applied.

In horse-grooming treatment, the feeding of raw nettles chopped and mixed in the bran, is an old groom treatment for encouraging the attractive dapple marks on a horse's body.

Many horse authorities hold the quite possible opinion that *Acarus Scabeii Equo* is of spontaneous origin among the unhealthy. It is closely allied to mange of the dog. (See Dogs.)

STRAINED TENDONS   Rest for at least seven days. Apply frequent cold water applications and loose, water-soaked bandages. Later massage well into the area a liniment made from half a pint of strong brew of seaweed, to which two dessertspoonfuls of vinegar have been added. In cases of severe tendon strain a year's rest is necessary. Part of the resting treatment should consist of running the horse out at grass through one winter; the constant contact with the cold wet grass restores the tendon.

Another old farrier remedy is to apply a paste made from whitening (whitewash) and warm cow dung. Spread well around the affected area and lightly bandage.

A Spanish gypsy remedy is standing the limb in hot salt water for a good half-hour. Then friction with warm olive oil. Bandage with cold water-soaked cloths. The English gypsy specific is massage with a strong brew of comfrey; also bandaging with cold comfrey-soaked flannel.

LAMENESS IN COLTS, AND SPAVIN When colts become lame it is often due to the presence of an incipient spavin, possibly in very early form, or of local rheumatism. The preliminary treatment should merely be a long and thorough rest, then if the condition is due to simple causes, such as injury or bruising, the lameness will soon be removed.

If the trouble is, however, of a more serious nature, it will not respond to rest treatment and will increase sufficiently to enable recognition of the real nature of the malady.

If the trouble is found to be spavin, it is then serious, and may be beyond cure if much bony substance has formed. The colt should be given the following herbal treatment.

Treatment Internally give a strong brew of nettle leaves, also abundant seaweed and molasses in the diet, as both have a beneficial influence on the bone structure. External treatment: apply at least three times a day to the affected areas, cloths wrung out in hot nettle brew.

I know a North-Country *didikai* (half-bred gypsy) who has cured spavin with very strong poultices of turnip (see Foot

Fever), but most gypsies are of the opinion that spavin is incurable except by surgery.

There is a form of spavin known as bog spavin, for which the above treatment has proved excellent, when combined with long friction with a salve made from pulped comfrey leaves and any form of fat suitable to make the salve. Bog spavin is most usually found among cart-horses.

GREASY HEELS (and CRACKED HEEL) 'Everything', says an old horse journal, 'that has a tendency to excite inflammation in the skin of the heel, is a cause of grease.' Accordingly lack of exercise is a common reason for this condition; the fluid which accumulates about the extremities through long standing in one position, especially on unlittered damp concrete stable floors, and becomes unable to return, forms a source of irritation and inflammation, through its constant pressure. To complete the disorder it requires but unnatural heavy diet to be combined with the inadequate exercise. Dirty stable conditions underfoot will aggravate the trouble, as likewise will the stabling of horses with wet or muddied legs, after work in the fields, especially in clogging clay. Shire horses with their wealth of leg 'feather' are common sufferers. Legs must be cleaned free of mud on return from plough work. Horses put to sudden hard work after long inactivity, and burdened with an equally sudden change of diet, often develop grease.

Grease is not local, it is thoroughly constitutional, therefore must be treated internally as well as externally.

Symptoms The horse shows much restlessness and general unease. The irritation of the heels and adjoining parts causes the horse to be rubbing unceasingly one foot upon the other. There is swelling of the legs and exuding of an oily fluid. The discharge is offensive smelling, and sometimes fungoid growths develop.

Treatment As in treatment of fistulous withers, internal treatment is essential, but is generally entirely neglected.

Treatment should commence with a one-day fast followed by the usual recommended laxative diet of entirely bran mashes with molasses, pulped carrots, as much green food as the animal will take, and also a small amount of linseed. The animal must be turned into the fields, as green meat is an essential part of the curative treatment. External treatment: first shave the legs clean of all hair and then thoroughly wash them and the heels, using merely warm soapy water; then well wisp out with hay, using the hay brush to remove all dirt, scabs and accumulation of matter that may have collected there. Next make a linseed-groundsel herb poultice as follows: six ounces linseed meal scalded with sufficient hot water until it becomes a good thickness for use as a poultice; mix two ounces of finely chopped groundsel into this, or plantain herb, or St John's wort, can be used instead of groundsel. Bind the poultice mixture around the legs with the aid of an old stocking, which should first be drawn up the leg and tied securely to the hoof, being then turned down to contain the poultice in the hollow of the heel. Poultices cannot do their work unless kept moist, therefore, having applied a fresh poultice in the morning of each day, the entire washing and poulticing treatment requires to be repeated also every night until the foot becomes normal. As an alternate treatment an application of cleavers can be applied (see Cleavers, Chapter 2).

MUD FEVER or MUD RASH This ailment is caused generally by neglect, especially permitting mud to remain caked on the legs when the horse is brought into the stable after field work. It is also caused by too much washing of the legs and careless failure to dry them well afterwards. Many horse owners condemn all leg washing: they say mud should be allowed to dry on legs, and then should be removed by brushing. In the Balearics a farmer well known for his strong horses told me that he attributes their excellent working powers and longevity to the simple treatment of a once a week cleansing of their legs with vinegar. The vinegar is only very lightly diluted with water. This regular cleansing removes grease and is also a tonic for the tissues.

Symptoms Swelling of the legs accompanied by formation of pus-filled eruptions, mild fever. If the complaint is not treated promptly, the entire body will become highly feverish.

Treatment A short fast, laxative diet. The fever condition should be treated by internal drenching with yarrow. External washing with a brew of elder leaves and/or flowers and dock leaves, using equal parts of herbs – two handfuls to a quart of water. Or a brew of bramble leaves can be used. Playing a jet of cold water from a hose-pipe on to the legs is very helpful, but dry very well afterwards. A hoof and leg tonic is friction of both with a rough cloth soaked in a mixture of finely-cut ivy leaves infused in vinegar.

FOOT FEVER or LAMINITIS This is caused frequently from long travel on concrete roads; over-heating diet; stabling on concrete; or is an aftermath of incorrectly treated influenza and other allied ailments. The sensitive laminae and all the vascular structures of the feet become inflamed. Laminitis can also afflict horses out at grass, although it is more general among those which are stable confined.

Symptoms Much unease, demonstrated by stamping of the feet and also their abnormal posture. The horse also appears to be suffering from a general chill, shivering and developing a small rise in temperature.

Treatment Immediate removal of the shoes and poulticing with hot bran salt; a teacup of salt to a quart of bran. Natural sea salt should be used, such as Tidman's, obtainable from chemists. Alternative poultices are, linseed meal or turnip. Turnip poulticing is an old and very well proved farrier remedy, used as follows: white or common turnips are used, they must be boiled and well pulped, then applied warm on flannel; they must also be kept wet. About four medium turnips to one poultice. The poultice can be improved further by mixing one handful of powdered charcoal in with the mashed turnip. The poultices must be freshly applied at least twice daily, being fastened both above and below the fetlock to hold them in the required position.

As soon as the temperature of the feet is restored to a normal warmth, the shoes should be replaced, although the hammering thereof must be kept as little as possible, the horse must then be got out walking on soft wet (or watered) grassland, for half an hour thrice daily, and the feet when in the stable must be kept cold-poulticed, using now a mixture of boiled nettles and mallow leaves. A strong brew of the mixture is also good for treating milder forms of foot inflammation.

SANDCRACK   This condition is an aperture in the wall of the foot, beginning at the coronet. In the fore-feet it is most usual for the crack to be central; in the hind feet it is generally an inner side crack. The condition is generally caused from stabling on unlittered concrete; long journeys on hot tarmac roads in summer months; injury from stones, pieces of iron, etc. on roads; bad shoeing.

Treatment Place on a laxative diet. Externally treat as for laminitis (see above). Then plug the cracks with either of the following compounds – salt and pulped rosemary herb. Two ounces of salt to one pint of herb (made by steaming the herb in very little water until it is softened and then pulping well). This is a treatment much used by Spanish horsemen and gypsies. Or salt and Stockholm tar. Four ounces of coarse cooking salt stirred into one pound of Stockholm tar.

THRUSH This is a disease of the frog, which emits a foul-smelling discharge. The cause is generally damp and dirty stable flooring; accumulation of sour stable litter; general lack of care of the feet. Sometimes it is an aftermath of influenza and allied ailments.

Treatment Well wash the feet in salt water, or with cinquefoil brew, then treat internally and externally as for greasy heels.

MALLENDERS AND SALLENDERS These eruptions are caused generally in the same ways as greasy heels. Mallenders develop under the knee and sallenders inside the hock.

Treatment For internal treatment, see greasy heels. External: cleanse with a brew of rosemary herb. If the trouble is severe the eruptions must be poulticed, using either hot bran and linseed mixture of equal parts, or a plaster of hot pulped cooked carrots.

CORNS This trouble is usually found among horses with flat, weak feet. If suppuration has occurred, there must be a careful paring of the area all around where the corn has formed in order to free all pus accumulations. An opening should be left to ensure thorough and continuous draining of the place, and thus prevent the accumulation of further pus.

Treatment Stand the affected foot, or feet, in hot water, to which Epsom salts have been added. One pound of Epsom salts to two quarts of hot water. Then use a poultice similar to that advised for greasy heels (see above). Poulticing will be necessary daily for from two to seven days. The corns can be softened by applying as a rub the white juice expressed from stalks of fig leaves or the cut off shoots. This juice dropped into castor oil, one part juice to two parts oil. When the corn has been treated a bar shoe can then generally be fitted, and a plugging of tow and wood-tar used. Care must be taken to see that there is no pressure from the shoe on the corn area. Another herb proved to soften corns is ivy. Ivy leaves are pulped raw and steeped in vinegar, then rubbed in three times daily.

CAPPED HOCK This is most frequently caused by a bruise obtained in the many ways possible when the animal is confined in the stable; commonly by a kick. However, many horse owners uphold that the trouble is purely constitutional.

Treatment The swollen area should be treated with a cold brew of seaweed or of elder leaves, and then some oil, preferably linseed or castor, rubbed well into the area. The animal must be given thorough rest from work, and placed on a laxative diet, which should include a daily quarter-pint dose of linseed oil. Comfrey is an important remedy for bruises, also the common daisy plant, and mallow. Also banana skins, applying the soft, inner side.

BROKEN KNEES Treatment must be immediate after the accident, especially in the case of broken knees where severe gravel rash may develop, resulting in permanent scarring, if prompt attention is withheld.

Treatment Well wash the cut areas with cold water if out in the country, then make a plaster of bruised elder leaves and bind firmly over the place of injury. The animal should be kept in the stable for careful observation for at least one day, though it is better for his health to be out in the fields. Stables are not the proper places for the healing of wounds or the cure of disease; sunlight and air and morning dew upon the grass are the best healing agents.

The wounds should be washed regularly three times daily with a strong brew of elder leaves or a less strong brew of elder blossoms; or rosemary whole herb. A half-handful of plantain leaves can be added to the brew with advantage. Elder and rosemary have invariably given me splendid results in all types of wounds, many of them very severe: these herbs not only soothe and heal but are also an effective disinfectant and a fly deterrent.

If, in broken knees, the injury is deep enough to cause synovial fluid to exude from the knee joint, the cure will be a long one and much rest must be given. Absolutely refuse to allow anti-tetanus injections to be given as wound treatment; such injections have killed more animals than the wounds themselves would ever have killed.

An old groom remedy for broken knees, sent to me by Wendy Riley, and a very excellent one, is a paste of unsalted butter and very finely chopped parsley; one handful of fresh parsley to a quarter pound of butter. The herb is rubbed well into the butter, and the mixture is then massaged into the knees after they have been well washed. This prevents scarring and promotes speedy hair growth. The Arabs sprinkle the broken areas with powdered liquorice root. An old and effective farrier remedy, is an application of wheaten flour and stale beer, heated to the consistence of a paste, and held in place with a cotton stocking.

To grow hair on broken knees (and on other hairless places), pound up one handful of poplar tree buds, mix with castor oil, two ounces, and thick honey, one ounce, and apply twice daily for a period of 15 to 20 days or longer.

SWOLLEN LEGS   The swelling of the legs in horses is usually
of rapid development; that is, when they swell to the extent
of being classed as a malady. The cause is primarily strained
tendons (see above). It can also be caused by overheating
owing to an abundant and starchy diet; also abrupt changes
in diet following removal from field to stable; oversurfeiting
with water.

Symptoms   When swelling is of a severe nature heat is
usually present in the limb, and the animal manifests pain
whenever pressure is applied.

Treatment   Internal treatment is as necessary as external,
and should consist of a short fast followed by a laxative
green diet, and also drenching with a brew of seaweed,
approximately one handful of seaweed to one and half pints
of water. This brew removes excess fluid from the system
and also immediately tones up the glands. Knapweed
flowers fed in bran are excellent. So also are sloe flowers.
External treatment: a jet of water from a hose-pipe should be
played on to the swollen areas, for from five to ten minutes
thrice daily. Also very beneficial are cold packs made with
brews of either rosemary or seaweed with vinegar. A handful of either herb brewed in a quart of water. To three parts
of the herbal brew one part of vinegar is then added. A brew
of daisy plant is a famed French gypsy remedy. Mexican
horsemen use Yerba Mansa flowers and leaves, with good
results. I also used Yerba Mansa very effectively for all types
of swellings, for humans and animals, when in Mexico.
Hemp-agrimony poultice made with bran is good too. See
also the resting-out at grass cure given under strained
tendons.

DISLOCATED SHOULDER or STIFLE   This is caused generally
by a fall or excited rearing or kicking. I saw a cart-horse fall

and dislocate a shoulder at Appleby (Westmorland) horse fair. The cure was completed within a half-hour.

Symptoms The displacement of the bone can be felt, the animal shows much pain, and the area is very heated.

Treatment This must be immediate within the hour, before any hardening of the tissues sets in. Basically the treatment is not herbal, but it is natural and unorthodox. Lead the horse into a deep pool in a river; the depth should be up to the horse's neck, so that the horse is made to strike out fiercely in swimming stroke. This striking-out movement brings the dislocation back into place very rapidly. The horse is kept in the river for a further short period – five to ten minutes – for the benefits of cold water in removing resultant inflammation. Afterwards, the area is well massaged with boiled cabbage leaves and a little fat – preferably butter or olive oil. This is what I saw at Appleby Fair.

BRITTLE HOOF Mix one pint tar oil with two pints crude cod-liver oil, paint the hooves several times daily with this.

WOUNDS (see Cows)

TETANUS (see Goats)

TUMOURS (see Cows)

EPILEPSY This is largely a hereditary disease in horses, as with other animals. Because of the nature of the horse's work this disease is always a source of danger to the owner, as the sudden falling down of the animal, which is the chief symptom of the disease, and the wild uncontrollable kicking that follows, has often caused serious accidents.

Symptoms There are no definite symptoms, and it is difficult to recognize an epileptic animal, apart from there often being scarring on the body and limbs where the animal has injured itself whilst in the fits. The commencement of the epileptic attack is generally without more than a minute's warning; the animal halts in its work or its movement, twitches its ears and rolls its eyes, the next moment it is on its side upon the ground, kicking frantically and foaming at the mouth. When in a severe fit it will usually void urine and faeces.

Treatment A long period of rest from work. A light laxative diet, including plenty of nerve tonic foods such as molasses, carrots, watercress, water-mint, seaweed, blackcurrant or strawberry leaves and bran, and hops. Poppy flowers and seed heads calm excited horses and generally soothe the nerves.

There should be twice-daily drenching with a strong brew of skullcap herb, two handfuls of the herb brewed in three pints of water, and one tablespoonful of honey added; give one pint twice daily. An alternative and excellent nervine remedy is grated peony root, rosemary and vervain (the two latter should be the whole herb, finely cut) to make one handful, and then given in the feed. Give lime blossom (*Tilia*) to eat. A further soothing herb, and much famed as an epilepsy remedy, is valerian root; a heaped tablespoon of raw shavings, twice daily in bran feed.

RINGWORM, ETC (see Sheep: Scab) Mange and other skin ailments, even when of a parasitical nature, are frequently constitutional, and are not found among well-fed and well-kept horses; both are general to places where there is meagre diet and lack of cleanliness. Applied raw lemon juice is effective. It hardens and then seals off the air from the ringworm fungus.

LICE Internal treatment is also necessary for a cure. The bloodstream of the horse should be well saturated with garlic, given daily in strong doses while the lice are present. Give sea salt. External treatment: scrub the animal well all over with soap and water to which pine disinfectant and some soda have been added. Then rub in well a strong brew of quassia wood chips from herb suppliers and finally, when the animal is properly dry, dust well with derris powder or N.R. insecticide powder. Vinegar, used undiluted, will remove the nits (eggs) of lice very effectively: add a few drops of oil of eucalyptus. Powdered southernwood and wormwood are also excellent, or they can be used as a brew. Also a strong brew of walnut leaves is good. The Arabs use oil of eucalyptus mixed into a little ammonia (the ammonia obtained from camel dung) and hot water added. Two teaspoonfuls of eucalyptus oil and one tablespoonful ammonia to one quart of warm water. Rub well into the body hair, avoiding carefully the eyes. This will clear serious lice infestation. A further effective, old farrier, treatment, is four ounces of turpentine (genuine) mixed into one quart strong tobacco water.

POLL EVIL This is a constantly recurring fistula upon the head area and should be treated as directed for Fistulous withers (see above).

QUIDDING This ailment is caused through malformation of the teeth, the horse being unable to grind its food adequately; the food is spat back into the feeding trough, or passes out of the animal undigested in the faeces: this is especially noticeable with the grain foods. The trouble may be due to malplacement of the teeth, if they are unevenly set in the rows and make proper grinding impossible, or the edges of the teeth may merely have become jagged and unable to do their work properly. If there is misplacement then the offending teeth should be extracted. If merely jagged then the teeth should be filed, and points rasped and smoothed, to make flat grinding surfaces.

If extraction does prove necessary, then the horse should be dosed with garlic to safeguard against infection, both before and after the operation, and the gums washed twice daily with a strong brew of rosemary. And after the operation the horse should be fasted on water for one whole day, and the second day fed only on milk, honey, molasses and barley gruel. A light diet should then follow for one week, both to help the sore gums and to aid the digestion back to normality: steamed hay with molasses, boiled and softened cereals. A mash of scalded bran with pulped carrots and molasses is restorative and excellent.

Finally it should be stressed that great care and expert attention is required to ensure that the offending teeth are extracted and not the good ones, such error being over-common in treatment for quidding.

STRANGLES This is an ailment usually of stall-kept animals, especially town van and riding horses. If not treated effectively and promptly, it can terminate in glanders. Horses out at grass will also develop strangles.

Symptoms General unease, lack of appetite, speedy emaciation, with hollowed cheeks, breathing disturbed, throat area hot and tender. There is frequently watery discharge from eyes and nostrils.

Treatment Fasting and general internal cleansing with heavy dosage of garlic and laxative brews. Externally: a nosebag should be used, using steaming bran with a little eucalyptus oil added. The purpose of the bag is to keep the nostrils well open by steaming. Should the tumour or tumours break internally this will be of great service. The breaking of the tumours should not be attempted by poulticing, because poultices can, when cold, act as a repellant to the opening of the tumours, and thus retard the cure. The hair on all sides of the throat and the jaw area should be clipped closely, and the throat, and tumours between the jaws massaged three times daily with a liniment made from finely-cut garlic, cold brewed in turpentine. Brew for from four to six hours, keeping covered all the time. Approximately three good-sized whole roots (not merely individual cloves) of garlic to one cupful of turpentine. The nostrils should be kept well sponged out with garlic or elder brew.

When the disease has been allowed to progress so far as to generate high fever and inflammation of the disease areas, then glanders is a possible termination of the malady.

GLANDERS This has become a rare disease, the cause of which has never been properly ascertained. It is almost unknown in England nowadays. As with foot-and-mouth disease, it is not found among healthy animals, but is a product of overcrowded stables, where poor foods and stale water are the rule. For that reason it is classified as epidemic. It is frequent enough among stall-kept van horses of the big towns. *It is contagious to man*, and can prove fatal. Most affected horses, except very valuable ones, are destroyed immediately.

Symptoms The copious discharge and the appearance of the typical abscess help to distinguish glanders from ordinary sinus trouble.

Treatment Garlic has long been the specific in the eastern countries for treatment of this ailment, and it is with garlic that the gypsies speedily restore to health and then are able to re-sell horses condemned with glanders. They combine knapweed herb with the garlic in their treatment, feeding two or three times daily in bran several handfuls of finely cut knapweed flowers and wild garlic plants. Rue being so powerful as neutralizing poisonous matter, is also advised as an addition to the bran.

The horse should be fasted, dosed copiously with garlic, given plenty of honey as a restorative, and then put on to a very light and laxative diet which should include plenty of green food. If fenugreek seed is given with the garlic the disinfectant powers and healing properties of the latter herb are increased. Two ounces of fenugreek to four garlic roots.

The horse should also be given a daily morning and night drench of hot liquorice and nutmeg. Approximately eight ounces of liquorice stick dissolved in one quart of water, and two heaped dessertspoonfuls of grated or powdered nutmeg stirred in. External treatment: the swelling should be fomented twice daily with a strong brew, at blood heat, of elder leaves, blossom or twigs. A strong brew of ground ivy is also excellent, used internally and externally. Two handfuls of either herb make a brew when boiled in 1½ pints water. The internal dose of ground ivy for horses is three-quarters of a pint daily.

ADDER BITE (and SCORPIONS, INSECTS, etc.) Adders are numerous on Exmoor, and this is a Somerset gypsy remedy, applicable to all animals. Two ounces of pounded rampion root (wild, broad-leaved garlic), two ounces of pounded ivy leaves and two ounces of oil of turpentine, mixed well into four ounces of olive oil. First apply hot cloths to the bite, express the venom, then rub the remedy well into and around the affected area. Give also garlic internally, and rue. Rue is a well-known poisons remedy and must be one of the given herbs in poison treatment. A strong, burning herb, its dose should be limited to one dessertspoon of chopped rue, morning and night. Viper's bugloss is another famed snake remedy, hence its name.

The pulped roots of garlic or onion, steeped in vinegar, make an excellent application for treatment of *stings of all insects*, for bees', wasps', ants', and the serious hornet and black scorpion stings. Yellow scorpion stings may be fatal for humans and smaller animals than horses. The Arabs make much use of the allium (onion family) plants, used raw, for stings. Also the acid from unripe tomatoes, and the ammonia extracted from camel dung. Raw lemon juice is also helpful; and inner leaves used raw, of cacti. I use a herbal oil which I prepare from powdered herbs steeped in vegetable oil. I prefer such oils as corn, sunflower, sesame or (lesser) soya. The chosen herbs are rue, rosemary, southernwood and wormwood. Fill a pint bottle one third deep with these herbs finely pulped or powdered. Then add one tablespoon vinegar, finally fill up with oil to within two inches of rim of bottle (room must be allowed for daily shaking the mixture). Place bottle in hot sun for fourteen days or so. (I make my herbal oils every summer.) If no sun available then give long sessions in a warm oven. Excellent for bites, wounds and for proud flesh.

GRASS SICKNESS (and GRASS ALLERGIA) The horse has not the digestive system for consuming a mainly fresh grass diet. By nature the horse is a browsing animal, not a grazer, and likes to roam around, cropping at woody and leafy things, rough herbs, etc., similar to the goat. Give a horse a flat field of plain grass, fenced by wiring only, no hedgerows, and without trees or other shade, and that horse will never attain true health and vitality, and may well become ill. Grass sickness may come along.

Symptoms The symptoms of grass fever are very severe and

cannot be mistaken for any other ailment. There is frothing at the mouth, and the saliva is usually bright yellow or green. There is great nervous excitement and pain. Often whole or partial paralysis sets in, especially of the hind-quarters. In severe cases the horse can neither drink nor eat, and there is no bowel movement. The disease, at least by orthodox treatment, is considered mostly fatal.

Treatment This should be immediate and concentrated – all day and night for many days. Give the horse a strong drench made of two handfuls of sage leaves in a litre of water. Add a tablespoon of anise seed (or dill or fennel), a tablespoon of honey and a teaspoon of ginger powder. If sage is not available then try wood sage or a half teaspoon of essence of peppermint to two cupfuls of warm water. Give any of the drenches warm, with 1 teaspoon of honey added. Give alternate drenches of a strong brew of poppy flowers or heads, hops, or lime blossom; poppy is preferable. If southernwood and/or lemon verbena (Luisa) are available, add some too. Absorb the internal fermentation with charcoal, twenty tablets night and morning, of the type sold for human use. Make sure it is wood charcoal and not the cheaper bone charcoal. Or finely powdered wood ash can be given made into balls with honey. Two dessertspoons of charcoal wood ash powder can be given morning and night. Externally apply to the bowels area and to the whole belly area, hot cloths wrung out in a brew of sage, thyme, or rosemary. If not obtainable then use a strong brew of hot common tea as an application. For treatment of the paralysis, if this develops, see Goats.

HEART STRAIN The heart of a horse is often strained following long sessions of overwork when ploughing heavy land, hauling timber or other heavy weights, or following long hours in the hunting field or, above all, on the racecourse.

A quick pick-me-up after strain is a warm bran mash with molasses, also a handful of raisins (washed to avert danger from chemical spray) or balls of thick honey with raisins. The well-proved heart tonic herbs are rosemary, sage and viola tri-colour, also known as heart's-ease. I learnt of the use of heart's-ease from a Suffolk postman who had much success with racing pigeons. He always eased their hearts and generally revived them on return from long racing flights by giving them several teaspoons of viola tri-colour syrup. I have since much used this herb as a heart tonic for all types and kinds of animals, including my winning racing Afghan hounds.

Coriander, the whole herb or the seed, is also a valuable heart tonic, although little known as such. A good tonic dose would be several handfuls of the herb fresh or dried, or a tablespoonful of the seeds once daily for a month.

Other powerful heart tonics are lily-of-the-valley (the flowers and roots, in small amount only, it being a strong herb), cayenne pepper, marigold flowers, and honey.

Treatment   A handful of any of the above herbs (a half handful or less of the lily) either plain or mixed, given in a bran mash with molasses or honey; one dessertspoon of the mixture night and morning. Cayenne pepper, one small teaspoon twice daily, mixed into milk and then added to the bran mash. Cayenne pepper is also a proved remedy for heart attack. Further heart relief is provided by the removal immediately of saddle or harness and, when back in the stable, a gentle massage of limbs with three parts of water to one of vinegar.

Foals

The remarks on the subject of calves are almost equally applicable to foals, especially the remark that the health of the foal should rightly be given thought and care before the service of the mare and throughout her pre-natal year.

The ailments of the calf and the foal are very similar: worms, scouring, skin ailments and so forth. Thus for the common ailments, Scour, Worms, Skin Diseases (see Calves): for Navel Ill (see Lambs). The foal is generally far healthier than the calf, owing to the more natural way in which foals are reared, nearly always getting the mare's milk and not being subjected to harmful bucket rearing, or given equally harmful milk substitutes.

Foals are healthier when born out in the fields, some form of shed shelter being provided for mare and foal, especially when the weather is adverse. Field-born foals are hardier than stable-born, and develop better legs and feet. The mare also keeps in better health.

FEEDING The early months of the foal's life, as with most young things, and especially where strong bone is an essential for the animal's usefulness in the service of man, are the most vital. For if good growth is not made then, it will not be achieved in the animal's lifetime. When foals are meagrely fed during the first months of their life, firstly through the mare not getting adequate or natural enough food, and secondly when good weaning foods are not forthcoming, then not only is growth checked but also full development of the digestive organs, so that should the foal get ample food later in life it will not have the power to utilize it, and it will prove of no avail.

Weaning should always be gradual and is dependent always on each individual case. But in all cases, unless the mare is sickly, it should not commence before the foal has reached four months of age. The foal will benefit if allowed to run with the mare and feed from her at least into the sixth month, and if the mare is very healthy and has not been served again immediately following the birth of the foal, then feeding into the ninth month or to the end of the full year, is wholly beneficial. The milk that the foal is taking after the fourth month is a supplement to the other foods that it will then be getting.

The chief rule of successful weaning is that it should be gradual. The foals, apart from the grass that they are taking at their mothers' side, should be encouraged to take a little of her daily feed of oats, bran, molasses, pulped carrots, etc.

The mare should be taken away from the foal by very gradual stages, and she should be allowed back with her foal every night so long as she will tolerate it feeding from her.

Feed for Foals Once the foals are weaned and on to solid foods they will require generous diet to encourage them to make maximum growth. An average diet for an average breed of foal would be: a basic feed of as much as it will eat hungrily of bruised sweet white oats, with half a quart of chaff; a gallon of bran with two tablespoonfuls of molasses; half a gallon of pulped carrots with a tablespoonful of powdered seaweed to aid bone formation and grow long, strong mane and tail; two handfuls of sunflower seeds, two handfuls of linseed meal. Give also nettle, raw, shaken in a rough cloth to reduce its stinging; several handfuls. Great attention must be paid to the pasture, seeing that it is young grass and rich in vital herbs. Good spring or brook water is as important as food for the health of the foal and for the production of rich blood. This is accepted by horse-breeders in many parts of the world, including England, who insist on a natural water supply for their horses, finding that perfection cannot be attained on lifeless water pumped through lead pipes. The wonderfully skilled horse-breeders of Arabia who have produced that superb creature the Arabian horse are great believers in sweet milk for foals and adults, long after weaning, and certainly an occasional drink of milk diluted with hay tea and some molasses added, makes a fine tonic for growing foals.

The Arabs also give honey to their best pure-bred Arabian foals; about two tablespoons per day per foal. If nettles and dandelions are not growing in the pasture they should be gathered and added to the diet at least three times per week, fed chopped, raw, with the carrots, about six handfuls of each, as they are an important aid to strong nerves and red blood. French herbal tonics for their famed racing colts are hop shoots, marigold flowers and strawberry foliage (strawberry foliage not sprayed). Such tonics are fed also to the best of their adult stock.

Winter diet should be hay, silage, sliced or pulped roots, and a moderate amount of crushed wheat and barley, well mixed with a small amount of chaff to roughage, and a daily gallon mash of bran and molasses and linseed meal, to which should be added any winter tonics and blood cleansers such as sliced carrots and swedes, beech mast, crushed rose hips and hawthorn haws, watercress, seaweed powder, a small amount of aromatic seeds, such as anise, dill or fennel. Ripe apples and pears can be given in small amounts.

Over-exposure should be guarded against, because cold saps the energy of the body and thus retards growth, but foals do better if wintered out, and given some form of shed shelter; hedgerows must be thick if foals are to stay out in the fields, as they are natural wind-breaks and shelter providers. Naturally wintering out is dependent on the breed of foal and the climatic conditions. A cart-horse foal would do well in Europe, but the fine-skinned English thoroughbred, almost without coat, would have difficulty in surviving, though some have been so reared in southern England.

For ailments of the foal, see the section on Calves, and treat exactly the same. For injuries to the limbs, treat as advised in the section on adult horses.

The breaking of foals to harness or saddle can spoil the best of rearing care if not done intelligently. The gypsies are among the finest horse-breakers in the world, and their own animals are singularly sound of nerve and highly intelligent. Gypsies are said to be cruel horse-breakers, but I have not found that to be true. I have found the Romanies to be skilled and courageous with all animals, from wild animal taming to horse-breaking, and I have watched them at work in many parts of the world. This is not a popular opinion. I realize, but it is the truth as I have found it.

Lynda Temple, 23 Roedean Crescent, London SW, England, writes:

> The young horse, part Arab, Roedean Rhythm 'n' Blues is a family horse, bred by my sister, Susan, and me, but owned by our two younger sisters, Mandy and Nicola. As a two year old, Rhythm 'n' Blues has been shown lightly, and apart from winning many firsts, we took him to the East of England Show at Peterborough, where he won his class, competing against three year olds, therefore qualifying for the Anglo and Part Arab Championship which to our delight he won; this in turn qualified him for the Supreme Championship, again all the Pure-bred Arabs, and we could not believe it when the judge pulled him forward and made him Supreme Champion – so now J de B-L, his full title is Champion Roedean Rhythm 'n' blues!

342

Is he the first N.R. horse champion? He was presented with the cups which he won by Princess Alice, Duchess of Gloucester.

This letter makes a fitting high note for the ending of this Horses section. And by strange coincidence the first N.R. champion *dog* – first of the many hundreds more which were to follow – was my brother Nissim's blue Harlequin Great Dane of an almost similar name: Ch. Blue Rhythm of Barlowmoor.

The Temple sisters have had impressive success with their Anglo-Arab horses. Over ten years they have raised, and shown, many generations of N.R. horses, conditioned with the N.R. Gruel for the mares and foals, and the seaweed blend for all their horses, young and old. Later, in time for this sixth edition, a message from the Temples that their horses 'are still doing brilliantly'.

Donkeys

All that has been said for the horse applies also to donkeys; and they have mostly the same ailments.

Donkey foals are hardier than horse foals and can stay outdoors the year through with merely some overhead shelter from rain or snow. They like a rougher and more woody diet. Will eat prickly and thorny foods with relish. Indeed, a soft and over-lush diet for donkeys is detrimental to health. The wild donkey comes from an arid climate of sparse vegetation, and this animal has a constitution built for such a diet. Donkeys also enjoy waste fruit peels and berries, discarded foliage of salad greens and vegetables, carrots, carob pods, some crushed grains, and seeds of all kinds from thistle to sunflower. They like stale bread and are addicted to honey! Kathleen Hounsell of Berkshire, England, agrees:

'It seems all animals love honey! Our donkey would fight to the death for her honey. She actually growls over her bowl until all the honey has been eaten.' Donkeys are associated with thistles, a rough and prickly diet, but as thistles are known to give endurance to those who consume them, some of the donkeys' sterling qualities of character and capability for hard work may be rooted in thistles!

7

Herbal Treatments for Poultry

Commercial poultry are the most unhealthy of the domestic animals, doubtless because they can survive into adulthood on the most artificial of rearing methods. The eggs obtained from poultry living in a state of semi-disease have little health value to impart to the human consumer. Scientific analysis may prove such eggs to have vitamins and minerals, but science fails badly in nutrition: note the discredited calories system, which was supposed to solve the problem of calculating adequate human diet. The orange yolks of eggs laid by the free-ranging, natural-living, farm hen, contrast remarkably with the pallid yolks of the eggs laid by the battery-house hen, as does the vivid comb of the former and anaemic comb of the latter. Battery-house-produced eggs habitually have paper-like shells, and the eggs have not the healthful, sharp, tangy odour of the naturally-produced farm egg, but are frequently sour smelling. In my experience a sweet-smelling battery egg is a rarity, especially after opening and exposure to air for some hours.

This will not be a long section on the treatment of ailments of poultry, because nowadays it is habitual to slaughter the unfit; only in the case of valuable selected breeding stock is there any general exception to the slaughter rule. Yet, as in the case of the larger farm stock, herbs have restored to excellent health numerous poultry condemned as incurable.

Poultry, to attain and maintain total health, require daily

quite large amounts of live protein, in the form of worms, flies, beetles, etc., which they would collect to the benefit of the land in the normal free-ranging, while at the same time further benefiting the land with the healthful manuring of their mineral-rich droppings. The greatest error in modern poultry-keeping is the overfeeding of stock on highly rich cereal concentrates, usually waste products of the food refiners' factories. Such feeding, as with all unnatural feeding, soon produces an artificial and depraved appetite, and the birds become sluggish and flabby, and wait around the feeding troughs for the food concentrates instead of seeking their own insect and vegetable diet in the pens or fields. Furthermore, poultry fed unnaturally soon produce over-acid droppings, which sour and burn the earth instead of healthfully manuring it. The scratching of the earth by the ranging hen is also most helpful to soil fertility.

Overfeeding of poultry, which are habitually spare feeders, must be strictly avoided. Birds that are over-fat do not moult well, and they are frequently infertile and nervous.

Feather- and egg-eating, and other depraved appetites, are largely resultant from idleness. Hens should be kept scratching at the earth.

Poultry require an abundant supply of natural water to achieve total health. Newly hatched chicks also need water, although provision of this is often entirely neglected. A dust bath is another essential for health, and a supply of grit should always be available as an important element in the daily diet. When birds are kept on clay soils the provision of grit is of especial importance, and oyster shells should be included in the grit. Supply poultry with old mortar, chalk, crushed egg shells to give hard shells to the eggs that they lay.

Some shade should always be provided if the poultry are confined in runs. Woody shrubs are beneficial, as the hen, being of the bird family, loves to roost off the ground. Birds which are able to roost in trees will come through the winter in excellent order, whereas other birds confined in damp and draughty poultry houses will develop colds, rheumatism, tuberculosis.

In the poultry houses sand is the best floor covering, with sawdust in wet and cold weather seasons; the sawdust preferably being of pine wood. Use powdered lime to keep the place sweet.

Certainly the best way to get the maximum health in the chicks is to hatch them under the hen. The shell of the egg is porous, and throughout the sitting the young and growing chicks are receiving healthful radiations from their mother's body and thus leave the eggs at hatching-time lusty and strong of nerve. The hen also possesses the wonderful natural gift of health selection: she will put out of her nesting box the unfit eggs. Artificially-hatched chicks generally begin life with weakly lungs as a result of intake of paraffin fumes both while in the egg and when being reared in close proximity to the heaters. Incubators heated by electricity do not cause the same pulmonary troubles.

If runs are used, and the birds have not the liberty of the fields, there must be careful supervision to ensure that the earth does not become sour, and bacteria- and worm-ova infested. Frequent resting, with digging and liming of the runs, is essential to prevent sourness. The growing of a crop of quick developing mustard is an excellent disinfectant for poultry runs when dug in green. Some salt and soot should also be applied during the cleansing.

When poultry have to be confined, a scratch run should be provided. I saw a very good demonstration of this on the Soil Association's experimental farms at Haughley, Suffolk.

Scratch Run The run, enclosed in wire-netting, should be

well littered with crude straw, hay, leaves or reeds. The poultry are then introduced into this run. Twice daily, grain foods are sprinkled into the litter, several handfuls per hen, of wheat, or oats, or millet, or buckwheat, or a mixture of the grains, and some green vegetables and herbs. Roots sliced in half, mangolds, turnips, etc. and some cabbage stalk and roots, provide important minerals and furnish excellent pecking exercise. The litter only requires to be changed once or twice yearly. The poultry with their scratching as they seek the grain, break up the straw or other litter to a very fine texture, making wonderful compost. Some canvas roofing may be necessary in very wet weather periods to prevent the litter from being made permanently rain sodden, and thus harmful to the poultry.

To preserve eggs   To preserve eggs rub all over with grease or butter to seal them. The French method is to varnish them with a preparation of olive oil and beeswax. This will preserve eggs for two years. Four ounces of beeswax should be melted slowly in eight ounces of olive oil and the eggs dipped into the mixture when still warm. Care should be taken to see that all parts of each egg are well immersed. Wipe with a soft cloth, and then carefully store in airtight jars or tins, filled with coarse sea-salt or powdered charcoal, all eggs completely covered and not touching each other, small ends (point) downwards. For successful storage eggs must be fresh laid: keeping time about one year.

Diet

An average daily ration of concentrated foods for a laying pullet should be two ounces of corn (mixed cereals) and two ounces of bran and chaff mash with molasses, plus a small amount of flaked roots, such as carrots, potatoes, etc. Tree fruits are also important during the winter months to provide heat and energy: berries of the hawthorn and rose, nuts of the beech, acorn, chestnut, the nuts crushed or flaked. Some seaweed is a very important aid to glandular health, and thus to maximum egg production, for reproduction is closely linked with the health of the glandular system, and therefore this food should be provided daily. A pinch of powdered seaweed per hen is the proved sufficient daily ration. It is the best and most potent source of natural iodine, and very rich in most other minerals. N.R. Products can supply an excellent powdered seaweed, made further minerals-rich and tonic by the addition of dried nettles and comfrey. This mixture has been long and well proved as a natural stimulant to keep laying poultry of all kinds. Hens of poor or zero egg production have been restored to useful producers. Poultry-keepers living by sea and woodland, can gather, dry and powder such a mixture themselves. Weeds, grass, nettle, lambs-quarter, goose-grass, etc., fed with their roots, are a vital food.

Abundant green foods should be provided, both vegetables and herbs; sprouts, cabbage, watercress, all mints, wild peas and vetches, and parsley are especially good; so also are clover, chickweed, cleavers, comfrey, all plantains and lambs-quarters (also called fat-hen of the Chenopodium family), groundsel, poppy, flax, shepherd's purse, thistle heads, dandelion, fennel, dill and wormwood: these last three are powerful tonics and appetizers. It is largely the green diet which gives the healthy orange hue to egg yolks. Peas and beans, green, are rich sources of protein and are an excellent tonic in the winter months and are most beneficial in maintaining steady egg production. Potatoes are fattening, providing they are fed whole, in the skin, and mixed with some suitable roughage such as chaff or bran. One part roughage to four parts potato. Mullein roots are also fattening; the roots should be grated.

Feed also chopped rue, an old-fashioned but excellent poultry tonic, for chicks as well as for adults. Chop the rue finely and mix into a bran mash. All these things listed can be used also for pigeons and game birds. Cut in their flowering season, for feeding fresh, and for drying, the following herbs, vital for poultry and game birds: heather, clover, willowherb, meadow-sweet, rose bay, flowering reeds. The seeds of all these are also valuable.

Chicks

The best feed for young chicks is finely ground, organically grown cereals, mixed with a little powdered slippery elm bark, and finely chopped green food such as chickweed, groundsel and especially watercress. The chicks should be ranging daily with the hen, and obtaining adequate insect protein, but failing this, they will require a daily one-ounce ration of fishmeal, and/or a little milk, to supply active protein. For special chicks, shredded raisins are highly beneficial, also fresh peas, nettle seed, millet seed, sunflower seed, and most seeds of edible plants, as they are Nature's finest food concentrates. A few drops of cod-liver oil mixed into the cereals, and a half pinch of seaweed powder per chick, provides the perfect diet. For backward chicks raw egg can be added to the diet, also raw milk, and the aromatic herbs such as fennel, dill, mint, anise.

Finely chopped garlic and onions are excellent for chicks, being both disease and worm preventive. Likewise rue has similar properties and is even superior to garlic for poultry use.

Hatching

To test a hen's sitting intentions she should first be placed on some hard-boiled eggs. If she then broods them she can be

entrusted with a clutch. Eggs are best set at the time of the
new moon. Hens should be set after dusk as they then take
better to the nest. The best nests are those made from
wickerwork as such material allows fully for ventilation and
moisture absorption from the ground, both very important
for healthful hatching. In dry seasons the eggs must be
sprinkled with tepid water three times weekly when the hen
is off the nest. Ducks and geese require more frequent
sprinklings of the eggs, five times per week is advisable in
dry seasons. A thick sod of turf is a useful retainer of
moisture, and can be put with advantage at the bottom of the
coop.

COCCIDIOSIS This is an ailment of the intestines, quite
common in poultry, especially where there is overcrowding,
lack of exercise and not access to green food.

Symptoms Faltering gait, anaemic comb, mucus at corners of
eyes, general debility. The chicks produce blood-stained
droppings and usually show roached backs.

Treatment A fast of one day on water only. Give drops of
senna brew, one and a half pods soaked in one dessertspoonful of water, a few grains of powdered ginger added. Give
half a dessertspoonful dose, using a pen-filler, per hen.
Chicks, one teaspoonful.

Give garlic, either one flaked clove (clove is a small section
of the compound root) or half of a N.R. Herbal Compound
tablet per hen, same amount, but given crushed, per chick.
Continue the herbal treatment for an average of ten days.
Garlic is also an important preventative of this disease and
will check infection in the pens. Raw wild garlic can be used
with excellent results. Professor Perek, DVM of the Agricultural Faculty, University of Jerusalem, Israel, told me that one
of the most interesting coccidiosis cures known to him was

achieved by a workman who took away with him some infected poultry and cured them with garlic. The others, not treated by the workman, died.

In cases of severe exhaustion give drops of warmed honey (using a pen-filler). This is applicable for all poultry treatment; honey is an immediate restorative. Drops of sweet red wine are also life-saving.

Diet following the fast should be laxative. Bran and molasses mashes, plenty of green food, especially chickweed, groundsel, rue, hare's lettuce (sow-thistle), mustard tops, comfrey, garden lettuce and all cresses, also grass seeds. Buttermilk is very helpful and is worm expellent . N.R. Garlic as a basic remedy features in most of these poultry treatments. The same dosage is given throughout as in coccidiosis treatment. When N.R. Herbal Compound tablets are used (of five herbs, garlic, rue, wood sage, etc), use instead of garlic root. In coccidiosis all poultry must be moved to entirely fresh land after cure, and the old ground should be heavily limed. Fumigate the poultry places by burning cayenne pepper powder or juniper. (See Cleansing of Farm buildings, Chapter 2, p. 178).

FOWL PARALYSIS This usually affects legs, though sometimes wings or feet.

Treatment Fasting and laxative diet as stated for coccidiosis. Give plenty of molasses in the diet, also seaweed powder and aromatic herbs such as sage, thyme, rosemary, dill. Give garlic. Externally: apply hot cloths soaked in mustard water.

FOWL POX This is generally caused through the same rearing faults as lead to coccidiosis. Garlic is a great preventative and curative.

Symptoms Yellow mucus discharge from mouth. The

appearance of clusters of warts on the comb, at the beak edges and under the wings.

Treatment Garlic applied internally, and externally as a lotion upon the affected areas. Fast for one day and then follow with laxative diet. Give two drops of eucalyptus oil daily, per hen, using a pen-filler.

All poultry must be moved to entirely fresh ground *after* cure, and all premises well fumigated.

FOWL PEST (also known as Newcastle disease) This disease is notifiable, and destruction of poultry – as in foot and mouth disease – is the general order. Garlic is a specific for prevention and cure. Overcrowding, sour earth, unnatural diet, are the chief accumulative causes.

Symptoms This disease often first shows as a common cold. Then an unusual dripping discharge from the beak begins, followed by rapid death. In the Eastern countries the combs usually turn black and the birds smell very offensive.

Treatment Treat as for coccidiosis. Wash out the beaks with diluted eucalyptus lotion. One drop of oil of eucalyptus to one teaspoonful tepid water: a little salt can be added with advantage. A well-proved Turkish peasant treatment which I have used successfully myself when in Turkey, is ground raw garlic mixed with vinegar, two teaspoonfuls of herb to one of vinegar twice daily, poured down the beak in half-teaspoonful doses. Also olive oil is given night and morning, one small teaspoonful twice daily. I also prescribed honey.

TUBERCULOSIS Slaughter is the general rule for this disease. Garlic has cured many cases, but as with all forms of tuberculosis, treatment is lengthy and time absorbing, and in the case of poultry, slaughter is generally considered as the most practical end to the ailment. Prevention is the best cure, good natural diet, sunlight, clean earth, avoidance of all over-crowding in the pens and houses.

Symptoms General wasting, accompanied by leg weakness; appetite irregular. When the disease becomes advanced, droppings have a fetid smell and are of green-yellow colour and appear greasy.

MEGRIMS or GIDDINESS The birds reel around, staggering and often falling.

Treatment Double their seaweed minerals ration, and dose them several times a day, forcing down their beak, the following mixture: castor oil one tablespoon, powdered ginger one quarter teaspoon, syrup or brew of poppy heads, reckon four poppy heads (small wide ones) to a half cup of water, per bird, one teaspoon, liquid honey one teaspoon – giving this mixture in teaspoon dose each time.

TYPHOID The chief cause of this disease is unclean blood-stream resultant from artificial diet. Overfeeding with cereal meals should be avoided especially during the summer months.

Symptoms The legs and beak feel very hot to the touch. Droppings are loose and very fetid. In the case of chicks, if they are not given immediate and thorough treatment, they will die.

Treatment Fasting. Garlic. Also half a teaspoonful of lemon juice per hen twice daily, dilute with the same quantity of a brew of sage.

Add finely cut rue and/or sage leaves to bran and molasses mash. Transfer all poultry to new ground.

WORMS These pests are a common result of artificial rearing, both in diet and housing. The free-ranging farm hen is singularly free from worms; the commercial exploited hen is rarely without them.

Symptoms These vary, varying also with the type of worms present.

Symptoms may be mild or sufficiently severe to cause death. Plumage, especially of the wings, is loose and open, eyes dull, often showing discharge. Droppings are often blood-stained; they are also irregular, due to either diarrhoea or constipation. The vent is much soiled with faecal discharge. There are many kinds of worms infecting poultry, both adults and chicks: round, tape, hair, pin and gape worms. Worms are best treated for removal when the moon is waxing full. They are then more active and not buried in the tissues or organs.

Treatment. Round-worms Merely give a course of garlic for ten days; approximately one to two flaked cloves, or one or two four-grain tablets, daily per hen. Also add to the diet finely grated raw carrot, chopped garlic and onion, bramble leaves, elder leaves, wormwood, wormseed, cotton-lavender, rue, hyssop, as available, all of which are worm expellent. If worms persist, then give fasting and laxative treatment. Plenty of raw parsley given in the diet will remedy the ravages of anaemia. N.R. Herbal Compound tablets are recommended, or powdered cayenne pepper made into pills with flour and honey is a powerful remedy when given after a whole day's fast, giving one large senna pod soaked in one dessertspoon of water, per hen, on the night of the fast. This will purge soon after the pills are given if the pills are used early. Pills are made from a full half teaspoon pepper, to equal of wormwood, rolled in thick flour and honey to bind them.

Tapeworms Treat as for round worms; but if the trouble persists, then give a one-daily dosage of grated male fern root, half a teaspoonful, mixed in bran with a little castor oil and molasses added, or give the cayenne pepper treatment.

Hairworms Dosage as for round worms, but if trouble persists then give three drops of oil of eucalyptus in a little tepid milk per hen. Repeat this treatment for three days.

Pin-worms These affect the lower bowel generally. Give garlic internally, and the worms can also usually be reached by a rectal injection which should be a strong solution of garlic or mustard water. A little soap can be added to the solution with advantage. Strong oil of peppermint, half a teaspoonful to one pint of tepid water, or quarter teaspoon eucalyptus oil instead, can also be used as a rectal injection.

Gape-worms These are mostly general to chicks, and are accompanied by inflammation of the trachea. The small worms bury themselves in the windpipe in a similar way to those in calves and lambs, and thus cause the chicks to cough continually, alternated with much wheezing and stretching of necks and opening of beaks.

The same treatment as for round worms should be used internally. The gaping chicks can also be given small pieces of bread soaked in spirits of camphor.

Externally, a feather dipped in castor oil and oil of turpentine equal parts, can be moved up and down in the windpipe to eject the worms.

Or a mixture of four drops eucalyptus oil to half-pint castor oil, well mixed, can be used instead of the turpentine.

In the treatment of worms the mere expelling of the worms is of little use if faulty diet is to keep the intestines sluggish and unclean and provide the conditions for further worm infestation. Full attention must be paid to a cleansing and laxative diet, which should include plenty of seeds. Also the birds when cleansed of the worms must be transferred immediately to fresh ground in order to prevent re-infection from worm ova or tapeworm segments embedded in the ground of their former pens. Gapes are often closely associated with skin vermin.

VENT GLEET This is an infectious ailment; infected birds should be isolated and their pens well disinfected.

Symptoms Yellow discharge from vent, fetid and gluey, matting the feathering.

Treatment Fasting, laxative diet, use of garlic. Externally the vent should be douched with a strong solution of garlic, or with N.R. Insecticide powder in solution, this being a powerful and safe herbal disinfectant.

SCALY LEG This is caused by a minute parasite. The legs should be well scrubbed with soapy water to which a little ammonia has been added. Then a strong solution of garlic brew, plus a pinch of cayenne pepper and vinegar, equal parts, should be rubbed well in twice daily. An old farm remedy is to dip horsetail grasses in a bottle of paraffin oil and scrub the legs well with the paraffin-soaked plants.

BROKEN LEG This is quite a common occurrence in poultry, especially when they are confined and are not free ranging. the broken legs of birds mend easily.

Treatment Make splints, preferably of elder wood. Bandage firmly. Stand the leg in a cold brew of comfrey leaves and mallow leaves three times daily. The water should come well above the place of breakage. Also give one teaspoonful

357

of the comfrey brew internally morning and night.

LICE, FLEAS, MITES, SCABIES (see Sheep treatment) All woodwork in poultry houses should have regular treatment with a blow-lamp and creosote, and the runs should be limed and fumigated yearly with cayenne pepper. Derris powder and powdered quassia chips should be added to the dust bath once weekly. Coal or coke cinders with powdered charcoal added make a good dust bath. Also dusting with tobacco is excellent. When dusting hens for vermin destruction, they should be held by the legs and suspended downwards so that the feathers will open easily and let in the powder.

The feathers should be turned the wrong way for dusting.

Young chicks should have a little oil of eucalyptus applied round the neck, under the beak, and rubbed into the top of the head – avoiding the eyes. These are the areas mostly infected. N.R. Herbal Protection powder is reliable both in dust baths, and dry or in solution for applying to the plumage. In Greece, the sticky herb elecampane, and the pungent herb fleabane, are put into nesting-boxes to deter fleas. Mouse and rat holes are blocked up with the prickly foliage of asparagus herb.

BACILLARY WHITE DIARRHOEA This disease can be severe and result in heavy losses amongst the chicks. It is more general in the spring and summer months.

Symptoms The droppings are white and liquid, and with the chicks, the passing of the droppings evokes shrill cries.

Treatment As for Coccidiosis. But give also a thrice-daily small feed of powdered slippery elm bark and honey, with warm milk. Much attention should be paid to disinfection of the houses and runs.

COLDS   This is a form of bacterial croup and is closely allied to influenza of humans, the chief cause being faulty and over-clogging diet with resultant heavy mucus accumulations. Another cause is overheated, ill-ventilated houses.

Symptoms   Eyes sticky with mucus, also mucus-clogged nostrils. Breathing laboured, appetite very diminished.

Treatment   Give plenty of garlic internally. Fast for one day, then laxative diet. Later diet should include daily cod-liver oil and plenty of chopped onion and mustard greens. Give inhalations of eucalyptus oil turned to vapour in boiling water. Also give finely chopped shoots of spruce fir in bran mashes with molasses added. Give teaspoons of strong sage tea.

CROP BOUND   There are many causes of this condition, the chief one being indigestion caused by coccidiosis, worms, fibrous vegetable matter, pieces of wire, twine, etc. Also blockage of gizzard or intestines from tumours, parasitical worms, retained egg yolks, foreign bodies.

Symptoms   Area of the crop is very hard and protruding. The hen shows disinclination to eat and there is often a staggering gait.

Treatment   Make a brew from half a teaspoon of powdered gentian root, brewed in one small cupful of water. When brewed add one tablespoonful of milk, two teaspoonfuls of olive oil. Divide into two parts and give the second part two hours after the first.

A full teaspoonful of linseed oil is another good remedy.

A simple operation is the cutting open of the crop, removal of the contents, sprinkling the clean crop walls with one teaspoonful of black pepper, sewing up again with ordinary needle and strong thread. Thereafter give plenty of finely chopped sauce-alone (hedge garlic) herb in the diet. Give also garlic and rue.

EGG BOUND   This is generally caused through glandular deficiencies, the best safeguard against which is the daily provision of seaweed and plenty of free exercise in sunny pastures. Feed also chopped up goose-grass (cleavers) in bran mash.

Symptoms   The abdomen becomes very blown-looking. The hen often adopts a peculiar squatting posture with the vent upon the ground.

Treatment   Inject some olive oil into the vent. Then apply hot cloths, and after several minutes endeavour to manipulate the blocking egg with the finger-tips. Break up the egg to help its removal. Also give an internal dose of castor oil, a small teaspoonful with a pinch of ground ginger added.

DROPPED VENT (PROLAPSE)   There are several causes, the chief ones being the retention of soft-shelled egg or eggs, disease of the reproductive system, degeneration of the muscular system and inability to stand the constant exercise of egg-laying, often promoted to excess by use of chemical stimulating laying meals, salts, powders, etc., and the cruel method of prolonging laying hours by use of artificial lighting after the normal dusk roosting.

Symptoms   Area of the vent protruding and hanging.

Treatment   Massage with grease the protruding organ, and then carefully press back into position. Place a pad of cotton-wool soaked in the astringent and muscle-toning witch hazel extract, and then lightly bind. Fast for one day, and then feed a very light diet, entirely of greens, bran mash, molasses and buttermilk. During this treatment stop feeding seaweed, as egg-laying is not to be encouraged until the condition is remedied.

CROOKED BREAST-BONE   This is due to dietary deficiency, and is closely akin to rickets. Bad housing, with lack of sunlight, is another contributory cause.

Treatment   Give a very mineral-rich diet, which should include whole-grain cereals, especially oats, organically grown, linseed, sunflower seeds, molasses, seaweed, grated raw carrots, plenty of chopped parsley, watercress, cod-liver oil. Beneficial herbs are cleavers, burdock, mustard, groundsel, chickweed, rue, comfrey, thistle heads, bramble fruits and pulped holly leaves. Give N.R. Gruel.

Provide plenty of exercise on dry, sunny land.

FUNGUS or PROUD FLESH   This is usually caused from pecks when hens are over-confined. Treat the places with the following mixture: burnt alum two tablespoons, castor oil one tablespoon, vinegar one tablespoon, thick honey to mix. Apply to the affected parts.

LAMENESS   This can be caused by many things, but is most generally due to the same causes as crooked breast-bone. Other causes are – parasitical worms, layer's cramp, intestinal disorders, severe coccidiosis.

Treatment   As for Crooked Breast-bone. If worms or coccidiosis are the causes, then the treatment given for those ailments should be followed. Feed plenty of garlic, wormwood, chickweed, rue and groundsel, also some mustard seed and nasturtium seeds.

GIZZARD BOUND   The fibrous matter of coarse grasses can accumulate in the gizzard, blocking it, and cause birds to waste away. This can be prevented by keeping careful super-vision in the late summer months when herbage becomes rank, also providing plenty of grit in the pens, and if the condition should manifest itself, then the provision of olive oil – or some other oil such as linseed, corn or peanut or rapeseed – is a necessity. A small teaspoonful twice daily. Give also powdered charcoal, as much as the birds will take.

Apply hot cloths externally to give relief to the distended skin, first dipping the cloths in yarrow brew, used hot.

EXCESSIVE MOULTING When moulting becomes so excess-ive as to expose large areas of bare inflamed flesh on rumps, throats, etc., this is often due to lack of protein or acute vitamin deficiency. All the aromatic herbs such as dill, anise, fennel, taken internally, are good for plumage growth and especially good are all the algae family – the seaweeds, kelp, bladderwrack, and dulse; also maidenhair fern, nettle, cleavers, and all the onion family including garlic. Externally rub in a lotion of a brew of burdock root with castor oil, two parts of burdock to one part of castor oil. Or a brew of the foliage of wild daffodils. Rosemary brew mixed with a little vinegar, two tablespoons to one pint liquid, is a proved excellent plumage tonic, or southernwood instead of rose-mary. Excessive moulting can also be caused by an unnatural confined life. The birds cast their feathers and pull them out in their boredom.

LARYNGO-TRACHEITIS This is primarily a disease of artifi-cial rearing conditions, and is rare among farmyard poultry getting free range exercise and abundant fresh air and natural foods. Paraffin heaters are especially harmful in the poultry houses, eating up the vital elements of the air and in their stead discharging noxious fumes.

Symptoms Congested and swollen combs of a blood-red hue. Breathing is gasping and there is a rattling in the throat and fluid discharge from the beak.

Treatment As for colds (see above), but treatment must be immediate and more intensive. Give drops of honey as a stimulant. Give very heavy garlic dosage and inhalations of eucalyptus oil or pine. Inhalations of elecampane plant are also very beneficial.

The eyes, insides of beaks and nostrils, should all be bathed with weak garlic solution.

BLINDNESS Bathe the eyes with a weak solution of raw lemon juice (see Lemon, Chapter 2), or with rue (see Rue). Feed raisins as a tonic.

Chicks

As with the young of the larger farm animals, provision for chicks should begin with the embryo. The hen's eggs for hatching should be from birds not less than eighteen months of age, eggs from very young pullets producing weakly chicks and a tendency to a predominance of cockerels. The cock should run with the hens for a whole month before the fertility of the eggs can be counted on.

The brood hens should be in vigorous health, with heavy plumage, and slightly fat, all to give added warmth, comfort and vitality to the eggs during their daily contact with the body of the sitting bird.

The nests should imitate the natural hedgerow nest as closely as possible. April and May hatched chicks are the best.

The early feeds of the chicks should be powdered whole-grain barley, moistened with a little buttermilk. Some slippery elm bark and calamus root, powdered, added to this, are highly beneficial. Or N.R. Gruel, which is basically slippery elm with added nutritious herbs and grasses for internal health and external strength. There should be no tempting of the chicks to take over-early nourishment. Their natural appetite must be allowed to assert itself. Chicks from the hour of hatching are supplied by Nature with an emergency ration of yolk, sufficient for three days.

Egg custard, with chopped onion, dandelion and parsley added, is also excellent when prize chicks are wanted. Put in some honey for extra health.

The grass in the coop should be kept cut short. Their feed for the first week should be given on wooden boards, to facilitate their eating. After the first week they should be let out with the hen. Early freedom from the coop, plus early hours, soon after dawn, is one of the secrets of healthy chicks. Also to encourage them to seek their own food they should not get their first feed until they have ranged for one to two hours. Fresh water must be available at all times. Sunlight is one of the most important requirements of chicks.

A good tonic is liquorice powder mixed with whole wheat bread and milk and a little honey. Also a ration of seeds, such as grass, rape, celery, mustard, anise, groundsel, shepherd's purse, thistle, etc. Raisins are an excellent tonic. Powdered seaweed can be given after the tenth day, a small sprinkle per chick.

The chicks should only get as much as they will pick up within the half-hour; surplus food should be removed, as it will only sour, encourage vermin, and cause scouring. As with all young animals, for possession of true health they should be kept hungry.

The ailments of chicks are closely allied to those of adult poultry (see above). Diarrhoea may be troublesome in the summer and should be treated by a half-day fast, and one and a half days on a diet of milk and honey, slippery elm, dill, and arrowroot, all three provided in N.R. Gruel. Give a teaspoon of raisins daily per chick. The raisins are not essential to the treatment but aid it. Powdered charcoal, grated raw apples, dried or fresh bilberries all heal diarrhoea.

Other tonic foods are hemp, millet, sunflower seeds, fenugreek seeds, fennel seeds, rape seeds, flaked nuts, pepper, ginger and paprika (genuine).

Ducks, Geese, Turkeys

All these birds are far healthier than the average breeds of hens, unless subjected to mass commercial rearing. Mostly they are spared the unnatural conditions of the battery house, and it is more general for the eggs to be hatched out naturally under birds, for artificial hatching has not proved very successful with these types of birds.

Their diseases are fewer than found with chickens, and those which do occur should be treated similarly to chickens, but larger dosage are given owing to the more powerful constitution of these three types of birds, and their greater size. Double the poultry dosage for geese and turkeys.

Ducks will sometimes develop a form of toe corn, which must be treated by soaking the feet in hot Epsom salts solution, two ounces to one pint water, then pinching out and dressing with a lotion of elder leaves – the lotion applied hot.

For convulsions in ducks, give them a pinch of black pepper mixed with butter. Add a half teaspoon of peony root, finely grated, into the bran mash, or one teaspoon dried skullcap herb.

Ducklings sometimes suffer from staggering gait or weak legs and should be given similar treatment to poultry with crooked breast-bone (which see).

Ducks keep in better health when they have access to

water. In the case of provision of artificial water for the young ducklings, care should be taken in the early days to guard against the ducklings drowning themselves; there should always be a high stone available for them in the water container.

The ducklings will take much the same diet as the poultry chicks, but more abundant green food should be provided, especially cresses and water-mint.

In addition they require their food slightly more moist than poultry chicks.

Ducks and geese are unsatisfactory mothers in the domestic state, but excellent when in their wild environment. Because they are such erratic mothers in captivity, both ducklings and goslings are best raised by hens.

Goslings can also be given the same diet as the ducklings. They, too, require a more moist and a more green diet than the poultry chicks. Goslings when healthy will be found to be very foward, and brooding can be dispensed with often as early as the tenth day. The best of tonics for young goslings is the herb cleavers, sometimes known as goose-grass because of the fondness shown for it by geese. It should be fed slightly dried to remove its adhesive characteristic, and chopped small.

Turkey chicks are the weakest of all the bigger birds; indeed their poor health record is only surpassed by that of poultry. Doubtless the over confined and generally overcrowded life of the adult birds in commercial rearing is responsible for the unsatisfactory health of the chicks. In Mexico and Israel I have seen wild turkeys in wonderful health; their running speed is remarkable and so powerful that a swift dog could not overtake them. In the wild state they are often in the trees, and quite probably the failure to provide trees or shrubs in modern poultry runs is one of the basic causes for the lung disorders, nervous ailments, and generally heavy mortality of turkeys from the common poultry ailments of the present day. In Spain I have seen large numbers of free-range turkeys around the farms, and all of them notably hardy and healthy birds.

Turkey chicks can be reared satisfactorily with their mother.

They do best if kept on egg custard, with finely chopped onion and cresses, for their first five days; finely ground barley can then be introduced. By the tenth day they should also be getting other cereal foods and N.R. Gruel, mixed seeds and abundant green food, including finely chopped grasses, dandelion and nettle, and some red clover. The best turkey tonic is wormwood herb; it promotes firm strong muscle and generally improves appetite. A little raw milk is a good form of protein for the young poults when they are confined. A very old and very satisfactory (seventeenth century) rearing food for turkey poults is as follows: 'Paste for weak turkey chicks. Eggs boiled fairly hard, nettles and parsley, all chopped up and moistened with wine.' The poults are very forward and can be let out into the fields to feed when they have reached ten days. But they must be kept dry, for turkeys are birds of warm, dry plains.

So far as the ailments of ducks, geese and turkeys are concerned, they are very similar to chicken, being worm, pulmonary disorders, intestinal disorders, and external parasites. The given poultry treatments are all applicable to the other birds, only the dosage should be increased according to the size of the bird. However, it is considered that the bigger birds are hopeless to treat when afflicted with disease, and that it is a better policy to slaughter than to waste time in doctoring. I have not been able to find reason for this general attitude to disease. I have found that all the domestic birds, including pigeons, react highly satisfactorily and speedily to remedial treatments with herbs. Geese are especially excellent and highly intelligent patients.

Finally it should always be remembered that geese and turkeys are wide-range grazers, and their health will degenerate if they are over-confined. They do especially well when allowed to graze the stubble fields; and geese, when grazing, encourage the growth of excellent quality fine grasses. Turkeys are fundamentally green feeders, and during their periods of heavy growth should have access to rich plants such as lucerne, red clover, sprouting corn and other cereal crops.

Powdered seaweed is an excellent tonic for all breeds of birds, especially when laying and during moulting.

The herb spurry, also dried nettles, are the most important for fattening birds. Chickweed, groundsel, cleavers, cresses, vetches, marigold, comfrey, wild garlic, mullein roots, and the aromatic herbs such as thyme, marjoram, sage, for conditioning. Garlic, rue and vervain as worm preventative and immunizer against infectious ailments. Ann Barrington, The Lodge, Great Bealings, Woodbridge, Suffolk, England, wrote, 'Your garlic and seaweed powder advice worked wonders on sick hens. All other advice was to wring their necks!'

All the domestic birds require an abundance of fresh natural water. Also a good daily ration of whole-grain, organically grown cereals with plenty of heart; they will not make normal growth or lay heavily if fed the modern pappy cereals which are stimulated into growth by artificial chemicals. They also need to graze on healthy land, rich in natural compost, and therefore teeming with vital insect life. They will not do well on grassland and in orchards saturated with the modern weed-killers and other poison sprays, and beware of modern slug and snail killers; fatal! When I look upon the moulting grey-hued turkeys of the modern poultry farm, I like to think back to the swift-limbed, glowing-plumaged wild species of the sage-clothed foothills of Mexico which I knew, and acknowledge the superiority of Nature.

8

Herbal Treatments for Sheep-dogs

No farm is complete without its sheep-dogs, guarding the premises, herding the sheep and cattle, killing vermin. And yet nowadays, especially in Europe, the sheep-dog receives the worst care at the hands of man of all the domestic animals (except for the poultry which are imprisoned in battery houses). This has come into being more through man's ignorance than his unkindness.

I shall try and explain why the present-day sheep-dog is getting such poor treatment. It is largely a question of feeding. Man himself is what he eats: daily, in his choice of foods he either feeds good health or future ill health to his body. The domestic animals, under the domination of man, are likewise dependent on man's care for their health or for diseased bodies. The grazing animals are partly able to forage for themselves on the moorlands and in the fields, but the dog is almost entirely dependent upon what his master gives to him. If the dog goes hunting and killing his food for himself he frequently gets punished for such transgression of the safe domestic code. Now as the dog feeds with man, if man's diet is devitalized and unhealthy, the canine diet likewise suffers from such defects.

The past diet of the sheep-dog should be compared with present-day diet. In the past, farmhouse fare was largely stone-ground wheatmeal or oatmeal porridge and bread, potatoes boiled in their skins, farm butter, whole milk, farmyard-laid eggs, rabbits, hares, home-grown vegetables, and other such simple fare. The farm dogs got the left-overs from such a wholesome diet, and there was plenty of milk and buttermilk for them. They were able to gorge themselves from the meal bins. The hens laid their eggs around the outskirts of the farm and many thus came the way of the dogs which found hidden nests. Rabbits had not been exterminated by gassing them in their burrows and other such modern warfare, and were plentiful in the fields, and the dogs got them regularly in their diet. (Nowadays if they are not exterminated but trapped for sale to the shops, they fetch such high prices that they are generally considered as far too costly to feed to the farm dogs.) Furthermore stock is seldom home-killed, and thus the dogs no longer get the excellent grass-filled paunches, the hooves, eyes, and other vitamin-rich offal. Sheep-dogs do much the same hard work as in former days, but they do not get the same nourishing diet.

Consider the diet of the modern sheep-dog. It is largely white flour dog biscuit of some proprietary brand, soaked in water or bone broth. Watered milk, cooked bones, and the unhealthy table scraps from the modern farm diet of white bakers' bread, peeled potatoes, white flour products and tinned foods. The sheep-dog gets little else on the many farms where I have watched them feed. The only exception is that they do, on some farms, get flaked corn, bought in for the cows and sheep.

My concern for the modern sheep-dog brought me a letter from a farmer in the Welsh hills, Merionethshire (now Gwynedd), in which he deplores the shocking condition of so many of the renowned working sheep-dogs in the Welsh hills. 'It is truly a cause of shame to many of us to see these useful dogs in such poor condition ... The sheep-dog is entitled to every consideration as to his physical condition, and I believe would enormously repay his master if the latter

could be enlightened about correct diet, of organically produced food.'

Every labourer is worthy of his hire; this is an old saying,
and the sheep-dog is a loyal and tireless worker, and is
worthy of a well-balanced diet to keep him active, disease-
free, and of long life. In my canine veterinary work I have
proved very positively that the dog, provided he is fed correctly, is an animal easy to keep in perfect health and entirely
disease-free. I personally reared eleven generations of an
exotic breed of hunting hound, the Afghan hound. My strain
of dogs, 'Turkuman', was renowned because it was disease-
free in a breed considered as being extremely hard to maintain in health. In the many generations I had no disease
although my veterinary work subjected my hounds, adults
and puppies, to constant and many infections. Several of my
Afghans have since travelled across the world with me, from
climate to climate, often in tropical places of intense heat, and
meeting with many new and infectious canine ailments in
foreign countries, especially skin vermin and worms, but
they also have remained disease-free. Only tapeworm was
ever troublesome.

Before I completed my canine rearing work I exported one
of the fifth generation of Turkumans, to the USA, to be
covered by Sunny Shay, of Grandeur Afghans, for Sol Mal-
kin, then editor of *Publishers' Weekly*. In that country, where
show-ring competition is so high, Turkuman Nissim's Laurel
became not only the greatest winning champion Afghan of
his time in the USA, but also the First Hound of the many
other hound breeds present in that country: he won the
entire Hound Group of Westminster Show (a show on the
level of Britain's Crufts), and was the first Afghan hound ever
to win that honour. Since then he has sired fourteen American Afghan champions.

Many of the Turkuman Afghans became champions in

England, also. It was mainly Natural Rearing and diet which gave physical superiority to those hounds, making them attractive to judges.

In this section on sheep-dogs I shall give simple directions for the provision of a well-balanced diet to maintain farm dogs in total health, and the herbal remedies for curing the common ailments which afflict farm-dogs, and which will continue to afflict them unless a correct diet is provided.

I give as introduction to this section the well proved and much followed canine diet for adults and puppies, which is known as the 'Natural Rearing' diet, and has produced generations of disease-free dogs in famous kennels in all parts of the world. I evolved the diets for the raising of perfect show stock, and they can be simplified for the farm dog. Also I shall discuss the question of meat-feeding for sheep-dogs separately, after giving the proved canine diet for the prevention of disease.

N.B. This Natural Rearing diet is taken from my book, *The Complete Herbal Book for the Dog*, first published by Faber and Faber, England, in 1955. The book has been translated into many languages and has been published in many countries. Swiss veterinary surgeons translated the editions for Albert Müller, Switzerland; Herr P. M. C. Toepel, the famed international hound judge, wrote the introduction to the Dutch edition for Beaphar, Raalte, which was published by Joppe, Holland; Duell, Sloan and Pearce, New York, published the American edition in 1961.

A new, revised and enlarged English third edition was brought out by Faber and Faber in 1971, and Arco Publishing Co, New York, published that edition in the USA. Fabers published a thoroughly revised fourth edition in 1975. A fifth edition in 1985, retitled *The Complete Herbal Handbook for the Dog and Cat*, was followed by a sixth edition in 1991.

In his introduction to the Dutch edition, P. M. C. Toepel, author of the Dutch Canine Encyclopaedia, stated that when judging at Crufts Championship Show, 1937, he saw two outstanding black male Afghan pups, brothers. He gave them high awards. 'Those pups stood out from the rest, they looked more vital.' That was Toepel's first meeting with N.R. dogs.

Later, in 1938, one of those winning brothers became mine and was given the name Turkuman Bamboo. He was the founder of my own Turkuman Afghan Kennels.

Natural Rearing Diet

The paramount rule in canine diet is raw foods: it is the cooking of foods which is responsible for at least 70 per cent of the disease found in the canine race. In cooking, not only are most of the life-giving elements destroyed (what farmer would ever sow his fields with cooked seed and expect living crops to result?) but the entire composition of the food is also altered. Consequently the internal digestive organs cannot then be used to their natural extent, cooking having already semi-digested the food, and thus the very strong digestive juices with which the dog is supplied, also the strong and muscular stomach and intestines are left only partly exercised, and therefore soon weaken and become unhealthy. Much meat is cooked nowadays through the mistaken belief that cooking is necessary to destroy the disease bacteria which may be present in knacker's meat, especially when most of such meat is classified as unfit for human use. However, the nature of the dog's internal anatomy is such that it is well able to destroy all disease bacteria, worm ova, etc. in the normal process of digestion. The dog in the wild state was created for the work of scavenger, preying upon sick and unhealthy animals and rotting carcasses; naturally it would be the unhealthy or infirm animals which would fall victims to the dog packs.

The dietary rule of next importance is the realization of the fact that the dog has far greater difficulty in digesting cereals than flesh foods; and therefore the natural food, meat, ought to form 70 per cent of the diet, the percentage of cereal fed should be kept apart from the meat and given as a separate feed. Working sheep-dogs require a light breakfast, no mid-day meal, and a main meal in the evening. It is not good for any animal to perform strenuous work on a full stomach.

The third dietary rule, also of much importance, is the regular resting of the digestive system through fasting; remembering that in the wild state enforced fasts are entirely natural to a carnivorous diet, no flesh-eating animal being capable of killing prey with absolute regularity whenever hungry. A meat diet does accumulate toxins, and regular fasting is necessary to allow for their frequent expulsion from the digestive system. Every puppy from weaning up to four months of age should have a regular weekly half-day fast, and a monthly one day's fast. After four months of age more frequent fasting is necessary. Every adult over two years of age should be fasted regularly one day per week; such fasting is natural to the dog and is necessary for complete health.

Note Watered milk with honey is permitted during dietary fasting, and some raisins if the dog appears very hungry.

Natural Rearing Puppy Diet

Puppies reared according to the laws of Nature are always far superior in every way to stock incorrectly reared on the usual unnatural canine diets, and have been found to possess extra-ordinary resistance to all disease. Natural rearing gives excep-tionally strong bone, dense body hair, heavy muscle in place of fat, and always sound nerves. The usual puppy ailments do not occur when natural rearing is strictly followed. The four main rules of natural rearing are: Correct natural diet of raw foods. Abundant sunlight and fresh air. Abundant free running exercise. Hygienic kenneling with use of earth and grass runs to give contact with the vital radiations of the earth: no concrete runs to be used. Of course, house-sharing with owners is happiest for all dogs.

NATURAL REARING DIET (FROM WEANING TO FOUR MONTHS) (For average-size breed puppy, such as the working sheep-dog. For big breeds and terrier breeds increase or decrease accordingly.) No puppy should be given other than milk foods until nearly four weeks of age.

8 a.m. Fluid meal of raw milk (cow or goat), not dried and if possible not pasteurized milk, strengthened with honey and preparations of powdered slippery elm bark (such as N.R. Tree-barks Gruel, obtainable from Larkhall Natural Health; for address, see p. 448). Some raisins are helpful.

Midday Whole-grain, flaked wheat, barley, oats or rye, soaked in cold milk (sour milk is excellent for this); a teaspoonful of flaked fat – such as butter, or a little corn- or sunflower-oil, less than half a teaspoon. Avoid margarine of any kind. It is of hydrolysed fats and extremely indigestible; it can kill dogs. Alternatively the cereal flakes can be soaked in cabbage- or nettle water. Barley being the most digestible of the cereals should be used first for weaning. A perfect cereal for growing puppies is two parts barley flakes to one part oat flakes (such as sold in packets for porridge making), or N.R. four cereals flakes – oats, barley, rye, maize, with dried herbs and vegetables added.

Note Many brands have the bran removed; in such cases it

must be replaced, a small sprinkle per feed, approximately one teaspoonful, all soaked in fresh cold milk. With this meal two or three slices of stale whole-wheat bread should be given.

4 p.m. Meat – approximately two ounces raw, shredded cow or horse flesh, or breast of mutton – the mutton bones of big size – may be given. Meat should never be minced as the powerful stomach muscles must be used for meat digestion. After ten weeks of age, meat should be given in pieces about the size of a teaspoon, increasing in size to about two teaspoons by the age of four months, and to amount, approximately, to four ounces per meal.

8 p.m. (Main meal) Meat – approximately four ounces (as above) to strengthen nerves, plus a sprinkle of bran for roughage. Add one heaped teaspoon of raw green leaves, such as parsley, mints, cresses, chives, dandelion, chickweed, radish, goose-grass (cleavers), and celery leaves. The leaves must be finely minced or chopped, to resemble the form they would be fed compared with the prey which dogs kill. Fine form is essential as dogs digest cellulose with difficulty. Greens can also be mixed into cereals. Give a sprinkle of powdered seaweed. Give raw bones with every meat meal. Flesh without bones is unnatural. *Never* feed pig flesh or bones. The pig is a carrier of canine (and human) dangerous tapeworm.

Allow plenty of drinking water, during weaning included (important). Do not use plastic or aluminium water bowls: shade water from sunlight. Do not prevent puppies from eating earth or eating excreta from any grass-fed animal – horse, cow, sheep, etc. – because such contains trace elements, minerals and some natural penicillin, and most puppies crave earth and herbs.

Diet from four to eight or nine months   After four months, omit 8 a.m. feed, and give only three meals daily – 12 noon, 4 and 8 p.m. By now the cereals allowance should have been increased to around three ounces and the meat to eight ounces. The *vital* (essential for whole health) *raw* greens should have been increased to one dessertspoonful. After eight or nine months, meals should be reduced to two: cereal midday, meat evenings. Remember of course to give the usual supplements such as raw chopped greens, seaweed, etc.

Note   Every puppy from weaning onwards should rest and cleanse its internal organs frequently by fasts on plain water only. A puppy should never be coaxed to eat. If food is not eaten up rapidly the puppy should be fasted for twenty-four hours. Large quantities of plain milk should not be given, but should be fortified with honey, treacle or thickened with cereals; this overcomes the tendency to create mucus.

The diet given here is for exhibition stock and can be simplified for everyday use. Also it is only for average-sized young stock doing average work. Older working puppies will require larger rations.

An important note.   The border collie, and most sheep-dog breeds, can manage with far less meat than advised on this diet; they can even work well on a meatless diet provided that their food remains natural, raw, and that all cereals are whole-grain. However, raw bones should be given. They are vital to carnivores for calcium and worms removal.

Some final dietary information. It may be claimed that foods other than meat are unnatural for carnivores and felines. Not at all! For example, it is told in the Bible that 'the little foxes rob the grapes'.

When such animals kill prey, their first choice is the stomach and intestines filled with grains, vegetables, fruits. All dogs enjoy fruits, especially dried ones. In Spain, I have seen dogs getting dried figs as a basic meal; in Tunisia, I noted that a basic diet of the Saluki hounds was dates. All dogs enjoy raisins, also dried bananas. As for nuts, all are enjoyed and are healthful.

As I pioneered seaweed for dogs (knowing they would get this from the intestines of animals) and honey, for well and sick animals of all kinds (both now in worldwide use for such), I now pioneer grated (powdered) *almonds* for dogs and cats (and children). This is a most powerful immunizer for all disease, better than vaccination. Fortifies the immune system. Learnt from Berber Arabs. Average amount: a heaped teaspoon most days of the week, sprinkled on food.

Diet for the Adult Dog

Midday 100 per cent flaked, whole-grain oats, corn, rye, barley, uncooked, softened with either raw or sour milk or vegetable juice. Corn puffs are much liked.

Whole-wheat, rye or corn bread or biscuits of same, also roasted whole maize flour, can be added to this meal. Raw eggs can be mixed into the cereal approximately four times per week. Likewise, some corn, olive, or sunflower oil, one teaspoonful.

Note Adult dogs should not be fed before midday because the hours from midnight to midday are strongly eliminative ones. In-between-meal scraps are harmful. Only dogs of the lighter greyhound breeds with small stomach capacity want a light morning meal of milk, cereals and dried fruits.

Evening (Main meal) Meat, raw in large pieces, never minced. Frozen meat is as harmful as cooked meat. A small quantity of fat should be included, plus one teaspoon wheat-germ flakes, one teaspoon cod-liver oil (winter), seaweed powder, and one heaped dessertspoon very finely chopped raw green herb, such as parsley, watercress, dandelion. The inclusion of the herb is important. Grated raw carrot can be added, and several dessertspoons of bran or flaked oats to replace lost roughage of the skin and hair.

When bones are given, they should be raw and fed after the meat. They should not be given on an empty stomach.

In-whelp bitches, nursing bitches, and invalid adults, are permitted an early morning meal of milk and honey which means they will be getting three meals a day. But do not overfeed; large pups would make birthing difficult.

Big, ample meals need to be given when the dam is giving her milk to her puppies.

All carnivorous animals need meatless days each week, four days or less on meat, and one day on fluids only.

No wild dog would be able to kill prey every day of every week. Appreciating this fact most of the zoos of the world fast the carnivores – lions, tigers, wolves – one day per week.

For the Natural Rearing diet it is recommended there be several meatless days each week, using instead milk, cheese (white), eggs, with cereal. One fast day should follow this, giving fluids only and a laxative the same night, also herbal antiseptic pills such as N.R. Herbal Compound, in the morning. This simple nature treatment wards off disease toxins, rests the digestive system and kidneys, always hard-worked on a meat diet.

Hungry dogs can be given a little honey in their water at meal times, or very watery diluted milk, or water from flaked oats or barley obtained by pouring hot water over the flakes and soaking overnight, or even a few slices of stale bread with some raisins.

Flaked cereals As their value is now appreciated, they are easy to obtain from local health food shops everywhere. Feed them raw, merely soaked in water or milk.

Fat of meat is baneful to the domestic dog and cat. Much fat is unnatural food. The wild prey which canines and felines killed when they lived free is never fat. Butcher's meat, especially if it is from animals raised by cruel intensive farming methods, is usually over-fat. Cut and throw away most of that fat! It is wasteful not to do so. *It is costly* to pay veterinary fees for treating dogs with disease of liver, pancreas and kidneys caused by over-much fat in their diet.

When eggs are given they should be fed raw with the meat. Large marrow-bones should be provided frequently. Paunches can be given with the meat. Offal such as liver, kidneys, should not be given. It is advisable to scald paunches well to kill worm eggs and cysts. Raw chicken legs and heads, well washed and carefully trimmed of their claws or beaks, are calcium rich and much enjoyed by dogs of all breeds, including the toy breeds. Washing is essential owing to the use of chemicals in modern poultry places.

Note on Meat   In hot weather raw meat can be preserved in salt water; or by burying in the ground, slabs of stone preventing contact of the meat with the soil; or by wrapping in a cloth well soaked in vinegar and water (two tablespoonfuls vinegar to one cupful water), some of which can be patted into the meat itself and is a harmless preservative. When preserving meat in hot weather I always bind around it strong-smelling herbs such as sage, rosemary and thyme. Big leaves of geranium and mallow are also excellent. Green leaves give coolness.

Stonehenge, in his book, *The Dog: in Health and Disease*, states that he has kept raw meat good for six weeks during the height of summer, merely by brushing the meat over with quicklime wash, and hanging it beneath a thick covering of tree foliage in ample shade. *Never* give canned meats. They are lifeless food and will clog the digestive system. As fat as they are cheap, they generally contain too much fat and sometimes really filthy by-products. All contain chemical preservatives, which are totally forbidden for the nature dog. Another harmful aspect of these meats is that they are usually highly spiced to induce over-eating.

Meat and the Sheep-dog   The dog is a carnivore by inclination and anatomy. The powerful dentition, including the tearing canine teeth, the small muscular stomach and short powerful intestines, are all suited only to a basically carnivorous diet. The dog can be kept in health on an entirely meatless diet, but it is far more difficult to keep a balanced diet that way, also, with cereal so costly nowadays, it is less economical. Trouble should be taken to contact a knacker and arrange for regular supplies for the dogs.

However, there is the age-old belief that meat feeding, especially raw-meat feeding, makes dogs savage and causes them to indulge in sheep-worrying. Now on countless occasions on my moorland wanderings in search of herbs, I have met with sheep-dogs away from the farms gorging themselves upon the rotten carcasses of sheep which have died of exposure in the winter months or as a result of a rock fall. Those dogs were not killers. They had not killed. They were merely eating carrion as their ancestors had eaten through countless generations of the canine race. Nor did those dogs return to their farms and begin worrying other sheep to provide for themselves further flesh diet. Training and instinct together, were sufficient to enable the dog to resist such temptation. I have met with killer sheep-dogs, and it is my opinion that most of them were cases of deranged nerves. Afghans, the breed of dog that I keep, are notorious by nature, and can pull down a cow with ease: all of them were fed with raw meat, and those which I trained to be able to give them their freedom in the countryside never killed livestock; a few of them were unreliable with poultry. It is a matter of training more than of diet; and the healthy dog possessing strong nerves and a well-developed brain, is far easier to train than the health-degenerate animal, product of a deficient diet. The Arab shepherds habitually feed the bodies of diseased stock to their dogs, and sheep-worrying is rare among them. In many farming books, including English ones, when writing about sheep-dogs, the fact is clearly stated that dogs are flesheaters, and that some meat should be given in the canine diet.

The sheep-dog, because of the stocky build and quite ample stomach capacity, *can* manage on a vegetarian diet, where dogs of the greyhound breeds almost cannot manage. Many types of dog are vegetarian from necessity. Even the carnivore wolf will eat tree barks and roots when prey for meat is scarce. However, if farmers refuse to give any meat to their sheep-dogs, then at least let them provide other raw protein. Raw eggs, oatmeal porridge, fish-meal, raw herrings occasionally, and some daily supply of fat. The Scottish mountain sheep-dog puppies reared on oatmeal porridge and raw milk are the best boned collie puppies that I have seen. On a cereal diet far larger quantities of food must be fed to the working adult dogs than the average half to one pound of raw meat daily and the balancing cereal, to satisfy the animal's appetite following hard field work. Twice the quantity of cereal must be fed to replace the meat. On the hill farms of the Pennine mountains where I have lived for several years, the basic diet for the collie dog is flaked whole-maize meal, soaked in hot water for several hours, and then mixed with household table scraps. New (i.e. fresh, whole) milk is also fed daily, and an occasional rabbit. The dogs themselves take new-laid eggs from the hedgerows, and help themselves to calf and poultry meal raw from the meal bins. The dogs also themselves find and eat raw sheep carcasses.

The dogs do well on this diet, which would prove over-heating were they not getting the daily hard work of sheep-herding. Raw bones are needed for jaw exercise and for tooth development; they provide immediate calcium and are necessary for roughage, and if dogs are deprived usually they will seek out their own supplies from neighbouring sources.

The healthy dog has a very small appetite in comparison with the unhealthy. That fact has been well proved. Less than two pounds of food, apart from milk, will satisfy the average working collie, providing that food is natural and wholesome.

I have written at length on the subject of canine diet, because it is a much more complicated matter than that of the food of the herbivorous animals or the free-ranging and grain-eating poultry. That the present-day diet of the average sheep-dog is faulty is well proved by the increasing ailments, fits, hysteria, diseases of the skin and worm infestation. The Merioneth (Gwynedd) farmer has only called attention to a matter which has been occupying the minds of the veterinary world for many years (see p. 371).

Internal Cleansing Treatment   The dog in disease must be subjected to the cleansing fast exactly as with the other animals, only the dog being a carnivore with a very simple internal anatomy can be given safely and beneficially far longer cleansing fasts than the herbivorous animals. The longest fast to which I subjected a dog was three weeks, on a diet of honey and water only; the case was a Dachshund with pneumonia complications and had been condemned as incurable by orthodox medicine. Following the fast he fully recovered. The main reason for fasting the dog is the presence of fever. There is a basic rule in the treatment of the sick dog: under no circumstances must solid food be given while fever is present. Nervous derangement or merely habit-hunger will often induce the dog in fever to eat proffered food, the results are nearly always severe complications of the nervous system often ending in death. In sickness the dog's temperature should be taken daily. If more than one or two degrees above the normal of 101.4°, the fast should be maintained. Meals of plain water should be given, or honey water: one heaped teaspoonful of pure honey to every cupful of water. *Note.* Quantities of herbs and foods given, are for an average-sized dog – border collie size. Decrease or increase amounts according to size of dog being treated. Honey is the most powerful restorative for dogs. It is the only known heart stimulant which is not a drug. Its beneficial and feeding properties are immense. It is a pity that such a wonderful life-saving substance is too costly to give sufficient to the larger animals, cattle, etc. when in sickness. Garlic provides an internal disinfectant, and should be given throughout the fast. Give this garlic either in the form of raw cloves, four to six small cloves make an average dose, or mashed to a pulp to aid their absorption, or one to two N.R. garlic-rue tablets night and morning. While an animal is fasting, a daily purge is needed; senna is advised. For an average-sized border collie, use four pods (Alexandrian) senna, one teaspoon of cold water to every pod and add a pinch of ginger. Soak for seven hours, then squeeze all moisture from the pods. If a little honey is added, dogs will drink the senna and not have to be dosed from a bottle. Break the fast when the temperature is normal, with a milk and honey diet for several days. Three meals of half a pint or less of whole raw milk, slightly warmed, with one dessertspoonful honey stirred in. Then bring the dog back to solid foods by thickening the milk and honey with flaked barley, and adding protein. The first protein feed is to be steamed fish, followed after two days by a small amount of raw meat. Whole-grain cereal meals, wheat and oats, can then supplement the barley; also stale wheaten bread can be given. This is the perfect diet for the treatment of the dog in disease; and it has stood the test of over forty years. Such a diet has saved the lives of thousands of sick dogs of all breeds, including many sheep- and cattle-dogs in Europe and other parts of the world. The diet is very simple; the accepted invalid foods have no part in it, eggs, meat broths, strong alcohol such as brandy; all are fermentative in the system, all should be avoided. Likewise yeast, except in bread-making, should be avoided in canine diet, when well or in sickness. It is highly fermentative in the system of carnivorous animals, and only has a place in the baking of whole-wheat bread in the ordinary way.

During the convalescent diet if there should be any form of relapse, especially return of the fever, then a short fast should be used again. In a very prolonged fever, when the dog begins to look very emaciated, then a mixture of honey and milk, also fresh-pressed grape or apple juice or sweet red wine, are all permitted.

Canine Diseases

The diseases which afflict the modern dog are manifold and so varied that mighty tomes have been written upon them. One has only to consult a comprehensive volume of canine disease, such as that written by Muller and Glass, to see what man has done for the health of the dog in his ignorance and his misunderstanding of the laws of natural rearing. In this sheep-dog section I am only giving the common ailments, such as one invariably finds listed in other books on farm stock, when sheep-dogs are included.

Many of the treatments given for sheep and goats can be applied equally well in canine ailments, and are indeed basic-ally the same.

I must, however, include the sad fact that, just as most

breeds have their specific hereditary ailments, so has the most famed of the sheep-dog breeds, the border collie. It is an ailment of modern times only, unheard of in the breed's past history.

EYE DISORDER, RETINAL ATROPHY The eyes become cloudy and dim-looking, the dog shakes its head and paws at its eyes. If the ailment is not checked quickly, blindness follows and, of course, the case can no longer work the sheep. Cure is not easy. *Prevention* is the best remedy, by a return to a natural diet. I have proved this, having checked blindness of this form by advising the N.R. diet and treatment of the eyes with the proved benevolent herbs. Although the ailment is said to be hereditary, I have proved that pups born to bitches with retinal atrophy, when the bitch has been put on to a proper whole-foods raw diet, have normal sight. For actual treatment of the eyes, see blindness in Sheep.

The keen-sighted eyes of the border collie are a gift from God, making this dog such a great help to mankind in the management of sheep flocks. Must man in his folly destroy this? Must he condemn this breed to blindness? Must they be lost then for ever, they of the beautiful traditional names which I have so often heard called over the moorlands of Yorkshire and Wales: Ben, Roy, Timothy, Meg, Moss, Fern, Bell, Ling, Lark, Linnet and many more?

DISTEMPER This ailment is known as the canine plague. It is the commonest disease which attacks the dog and is the cause of hundreds of deaths annually. And yet correctly treated by natural methods it is one of the most simple diseases to cure. Distemper inoculation has been much boosted, much used, and has proved a failure. All inoculative treatments are indeed proved failures, only kept alive at all by misleading statistics, which on paper make impressive reading, but which in true fact are failures.

A very large percentage of distemper cases sent to me for treatment in the years when I was specializing in that disease, were inoculated animals and invariably they had the disease in a far more complicated form than un-inoculated stock. My findings in this respect have been fully supported by other people treating sick animals.

In Israel, where veterinary treatment of animals is often very practical and sensible, I am interested to find that general veterinary opinion is opposed to canine distemper inoculation, it being considered that no sure vaccine has been found, and that distemper vaccination often brings disease to healthy dogs. Many veterinarians in Switzerland also uphold this opinion. Human cholera vaccination is also not advised in Israel.

Canine distemper is classified as a virus disease, and yet so far – as with foot-and-mouth disease – no specific virus has been isolated. The disease attacks the mucous membranes primarily. It is also supposed to attack the nervous system, but the nervous complications which afflict the canine distemper case are never a primary symptom of the ailment. They are always resultant from wrongful treatment, above all the feeding of solid foods to the dog when fever is present, or the suppression of the fever symptom with sera or chemical drugs – especially those of the sulphonamide group, which are lethal in the effect upon the canine species.

Symptoms Loss of appetite, cough, slight discharge from the eyes, followed in a few days generally by copious eye and nose discharge. The mouth becomes fetid, the eyes very bloodshot, and diarrhoea is often present. High fever develops.

Treatment The dog must be placed immediately on the

internal cleansing fast, already described in detail, kept quiet in a warm room with a window sufficiently open to provide change of air, or confined in an outhouse and given a deep hay bed. Twice daily garlic dosage, or N.R. garlic and rue tablets. The mouth and teeth should be cleansed with slightly diluted raw lemon juice – it is advantageous if the dog swallows some of the lemon juice. The eyes and nose should be cleansed with a little cold Indian tea, or brew of chickweed or mallow or balm herbs. No solid food whatsoever must be given until the fever is ended and temperature has been normal for several days. Honey-water may be given. If the dog will not take the honey-water, then balls of thick honey can be pressed down the dog's throat three times daily. Pure grape juice is permitted. When the fever is very prolonged – over ten days– some milk can be given three times daily. When the fever is over, the dog can be fed according to the daily instructions given in the internal cleansing treatment. If nervous complications should develop, treat as for hysteria (p. 396). This applies also to chorea.

HARD PAD (Canine encephalitis)   This is an allied ailment of distemper, and is sometimes known as brain distemper. Until the 1940s the disease was very rare, but has become increasingly common, doubtless due to the acceleration of canine health degeneration, resultant from wartime and post-war poor diet and general neglect, also to the growing preservation and adulteration of the foods fed to dogs, all of which starve the nerves of their essential nutriment. However, a very large percentage of cases classified as hard pad are purely common distemper. When dogs inoculated against distemper develop this very disease as they have commonly done since the commencement of distemper inoculative therapy, then it is policy for the owners to be told that the illness is not distemper at all but hard pad; likewise when dogs afflicted by distemper and treated with injections of sera, succumb to the disease, the owners are informed that the sera failed because the disease was not distemper but hard pad. Those are only the natural politics of all modern medicine, always excuses to cover the constant failures of inoculations no matter for what ailments they are employed. No animal of mine has ever yet been subjected to the harm of inoculations, and doubtless that is one of the basic reasons for consistent immunity to disease and outstanding health enjoyed by them.

Symptoms Much the same as for distemper, but mucus discharge is usually absent. A common and rather typical symptom of hard pad is an excessively moist nose. There is staring coat, ear flaps very hot, and the entire body is feverish. High temperature develops, and usually diarrhoea. It was always much later, and sometimes not at all, that the foot pads, and in some cases the nostril pads, thicken and become leathery, and finally harden and become almost without feeling, so that the dog walks 'as if on hot bricks'. With that stage are found the brain symptoms, staggering gait, and the animal emitting a constant whimpering which cannot be suppressed by command, and often ends in raging madness similar to pure meningitis.

Treatment The same as for distemper; the fast especially must be strictly followed, heavy and rich feeding being fatal in this ailment. For treatment of the nervous ailments a brew of skullcap should be given, one handful of the herb brewed in half a pint of water. Give a dose of two tablespoonfuls of the skullcap brew three times daily. The same treatment should be applied in other nervous complications such as fits and chorea.

If paralysis (see Sheep) develops, give also a course of N.R. Herbal Compound tablets. No suppressive chemical drugs such as bromide, luminol, and others should ever be used. Externally: the footpads, and nostrils, if affected, should be bathed with a strong brew of potato peelings.

PARVO-VIRUS (see also GASTRITIS) This is a gastro-intestinal virus disease which especially affects young dogs, though dogs of all ages may develop it. Veterinarians describe it as the most formidable disease which has come upon the canine race in the last twenty years. Personally, I consider parvo-virus to be the worst canine ailment of all time. The once-dreaded canine distemper disease is readily curable, as is hard pad, a disease linked with distemper. The peculiarity and the danger of parvo are that it can infect a contact within a day, even within a half day.

This disease became known as an epidemic in 1980 and it is to be found world wide. America, Europe, the Middle East – all report it and the casualties are hundreds of young dogs in each of the countries affected. Some veterinarians try and link parvo-virus with feline infectious enteritis because this ailment, panleucopaenia, is similar, and because they want to use on dogs the same vaccine which they use for cats. I am not going into the merits or otherwise of any of the parvo vaccinations as I never use vaccine or therapy for my own dogs. I advise all who believe in the natural rearing of animals to avoid vaccination as this totally unnatural treatment is linked by many observant persons (I also share their opinions) with the fact that vaccination can well be a root cause of cancer and diabetes, formerly unknown in the canine world and now, sadly, commonplace. The list of veterinary recommended vaccinations grows alarmingly. Once it was merely canine distemper vaccination; now we are advised vaccination for hepatitis/leptospirosis, streptococcal infection, and parvo-virus, plus suggested booster vaccinations every six months for all those ailments.

If all that vaccination money were to be spent on the provision of good, natural foods, from whole-grain cereal products to fresh, *raw* meat, the terrible health decline seen among modern dogs, including the border collie, would be halted. There is one protection against all canine ailments, new and old, and that is *good health*. My own Afghan hounds have been exposed to every known canine ailment, including rabies and parvo, and have remained immune and will continue to remain immune. I met parvo in Greece, saw many pups die from it, but the few who were on true N.R. rearing either never took the ailment or took it only so mildly that they recovered fully with no after-effects such as heart damage or sterility. I can truly state that I have not heard of any death from parvo from those thousands world wide who follow N.R. for their dogs. Some N.R. kennels had the disease mildly and an extract from one kennel report is at the end of this section.

Symptoms Parvo-virus takes two distinct forms, but it is a linked ailment because dogs on the same premises, at the same time, can be infected by one or other of the forms. The first form is cardiac and only attacks young pups, the most general time being immediately after weaning, from six to nine weeks, but can be extended to six months of age. The muscles of the heart are affected rapidly and acutely, and the pups collapse and die from heart failure. The other, more prevalent form, is a gastro-enteritis disease, also very rapid in its development. The details differ: many cases vomit and excrete much blood, others have only a foul-smelling, very liquid diarrhoea. But in all cases there is a morbid interest in water (as found in rabies); the cases want to drink, but seem to fear the water. When they do drink they vomit it back again very quickly. Usually there is high fever, around or above 104°, but fever may be absent. There is rapid and alarming dehydration, within very short time much flesh is lost, especially of the head area, the coat stares and the limbs weaken. Another typical symptom, again similar to rabies, is the changed look of the eyes: they take on a glazed and squinting expression, which can only be described as sinister and abnormal.

Treatment   This must be quick! Immediate, as with cases of poisoning and this, strangely, is the treatment which should be followed. Treat as one does with poison, and urgently, or death will rapidly result.

Here you have a truly deadly virus. Get rid of it at once and sweep it out of the body in which it has taken hold. The first cases of parvo I ever treated were in three Afghan pups. I did not know parvo-virus then and I suspected poison from the sudden unexplained vomiting and acute diarrhoea, much abdominal pain, and urge to drink but vomiting up of the fluid taken, and the glazed eyes.

It was a case of an immediate large dose of castor oil, to be followed by senna pods, which take seven hours to prepare in cold water infusion. That hasty treatment is to clean out the intestinal tract. Dehydration must then be checked by two-hourly liquid feeds of a mixture of honey, glucose and common salt, in barky-water solution, or alternating with the same in milk whey solution if available. I never advise force-feeding of any sick animal – fasting is nature's way of treating all disease – but in such a violent infection as this one the dehydration must be halted or the case will die. And the liquid being given is medicinal more than food.

A recent BBC programme, 'Science in Action', discussing infant diarrhoea, disclosed that modern medical policy had been reversed to follow a lead from Third World countries. There, where diarrhoea is so prevalent, it is not checked by drugs or clay products but allowed to run its course and dehydration prevented by the oral feeding of glucose and salt in water. Another programme reported that in Third World countries where parents could rarely manage to obtain vascular treatment from doctors for the control of dehydration in infants, oral treatment was the replacement – in water solution, salt and glucose to replace drainage of natural salts and minerals. I have added honey as it is an internal antiseptic and soothing medicament, as well as giving immediate help to the brain and the heart. (Again it must be stressed, especially in such a death-fighting treatment as this one, that the honey used should be pure, natural honey and not from bees fed white sugar to double their honey output, whose product is a substance not from vital nectar of flowers and fruits but one which is almost worthless.) In place of plain water, use fresh-made, not bottled barley water. Also essential is internal disinfection with the most vital of the ancient 'plague' herbs, advised throughout this book – wormwood, garlic, rue, sage – given in pill form or in home-made balls of flour and honey binding the herbs, to be pushed down the throat as they are very bitter. Also vital to the healing of the stomach and intestinal tract is a gruel which contains such soothing and strengthening ingredients as slippery elm bark, arrowroot, marshmallow root, corn flour, barley flour, in a solution of milk fortified with honey. For further soothing, the two herbs Luisa (lemon verbena) and southernwood, made into a tea: one tablespoon Luisa, one teaspoon southernwood to a large cup of water. Give by mouth, sweetened with honey.

Here is a parvo-virus report. I've given few reports in this book; there is no space for them and they would make the book too highly priced, but parvo is of such international interest I have made this one of the few exceptions.

From Mrs Christine Macdonald, 120 Meldon Court, Ryton, Tyne and Wear, England:

I must say firstly that I have never seen my lovely dogs, golden retrievers, in such superb health, and only since becoming strictly N.R.! Parvo-virus has been rife in this area (Newcastle). The vets were almost begging all dog owners to have the inoculation against parvo done, although reports were flooding in that it did not work. They were powerless to do anything and hundreds of dogs up to the age of three died in this area, pups under three months being worst hit.

My friend, who breeds German shepherds, and myself kept strictly to N. R. methods, refusing to consider inoculation, and while other dog owners kept their stock indoors to avoid contact with the disease (impossible as far as we could tell) we continued to give our dogs as much exercise as they were used to in order to maintain their high state of health.

As soon as our dogs showed symptoms we fasted them and used the Herbal Compound tablets and cayenne pepper, and castor oil and then gruel (tree bark, roots, etc.) and liquid diet. We took the most drastic action we could (I had not yet heard from you with parvo advice) – we went out to drastically improve their health and resistance as *quickly* as possible. My friend's dogs were worse than mine, with profuse bleeding in stools and dehydration, and the glazed and bloodshot eyes peculiarity. She had two pups, four months (second generation N.R.), one dog, eighteen months (second generation N.R.), two bitches, one five, the other seven years.

My own parvo cases, thanks to strict N.R., were very mild. One bitch pup of eight months, two young adults, one in whelp (recently mated). Diarrhoea was not too violent, but temperatures were high, and again typical parvo eyes symptom, glazed look and bloodshot. All my dogs recovered within four days, and with improved health and vitality.

[Later report:] The in-whelp bitch who had parvo had a beautiful litter of eight pups, all healthy and strong, and a credit to me and to my N.R. bitch, and to N.R. rearing in general.

HYSTERIA   This is quite a common ailment of farm dogs. It is caused by prolonged nerve starvation through an ill-balanced diet, especially the giving of white flour cereals in place of whole grain: and lack of sufficient protein. The flour preservative *agene*, used in modern baking, is a potent cause of hysteria. It is more general in the summer when the overheating of the system causes excessive irritation of the weakly nervous system.

Symptoms   Unmistakable. The dog sets up a frantic howling, and usually begins a mad running, generally bolting for some dark place where it cowers trembling in a corner. Urine and faeces are often voided involuntarily, as with fits.

Treatment   Internal cleansing. A fast of at least two days is indicated. Dosage with garlic and skullcap. Bathing the head with cold brew of dock leaves or wild poppy seed heads. A daily tablespoonful of black currant *purée* or rose hip syrup, have a beneficial nerve-soothing effect in hysteria cases. So has a strong brew of rosemary and poppyheads (two tablespoons finely cut rosemary and a half dozen poppy seed heads, to a half pint of water) give two tablespoons three times daily. (See also Valerian, p. 157.)

PARALYSIS   (see Sheep)

PNEUMONIA   This is often found as an after-effect of wrongly treated canine distemper, although the dog from severe chilling may develop the disease apart from any other infection. Correctly treated in its early stages it is readily curable. The same treatment is used for the other chest disorders, bronchitis and pleurisy.

Symptoms Fever, staring coat, disinclination to eat. The breathing is very painful and laboured, the dog usually keeps in a sitting position, head hanging, mouth kept closed with much puffing of the lips, panting lungs. Sometimes there is mucus discharge from eyes and nose. As the fever increases the eyes become very congested. Fever may reach 107°.

Treatment Fasting, with intestinal cleansing. The use of garlic, brew or tablets, three times daily: garlic is used not only to cleanse and disinfect the bloodstream and intestines, but also to expel the bacteria from the lungs themselves. Honey should be given generously throughout the treatment, to maintain energy without burdening the digestive system, and for the succouring of the heart, which bears much strain in pneumonia. Inhalations of eucalyptus oil or camphor oil, given in hot water, are also helpful. The dog can also be given eucalyptus internally, two to four drops poured on to a lump of sugar, given not more than twice daily. Vicks Vapo-rub, with its excellent herbal formula, provides much help, rubbed along the muzzle, throat and chest, three times daily. If the case is very severe the dog can be given a flannel jacket, or blanket jacket, with two holes cut in front through which to pass the fore-feet, the jacket then being fastened down the back with stout safety-pins. For extra comfort the jacket can be lined with Thermogene wool over the chest area. The dog must be able to get abundant fresh air through an open window. Keep the dog warmly wrapped but let its panting lungs get fresh air. The curtailment of air is one of the chief errors in pneumonia treatment. (For further advice concerning pneumonia treatment, see this ailment in the chapter on Horses.)

DIARRHOEA   This is usually a symptom of some other complaint, not in itself a separate ailment. Gastritis is a common cause of diarrhoea, brought on by over-eating or prolonged incorrect diet. Or the condition may be caused through worm infestations, especially wire or round worms massed in the stomach or intestines. Also it may be a symptom of distemper, when it is usually then found in acute form. Diarrhoea correctly treated, is not a difficult or prolonged complaint, and is often actually beneficial to the dog, insomuch as it serves Nature's method of removing toxic matter from the body in the shortest possible time. This diarrhoea should always be allowed to run its natural course, and should not be checked by unnatural means. Only if very prolonged should attempt be made to slow down the bowel evacuation by the use of healing and soothing, such as fresh bilberries, fresh (raw) apple purée, raisins, milk and honey diluted with barley-water, and the use of the very healing N.R. Gruel. That is where herbal treatment differs from orthodox; the latter immediately aiming at suppression of the bowel discharge, using such aids as opiates for drugging the intestinal nerves, or blocking the bowel tract with chalk preparations, or by the feeding of very starchy substances such as refined arrowroot, rice, cornflour, and further the suppression of water drinking. The unnatural treatments merely leave the bowels in a half-cleansed state, and thus produce perfect breeding conditions for the multiplication of worms and harmful bacteria. I advocate the opposite treatment; the encouragement of the bowel discharge by the use of aperient mineral waters, herbal laxatives, and also encouraging the dog to drink much water: cleansing enemas are also given if necessary, one quart of warm water being sufficient in the enema for a medium-sized dog. Such cleansing treatment is maintained until the bowel flow loses its putrid odour and assumes a natural colour.

Enema Add one tablespoon lemon juice to every quart of water, as an antiseptic. If there is evidence of pain during the illness, give doses of sage and wild poppyheads tea, with honey. Two tablespoons of the mixed herbs to one glass of water.

Symptoms Very loose faeces of a foamy nature, and quite liquid. The dog acquires an unpleasant smell, fever may be present or the temperature fall to subnormal. The dog refuses food and shows an abnormal craving for water.

Treatment Internal cleansing, continuing the fast until the bowel flow loses its toxic character. Plenty of garlic should be given, and brews of the aromatic herbs such as sage, thyme, marjoram. One tablespoonful of herb brewed in half-pint of water, two tablespoonful doses given twice daily; honey should be added. A daily laxative must be given, such as senna (see Senna, Materia Medica), or a tablespoon dose of syrup of figs (preferably Californian brand). Give two charcoal tablets, morning and night. Honey should be given daily as both food and healing agent, average amount two tablespoonfuls total throughout the day. When the bowel flow has normalized, the intestines can be healed and strengthened with slippery elm bark powder, which acts as an internal poultice, or N.R. Gruel with its base of pure slippery elm improved by other healing and nutritious tree barks and herbs.

The first solid food given should be flaked barley. Then follow carefully the feeding directions Internal Cleansing (see after Diets).

GASTRITIS This can prove to be a very serious complaint in the dog, especially when of the fine breed lurcher type such as kept on many farms. If the ailment is not treated promptly and carefully, the dog can die very quickly.

Long-term incorrect feeding – especially the feeding of hot food, a common error in the feeding of sheep-dogs – is a frequent cause of gastritis; also foreign causes, such as eating of sharp objects, such as glass, mixed in food taken from refuse bins, the presence of masses of worms in the digestive tract, or the eating of poison. (See Poisoning.)

Symptoms The dog vomits unceasingly, bile and white frothy fluid. Floods of orange-coloured diarrhoea sweep from the bowels. The dog is incapable of controlling its bowels. The breath is fetid, and the temperature is usually subnormal.

Treatment As for Diarrhoea. Additional treatment should be a brew of parsley leaves, made as follows. Half a cupful of finely chopped parsley mixed into half a pint of cold water and brought to the boil, simmered for two minutes. Add one dessertspoonful honey to the brew. A very long fast is often necessary. When the fast has ended use should be made of steamed parsley roots, well minced and fed with the cereal feeds of flaked barley. Use should also be made of slippery elm bark, as instructed in the diarrhoea treatment. A brew of fennel is also excellent. The dog should be allowed as much cool water as it desires, water being kept available both night and day. This provision of water is very contrary to orthodox treatment which forbids water in gastritis. The mouth of the dog should be kept free of fetid matter by twice-daily bathing with diluted lemon juice, one teaspoonful of juice mixed with two dessertspoonfuls tepid water. The gums and inner cheeks often become ulcerated in the acute form of gastritis: the lemon juice will assist healing, but it should be used in less amount.

POISONING   (see Goats)

INFECTIOUS SKIN AILMENTS: MANGE (see also Scab in Sheep)

MANGE   This is a severe parasitical disease which occurs in two forms, sarcoptic and follicular. It is quite common to the present day sheep-dog, due largely to the impure blood and unhealthy skin which arise from long-term devitalized diet.

Sarcoptic is the most common of the two forms and also more contagious than follicular, but fortunately it is the more readily curable. As mange attacks also the fox and the wolf, there is indication that it can be equally parasitical upon the quite healthy animal; therefore keep stock away from animals showing signs of mange skin disease.

Two kinds of mange parasites are small, louse-type mites, invisible to the naked eye. They burrow beneath the skin and increase with great rapidity. Cases of follicular mange often look as if they have been sprayed all over with gunshot, so numerous are the skin eruptions. The skin further turns elephant grey, hair falls and an unpleasant mousey smell becomes noticeable, death can result. Sarcoptic mange is unpleasant but less serious than follicular mange. It produces inflammation of the skin and intense irritation.

Treatment   This, understandably, should be external principally, but in order to effect a complete cure, the state of the dog's general health should be improved also, for the tough, vital skin of the dog in sound health offers more resistance to the mange parasites. It is usually the skin of sickly animals that is attacked. Some animal experts go so far as to say that mange can be cured entirely by corrective dieting and internal medicament. I consider that patient external treatment also is essential once the teeming parasites have established themselves in the skin tissues. Complete fumigation of collars, leads, grooming equipment, kennels and runs is essential.

Herewith are four effective cures for both forms of mange: all have been used widely with excellent results. All are non-chemical and do not contain grease, which I consider to be very detrimental in the treatment of parasitical skin ailments, for it protects the tiny parasites and also they feed on it.

Bathe the dog thoroughly before applying any of the following treatments, using both soap flakes and a bar of olive-oil soap (preferably). Repeat the bath once each week throughout treatment.

Herbal insect repellent alcohol lotion This is effective and entirely harmless. Indeed it is tonic to the skin and hair. Pour one half-pound weight herbal insecticide powder, such as my own N.R. products five herbs powder, or derris root powder or tobacco dust, into a glass flask big enough to hold two quarts (the big bottles sold with spring or purified water are suitable). Next, add two ounces of oil of eucalyptus and one quart of pure alcohol (or white beer can be used with very good results). Cork tightly to prevent the escape of the natural herbal oils released by the alcohol. Set this to steep for four days. Shake the contents well, morning and night. The lotion must now be filtered to prevent over-fermentation. Do this through a large funnel packed with cheesecloth or cotton. Have ready another large bottle capable of holding at least two gallons, or have two bottles capable of holding one gallon each. The alcohol can now be diluted with vinegar to a quantity of two gallons and yet retain its pungency sufficient to destroy the skin parasites. If there is any further fermentation later, it does not matter; it will increase the pungency of the lotion, and it is for external use, not internal.

Lemon peel lotion Save all used lemon halves and place them in a gallon container in the hot sunlight or pour hot water over the lemons. Let the lemon halves remain permanently in the water until they begin to turn mouldy, then remove and replace with fresh ones, squeezing out the old ones very well first. Do not throw away any of the old lemon water that then remains. Then add one part vinegar to every two parts lemon lotion. Rub the lemon-vinegar lotion well into all parts of the body. A little may be dropped into the ears. For a stronger lotion, add the juice of two lemons to every quart. (Keep the jar covered with a paper top – not greased paper.)

Garlic–elder lotion   Slice up three whole roots of garlic, consisting of about twenty cloves, and add to this two handfuls of finely cut elder leaves and stalks. Place in a pan with one quart of cold water, bring to a boil, and simmer slowly for half an hour. Keep covered throughout. Remove from heat. Do not strain. Allow to brew for at least seven hours, still keeping covered. The lotion is then ready for use. Soak large pieces of cotton wool or towelling in the brew and friction the entire body with this very well. Two or three tablespoons, dependent on size of the dog, can also be given internally, early morning and night.

Diet   There should be a short course of Internal Cleansing treatment (see, after Diet), and then careful following of the N.R. raw foods diet. I have also heard of good results, at least in sarcoptic mange, using Cooper's Kurmange bathing treatment.

ECZEMA   Is mainly Nature's method of ridding the body, especially the bloodstream, of accumulated toxins, collected in the body as a result of unnatural rearing methods. It is speedily curable by diet.

Symptoms   Inflamed and discharging areas of skin, especially prevalent down the back and around the base of the tail. The animal rubs itself against available hard objects, and its body seems very irritable. Discharging mattery areas form, and there is often loss of hair.

Treatment   A short course of internal cleansing. Followed by very laxative diet, giving very limited cereal and plenty of raw meat and finely shredded green herbs, especially watercress and brooklime. A brew of meadowsweet or nettle leaves is also excellent cleansing medicine. Two tablespoons twice daily. Externally, there should be application of a brew of blackberry leaves or tops. In very severe irritation, extract of witch hazel can be applied. All suppressive greasy ointments and calamine lotions should be avoided. Also of value, raw cucumber juice applied or elder blossom lotion.

CANKER   This may be caused through mucus discharge, as a cleansing effort of a toxic body, or a bacterial infection of the inner ear channels, or a form of mite which infests the ears.

Symptoms   The ears become very hot-feeling, emit a brown discharge, and unpleasant smell somewhat resembling that of follicular mange. The dog shakes its head unceasingly.

Treatment   Treat both ears always, even if only one is infected. Cleanse the ears with diluted witch hazel, half a teaspoonful of witch hazel to one tablespoon tepid water. This lotion is astringent and antiseptic. To heal the ears further a brew of horehound or rue should be used. One tablespoon of the finely-cut herb brew in one and half cups water. Stand for four hours, then strain and use tepid N.R. Insect Repellent (five antiseptic herbs) powder, made into a lotion; this is another proved cure.

EAR MITES   Treat as above, using horehound lotion. Add extra, two drops *only*, of oil of eucalyptus to every dessertspoon of the lotion. Eucalyptus oil is very burning (but very effective). If much discomfort is shown, pour a little fresh milk into the ear to neutralize the eucalyptus.

EYE ULCER and KERATITIS   When the eyes have become

infected by such complaints as keratitis (clouding of the eyes) and ulcers, temporary blindness often results. Also thorns pricking the eyes are often the cause of ulcers.

Treatment Internally garlic should be given, also daily one to two tablespoonfuls of carrot juice, obtained by pressing grated raw carrot through a square of butter-muslin. Externally make a brew of balm herb, bathe the eyes thrice daily, first removing all mucus deposits, external and internal, with a swab of cotton wool soaked in raw milk. Chickweed herb makes an excellent eye lotion, made the same way as the horehound, or a strong brew of quince seeds boiled for five minutes and brewed for three hours. Flaked valerian root, made into a lotion, can be added with benefit to any of the suggested eye herbs, as valerian soothes the eye nerves.

ABSCESS Found on any part of the body and commonly between the toes as interdigital cysts.

Treatment Internal cleansing treatment, using plenty of garlic. Hot fomentation with blackberry leaves brew or groundsel brew. Poulticing with bran is also excellent.

BLADDER DISORDERS (see Goats)

BROKEN LIMBS (see Sheep)

TUMOURS (see Cows)

WORMS Dogs are very frequently infected by worms. Worms are especially prevalent in animals getting a diet of cooked foods, which cause degeneration of the muscular tone of the stomach and intestines and also create mucus and other toxic deposits among which the worms can burrow and multiply. The two kinds of worm common in the dog are:

round worm, of which there are many species, and tapeworm, of which there are three common types. In many countries beyond Europe, there is also the hookworm and heartworms. Tapeworm in farm dogs is of danger to sheep, for segments of the worm, taken up when grazing grass where infected dogs have been, can encyst in the brain area of the sheep and cause the often fatal ailment, gid.

The ova of the worms enter the dog through the mouth, doing so from many sources: from infested ground (worm ova can lie dormant for years in the soil); from stagnant, or even from running water, to which other dogs or sheep or vermin – such as rabbits and rats – have access: from fleas which are carriers of a species of tapeworm: from worm-infected intestines of rabbits, cattle or poultry; or from the flesh of such animals when the worm is in the encysted state: and finally, in the case of puppies, taken in as ova from their mother's milk. It should be appreciated from the above details, that if such a minute creature as a flea can be a host for tapeworm, the larvae of the blow-fly and other meat- and carrion-eating flies may well be worm-carriers also, as may be the hairy legs of the flies themselves spreading the minute dried worm ova. Wild birds and also domestic poultry are often infected with worms, and their droppings, dried up to a dust-like consistency, and spread over grassland where dogs exercise, can form a very likely source of worms in dogs and other livestock.

All this merely proves that it is almost impossible to prevent a dog, especially a puppy, from absorbing worms into its system from one source or another during its lifetime. But what is possible is the prevention of the worm eggs from breeding to an extent which will create a state of worm infestation. The presence of a few round worms in the adult dog or puppy is no cause for alarm; it is only infestation which is harmful. Worms cannot continue to survive in a clean, hard-muscled stomach and intestinal tract, and will soon be expelled. The dog owner must aim at keeping the dog internally clean, through correct natural diet and internal disinfecting with herbs. Hygienic kenneling and exercise enclosures must be maintained always, and also cleanliness of the dog's drinking and feeding dishes.

Symptoms Staring coat, emaciation, ravenous or depraved appetite, eye discharge, biting at the tail area or dragging of the hind area along the ground. A cough is sometimes present, and in tapeworm the worm segments can be seen adhering around the anus like particles of rice, or as flat white or flesh-coloured objects, moving in the expelled faeces. Round worms are also to be seen in the faeces, singly, or in balls – when there is infestation.

Treatment Give a course of worm-expelling herbs, preferably in tablet form, as N.R. Herbal Compound. This will remove worms provided that a raw foods diet is followed to cleanse and tone up the system. The in-whelp bitch should be fed such tablets or garlic throughout pregnancy. In this way nursing mothers will be kept worm-free, and if the herbal treatment be continued after whelping and throughout the feeding of the litter, giving tablets and also fresh, finely cut herbs in the diet, the puppies will receive early worm treatment daily through the mother's milk. In the case of actual worm infestation a more thorough treatment should be given. The treatment is also applicable and harmless to young puppies. Fast completely on water for one day (puppies can have a little honey added to their water). A very infested puppy over six months of age or an adult can be given two days' fast. Each evening give a strong dose of castor oil, one dessertspoonful for a puppy between four to six months, and a much increased dose for older stock or a brew of senna pods (see p. 409). The following morning give a very large dose of

N.R. Herbal Compound or garlic tablets; an average dose would be six to eight four-grain tablets, or one to two whole flaked garlic roots, well pounded and then brewed in a little water. Follow this a half-hour later by a further dose of castor oil or one of the natural aperient waters such as Chelsea or Apenta, or a tablespoonful of Epsom salts, dissolved in sufficient hot water. Give the bitter-tasting saline waters by means of a long-necked medicine bottle. Twenty minutes later give a warm meal of milk-honey, thickened with slippery elm powder or tree bark food (such an N.R. Gruel) containing slippery elm and other beneficial digestive ingredients. Keep the case on a fluid diet of that food for the entire day, the following day thickening the food with flaked barley, and then finally restoring to normal diet. If the stomach and intestines are very inflamed as a result of severe worm infestation then the slippery elm diet can be maintained for two to three days. Modified dosage of Herbal Compound tablets or garlic dosage, two or three four-grain tablets, or the flaked root should be continued for several weeks following the worming, to disinfect the bloodstream and digestive tract completely, and to expel any newly developed worm ova lying latent in the body. Other efficient and safe worm-expellent herbs are mustard seed, one dessertspoonful of seed, average dose, ground into a powder and given in a little milk, then followed by castor oil. Or a brew of walnut leaves, two tablespoonfuls of the standard brew being given night and morning for several days, followed on the final day by a strong dose of castor oil.

All of the above treatments are applicable to tapeworm. But in very persistent tapeworm cases, capsules of male fern oil should be used, sold at chemists' for human use, half the adult prescribed dose being given to an average-sized adult dog. A teaspoonful of extract of male fern given in milk is a general dosage. Or a medicine can be prepared from the fresh roots of the male fern, as follows. Take two roots, and bruise well. Scoop out the hearts of the root, and take also a little of the external fibre, to make two full ounces, then simmer slowly in one pint of water until only half a pint of the liquid remains. To this, when cold, add an infusion of senna, made by infusing four large pods of senna in four tablespoons cold water for four hours. Then give two tablespoonfuls of the fern and senna mixture on rising and retiring, in conjunction with the standard worm treatment of castor oil and fasting already described. Or Epsom salts can replace the castor oil treatment. A large morning dose of two tablespoonfuls of salts is given and the dog fasted for one day to starve the worms. The following morning give the correct number of male fern capsules and thirty minutes later repeat the salts dose.

A further effective tapeworm remedy. Prepare dog as for standard tapeworm remedy, then give big dose of finely crushed, raw pumpkin seeds: 30 minutes later, 2 tablespoons castor oil. Repeat treatment for two mornings, if necessary to remove entire tapeworm.

The recommended cure for hook-worm in dogs is a course of thymol – the oil extract from the thyme plant. Four to six drops are given twice daily on lumps of sugar. A laxative diet, using bran, grated raw carrot with the meat, should be maintained for some time. A fasting thymol treatment can also be given. The case must be fasted for two days, no fat at all being given as thymol is very fat soluble. Half an ounce of sodium sulphate is then given to clear out the bowels, twenty to thirty grains of thymol are then given in capsule form. Skimmed milk is allowed during the fast. The same thymol treatment for heartworms. Give herbal compound tablets for prevention of heartworms. As heartworm is basically mosquito-carried (although personally I do not rule out the possibility that it is also spread by direct intake of ova from infected dogs in the usual way of worm propagation), attention should be given to protection from mosquitoes. This insect does bite dogs habitually and causes irritation and restlessness at night. During the mosquito months the bare parts of the dog's body, such as inner thighs and ear flaps, should have a light dusting nightly with a mixture of finely powdered bitter herbs, along the spine, too. Use a puffer container to spread the powder. This is objectionable to the mosquitoes but, of course, does not give total protection against them. Avoid screened windows as they create the airless atmosphere which mosquitoes prefer and window screens do not prevent the entry of the pests through the door.

It would require a separate booklet to go into all the detail of heartworm prevention and cure. This worm, once rare, has increased tremendously, and orthodox treatment of giving dogs a daily dose of lethal poisons, including such remarkable things as arsenic and strychnine, only weakens the infected dog along with the worms, and the worms increase in their weakened host. This is to say nothing of the fact that such terrible poisons destroy the nervous systems of the dogs and cause mental decline.

In addition to thymol, cayenne pepper (in tablets), rosemary, and all bitter herbs (wormwood, southernwood, gentian, rue, etc.) are proved useful deterrents of heartworm. Cayenne and rosemary are known to have direct influence on the heart and arteries. Tabasco sauce is a good way of giving cayenne pepper.

In concluding this very important subject of worm treatment, it is important to emphasize that all of the treatments given are entirely harmless. I am absolutely opposed to the 'blasting-out' process of modern worming with chemicals, usually poisonous ones. No cure is thereby achieved and the worms soon return to reinfest the weakened intestines further degenerated from the treatment. In herbal medicine the main aim is the cleansing and restoration of the digestive organs, so that the worms have no toxic accumulation in which to embed themselves and multiply.

Note Use of tabasco sauce: half a teaspoon well mixed into flour and honey, divided into pills. Four morning and night for several weeks.

JAUNDICE This ailment is commonly called 'the yellows', the name being given on account of the brilliant yellow hue which dyes the entire body surface, even the gums and the eyeballs. The causes of jaundice are many in the dog, and include: congestion of the liver, frequently brought about as a sequela of distemper or by a thorough chilling: blocking of the bile duct by the passing of a gall-stone or the entrance of a round worm. Jaundice alone is readily curable, but as a double distemper complication it is a very serious condition and may have fatal results. There is also a form of jaundice said to be caused by rats, typical cases of that type have been found, however, where no rats or mice could have been responsible. Serum injections are given for the form of rat jaundice with the admission of 'kill or cure the case': they usually kill. There is also preventive inoculation which is even more deadly to young stock in its after-effects than the notorious distemper inoculations. The one unfailing preventive against jaundice is sound rearing according to the laws of Nature.

Symptoms The dog becomes heavily pigmented with a yellow colour, even the eyeballs are suffused with yellow. Food is refused, the back is frequently roached, the bowels become costive, and pale-hued faeces are passed.

411

Treatment An immediate course of internal cleansing, with use of garlic; also a brew of one of the jaundice remedial herbs such as dandelion, toadflax, blue pimpernel, speedwell, fumitory and hops. Shred two tablespoonfuls of the herb and brew in half a pint of water. Give two dessertspoonfuls of the brew very frequently, every four hours. Or the herbs can be chopped fine and given in honey balls. Use all parts of the herbs. Externally: some of the herbal brew can be applied hot on flannel, placed over the region of the liver. Or a poultice of common mustard powder can be made, and applied hot over the liver region.

Note It must be emphasized that the entire success of the jaundice treatment depends upon strict fasting long enough for the congested liver to become cleansed and the bile to be cleared from the bloodstream and body tissues. Also no fatty foods should be given for many weeks following jaundice condition. Although this ailment is generally reputed as being fatal to the dog, very many cases have been fully restored to health following the herbal treatment.

LICE, FLEAS and other SKIN VERMIN (see LICE in Horses) Treat carefully with N.R. Herbal Protection powder, after bathing with soap, or make a strong solution of that powder (see MANGE). Also I have found a bath of Cooper McDougall's Kurmange good in the destruction of skin vermin. Rubbing the body with eucalyptus oil and ammonia is also very effective. One teaspoonful of eucalyptus oil and two teaspoonfuls of ammonia mixed into a half-pint of tepid water, and the lotion well rubbed into the body area, special attention being given to the neck area, ear flaps and base, the brisket, the back, and the base of the tail. But the entire body should be treated. Bathing in the sea is helpful.

The modern flea collars, because they work on a chemical

principle and carry health-precaution warnings, I suspect are more hazardous to health than the presence of fleas on the dogs. For years I used a non-toxic bathing block, called Canex, made in Israel; a total killer of fleas. But the weight of the block made it non-commercial for selling by post and it is no longer available.

Using the same principle of foamy suffocation of fleas and a herbal oil to compel them to hair surface, I have evolved a successful flea-killer which is harmless in use to all types of animal. Make a bathing lotion as follows: take a cupful of *non-poisonous* washing-up liquid, choosing one which claims to be 'kind to the hands'. (I have found Palmolive to be reliable.) To every cup of detergent add two teaspoons of oil of eucalyptus and mix well.

Now wet the dog thoroughly, soaking the hair well. Next rub some of the lotion deeply into the hair to reach the skin. See that all parts of the animal are treated thoroughly, especially the ears, but keep out of the eyes. If it does enter, soothe at once by pouring in some fresh (not Long-life type) milk. Rinse off the lather thoroughly and apply a second time. Allow the lather to remain five minutes, rubbing in well all the time. Finally, rinse off very well and partly dry the animal with towels. Then stand it on a sheet of white paper and brush its hair thoroughly to bring out the dead fleas. Search the hair for any fleas which may have escaped the lather; they will be in a feeble state and can be killed with ease. I regret the use of a detergent, but its bitter-tasting foam is needed for such a foe as the flea!

A pungent species of mint, named pennyroyal (*Mentha pulegium*, from the Latin, *pulga*, flea) was a former widely used fleas control for dogs and cats. The herb was bruised to bring out odour and then spread beneath and around dog beds and in kennels.

413

SORE PADS Concrete roads, gravel paths, flinty hillsides often injure the pads of sheep-dogs, especially when the animal is overweight or in a low condition with weakening of feet. Attention should be given to the diet too.

Symptoms The pads of the feet are puffy and inflamed, or cracked, sometimes very deeply, accompanied by bleeding. The dog shows reluctance to take exercise; appetite is also poor.

Treatment Rest the dog from exercise at least for several days. Bathe the pads with seaweed powder. Two tea-spoonfuls of powdered seaweed mixed into a half pint of hot water, and one dessertspoonful of vinegar then added; use tepid. Witch hazel extract should be applied to the pads when they are actually bleeding. Dusting with orris root powder completes the treatment, or finely powdered oatmeal can be used. In very deep fissures, pads of cotton wool should be soaked in an equal mixture of witch hazel and ivy-leaves brew, and placed around the pads, the foot or feet then confined in bootees made of wash-leather, and firmly tied. In order to prevent the dog from pulling off the dressing, if it shows inclination to do so, the dog should be kept on a short chain for one hour until the dressing has done its work, morning and night. The boots can also be lined with mallow leaves or traveller's joy (whole sprays of this climbing plant), friend of the travellers.

Puppies

Puppies from natural reared parents are easy to raise to healthy adults. After weaning, follow N.R. puppy diet (p. 375). All pups need, in addition to whole food, an abundance of sunlight, and ample space in which to develop and exercise rapidly growing limbs.

The spring is the natural time of birth for puppies. Spring litters are healthier and more forward than winter-born ones.

For Diarrhoea, Skin Ailments and Vermin, Nervous Ailments, Fits, etc., Canine Distemper and Hard Pad, see treatments given for the adult dog, modifying the prescribed dosage by half or less according to the age of the puppy.

MILK RASH   This rash affects unweaned puppies in the nest. It is an eruptive type of skin ailment, distinguished by profuse crusty sores which cover all parts of the body but do not cause any loss of hair. Nor does the rash seem to cause the infected puppies any discomfort or irritation. There is a general belief among dog breeders that such a rash occurs when the bitch is feeding her litter very well. I do not accept that opinion, but consider the skin trouble to be due to acid milk. I have never had such an infection among any puppies of the many breeds that I have reared.

Treatment   Give the puppies tablets of leaf-extract (chlorophyll), two four-grain tablets daily. Externally: friction the bodies of the puppies with swabs of cotton wool soaked in a brew of blackberry leaves. Some wild daisy plant can be added to the blackberry brew with advantage. Witch hazel extract, used full strength, has also proved an excellent remedy.

EATING FOREIGN BODIES   Puppies will eat wire, glass, tin, rubber, and other remarkable things, often out of sheer playfulness. The best remedy is a meal of bread and milk, followed by a strong dose of castor oil. For splinters of cooked bones – highly dangerous – small balls of sphagnum moss or even common moss or lichens should be rammed down the throat; a laxative dose to follow. Cotton wool can replace sphagnum when moss is not available.

VOMITING This should always be encouraged in the dog, for it is Nature's way of causing rapid internal cleansing. Dogs – and likewise puppies – eat couch-grass especially to provoke cleansing vomiting. Fasting for at least one whole day should always follow the vomiting of solid food; a half-day's fast to follow the vomiting of yellow bile, or frothy saliva type of fluid. If severe vomiting seems to cause distress, then the stomach should be soothed by the giving of flaked gentian root, or grated burdock root, one small teaspoonful in a quarter-pint of watered milk and honey. Follow on with barley-lemon-honey gruel or N.R. Gruel.

STOMACH SWELLING Frequent swelling of the stomach of a puppy following meals, often indicates worms, and the puppy should be treated for this complaint. If no worms are expelled and the swelling continues, then the condition is generally purely one of overeating. Stonehenge rightly says that 'art founded on experience' is required to fix the amount of food to give a growing puppy. The main test should be, the eating-up of all food eagerly, no after meal stomach swelling or scouring. Puppies should still remain lively and active after each meal taken.

RICKETS This condition is 100 per cent preventible. Rickets result from unhealthy and unnatural rearing conditions, both of diet and kenneling. Cooked foods in the diet, de-natured foods, lack of fresh air, sunlight and exercise, are all preconditions for rickets. Feed raw foods, provide sun baths and exercise, and rickets will be cured. Give much vitamin C in natural form and the vitality foods such as malt flour (raw), peanut flour, raw finely grated carrots; also flaked cereals, honey, raisins, oil of sesame and corn, the oils in small amounts, not more than one teaspoon daily; three or four raw (fresh) eggs weekly, dessicated coconut.

From Alice Bondi, 141 Well Street, East Malling, Maidstone, Kent:

> I acquired the border collie bitch, Kai, from a friend who worked her in Wales. I shepherded a large sheep flock in Scotland, using Kai with much success. I now work her *grand-daughter*, Kess, who in her outstanding stamina and ability shows all the benefits of a third generation Natural Rearing.

From Bill Hall, Preston, Lancs (the canine journalist and hounds expert):

> Juliette de Baïracli Levy, whose writings on the use of herbs and natural methods for the prevention and treatment of canine diseases is well known world wide: I recall with pleasure working with Juliette at our Crufts Show trade stand, to meet followers and critics alike of her methods. Our own belief in the value of herbal practice was founded then and *resulted in over thirty-five years* of dog breeding and exhibiting entirely without the use of orthodox preventative medicine.

Faber have published a book of great interest to keepers of herd-dogs, written by Iris Coombe, an expert on this subject and author of earlier books on shepherd dogs and their shepherd owners and trainers. Her book, *Herding Dogs: Their Origins and Development in Britain*, is very readable and informative and I highly recommend it to all who keep and love herding-dogs. There are numerous illustrations from photographs and drawings of herding-dogs, many of them now very rare. This excellent book makes me nostalgic for the years I spent during the 1940s in the beautiful and wild region of the Pennines near Cumbria, working with the shepherds and their border collies.

9

Natural Care of Bees

Of all the creatures that God created, the bee found most favour in his eyes.

Old Hebrew saying

Bees respond very well to nature bee-keeping, because they themselves are instinctive and highly skilled herbalists. From studying the ways of bees, one can learn much about the health values of herbs.

In the section on Honey (Chap. 1) I write about the importance of honey as food and medicine for man and the animals which man has domesticated. The wild bear, strongest of animals, he can kill any species of animal that he meets in combat – he has his own supplies of wild honey!

One of the main values of honey is that it is a healthy substance which imparts immediate vitality. In modern times, like so much else, honey is often low in vitality, because it is saturated with white sugar – commonly fed to bees to double the honey flow, and because 25 per cent of commercial beehives are suffering from some form of illness. Typical of man's greedy exploitation.

In clear-headed truth the exploitation of bees does not pay either in time or money. Leave the bees alone to manage their own kingdoms (in which management they are perfection in every detail), and the healthy hives will produce enough surplus healthy honey to justify the small amount of care required from the bee-keeper. (Such as painting and whitewashing the hives, supplying combs, and what *should be* done – the planting of a garden of bee herbs.)

Modern bee-keeping seems to be a deliberate disorganization of every bee community (kingdom) that the bee-keeper owns. The biggest crime of the bee-keeper is the killing off of the chosen queen of the hive. The heart, the love and the inspiration of the hive then dies, and the very tragic shock brings sickness.

The reason for such killings is that the bee-keeper wants to possess docile bees which he can rob without any of the famed bee warfare. The true queen is removed and killed (the all-wonderful queen bee) and a queen of a quieter strain is put in her place. The quiet queen then produces a strain of weak fighters. But the core of a hive's power is the fighting fury which protects the kingdom from such enemies as hornets, rodents, ants – and man. Better to keep the hives strong in warfare and for the bee-keeper to wear more protective clothing against bee stings!

I am convinced that the only improvement on bee organization is the use of a queen excluder, preventing the queen from laying larvae in the upper stories (supers) which make difficulties later on, when the bee-keeper desires to take away frames of pure honey without larvae mixed in the combs.

An excuse for feeding white sugar is that this is the best medium for the giving of medicine; but do bees need medicine from man? They are such wonderful doctors in their own right. If medicine *must* be given to bees, then at least let the medium be honey, which in itself is a great all-round healing substance. The acknowledged father of all medicine, Hippocrates, used hydromel – which is honey and water, as basic medicine for treatment of all the ills of mankind. It is said that when this great Greek doctor died, he who so loved bees and exalted honey, was kept company in death by a swarm of wild bees who settled on the great one's tomb and produced honey with which miraculous cures were achieved. Hippocrates also made much use of another honey mixture, oxymel, which is vinegar and honey.

A Spanish bee-keeper, who is famed for his excellent honey, feeds vinegar to his bees regularly. He told me that his bees have a passion for vinegar – wine vinegar. After all, such vinegar is only strongly fermented grape juice; apples and other fruits also produce excellent vinegar. When he has to feed sugar to the bees in his apiary in spells of bad weather, he thins down the sugar (or honey) with vinegar instead of water. Vinegar could be used in the Syrup of Sage Honey recipe that I give below, reducing the water to one pint and then later, when the syrup has cooled, adding half a pint of wine or apple vinegar to the mixture.

Syrup of sage honey Four dessertspoonfuls honey to every one and half pints water, plus a half cup finely chopped sage (more honey can be added if preferred.) If apple cores or rose hips are available, add them too; they prevent scouring.

Make a standard brew of the sage and water, keeping well below boiling point. Keep covered throughout. Allow to stand and brew until tepid, then stir in the honey. When cool, pour into the hive feeding trough. (Do not use brown or white sugar. The former causes scour, the latter causes general health decline.) Since writing this about sugar, I have been informed that old-time bee-keepers added a pinch of salt to brown sugar when feeding it to bees. The salt prevents the brown sugar from causing scouring.

Bees appreciate a little salt, especially in hot weather. Along the sea coast it is quite usual to see bees sucking salt from rocks. A bee-keeper in England noted that bees came in numbers to a sea-rock she had put in a bee drinking place to make a platform for them. The bees were always seen on that rock a long time. She felt sure they were sucking salt from the rock and to make sure, she took the sea-rock away and replaced it with an ordinary stone. The bees showed no interest in the new stone.

I myself observed that bees like whole-wheat flour. When I put flour out into the sun to be sun-warmed before mixing it in bread-making, the bees came to the flour, trod in it and flew away with their legs heavy with the flour. They were interested only in whole-wheat flour. I specially bought a little white flour to test them! They also make use of old wall plaster.

Finally, just as the farmer grows special crops for the feeding of his livestock, so likewise should the bee-keeper plant bee plants for his bees, whether he owns a mere couple of hives or a large apiary.

Here are favoured bee herbs, beginning with a general statement that bees love greatly all aromatics. Lavender, rosemary, thyme, santolina, sage, bee-balm (*Melissa*), basil, marjoram, and many more; bitters such as southernwood, wormwood and rue; all the mints, especially peppermint; all the rose family, especially the hedge roses, and blackberry and hawthorn; lovage, sweet Cicely and angelica; most of the borage family, especially the borage called bee-bread, alkanet, viper's bugloss and anchusa; the heath, especially ling and bell heather; scabious of all kinds; thrift (sea-pink) and the carnation family, particularly clove pinks; poppy flowers, too, are a great favourite. Of the trees, lime (linden) particularly; also elder, acacia, carob and olive; all the rose family, apple, pear, cherry, almond. Bees love ivy and honeysuckle, also the bitter olive-tree flowers.

A test for pure, good and powerful honey, is that it should burn the throat of the consumer (my father taught me this).

Honey heavy in white sugar content does not have any effect on the human throat at all. My herbal honey was so strong, that people eating it declared that hot pepper had been added! but they were able to take comb straight from my hives for themselves to test!

Care of hives is important for bees' health and comfort. Annual or bi-annual limestone treatment (whitewashing) of the outsides of the hives keeps the wood weatherproof and provides warmth in winter and coolness in summer. Treating the hives with paint prevents the wood from 'breathing' and makes them over-hot in the summer. Plastic wash, now often used in place of whitewash, fails on every count where health values are concerned and should be avoided. The only value of plastic wash is that it is more adhesive to the wood. Ordinary whitewash can be made longer-lasting by the addition of such things as a handful of coarse salt to every bucket of liquid wash, plus two tablespoons of cheap cooking oil, two eggs, some milk and even the inner pulp from cactus plants. A blue dye can be added, as it is known that bees favour the colour blue. Old-fashioned clothes whitener 'dollie blue' is suitable.

I have found that bees keep far healthier in winter when left with one super, instead of removing all for the winter season and crowding all the bees into the small hive proper and almost sealing off, the only exit. Such measures are believed to keep the bees warm, but this enforced confinement is unnatural and in contrast to the roomy tree-hollow, which is a usual choice of wild bees and in which they stay during all weathers, cold and hot. Those bee-keepers who are close to Nature know that there is never any time in the botanical cycle of the year when no bee food at all is available in tree blossom and winter weeds. There is *always* honey in the countryside, and the bees like to leave their hives during lulls in winter weather, to seek honey and use their wings.

Smoke from vegetable matter – aromatic plants and good-burning tree material of various types such as pine and juniper – is a great cleanser of woodwork. All supers should be smoked yearly and empty hives also smoke-cleaned.

When possible, place the hives under the protection of deciduous trees, so that they get shade during hot, sunny months and sunlight during the winter months when leaves are shed.

Since this book was first published there has been drastic deterioration world wide in the health and honey yield of domestic bees, caused by the greed and folly of modern bee-keepers and the use by many farmers of poisonous chemical sprays. A serious crime is killing an old queen and replacing her with a young one, often of a different breed. In Israel my neighbour used 'modern' methods. His colonies were wiped out by foul-brood disease: mine, near by, kept by nature's method, remained disease-free.

Finally, I quote from a bee-keeper friend near England's Forest of Dean, Douglas B. Oliff, Woodside, Lydney, Glos, who is famed for the excellence of his honey.

I tend to leave quite a lot of honey on my hives for the winter as I do not believe in feeding sugar-syrup.

For one thing it is so time-consuming, and I don't think that healthy brood will result from anything but natural honey. Thank heavens my bees seem resistant to most bee diseases, which I attribute to the fact that I never rob them of much of their hard-earned food, and am grateful for the amount of surplus that I can safely take from them.

My bees are now having their final fling of the season, working on the ivy. I should get far more honey if I exploited them, but I can't do so. I love them for what they are, all part of the household. I spend hours just watching and listening to them on summer evenings, hearing those thousands of wings fanning the nectar into honey. The lovely scents of flowers and tree blossoms wafting from the hives.

Selling honey: most honey is ruined by the fetish of removing every speck of wax, by heating and refiltering. I don't do this; mine is filtered only once (unheated) and thus contains a bit of wax and the odd pollen lumps, but it retains the natural essential oils and essences which heating destroys. The old people of the forest always buy some of my honey to store ready to cure winter ills.

10

Conclusion

In writing a book of this kind, by the time the end is reached there have often accumulated in the author's mind many thoughts which could not well be included in the earlier chapters. Generally such thoughts might not be appropriate in the foregoing text, or they need special emphasis and therefore are best at the end of the book. Or again they have arisen directly out of the writing of the book and therefore their correct place is at its conclusion. For reasons such as these a short concluding chapter is of service both to the author and readers.

I want to say first that it has not been possible to include all animal diseases in my book: such an attempt would make the book over-lengthy, and then it could not be considered as a handbook. Furthermore, new diseases are constantly coming forward as man's rearing of the domestic animals departs more and more from the natural. I have given the commonest animal ailments of farm and stable, and have included some uncommon ones when especially good herbal treatments are known for their cure. I hope that no farmer or horse-owner, obtaining my book perhaps for the treatment of some specific disease, will be disappointed at not finding it included therein, for it is easily possible for readers to work out their own treatments with the help of the Materia Medica chapter where many herbs are given suitable for further ailments, which I have not included. All disease treatment of animals is

425

basically the same, evolved from the unchanging laws of Nature.

A short fast, using a recommended laxative and a herb for disinfection of the blood and digestive system: garlic being the specific herb given in my herbal. To complete the treatment the reader has only to consult the herbs given in chapter 2 and select the one most applicable to the disease. It is thus that I myself have evolved many of my veterinary treatments: others can do likewise and feel sure of success.

I should mention that in my work the herb garlic has stood the test of time; it has given me over forty years of success in all parts of the world where I have travelled and worked with animals. The gypsy people consider that the garlic plant possesses magical properties; they strew the graves of their dead with its white flowers. But apart from Romany mystical beliefs, the practical scientists also recognize its medicinal value. Russian doctors make much use of the herb (and even some of the chemical-minded American medical leaders give it high praise).

Also I have found rue, rosemary and sage to be especially important herbs. Honey is also valuable as an extraordinary healing agent. It is a pity that its high cost often prohibits its use in treatment of the larger animals. But in special cases I advise its use despite the expense.

Also the importance of fasting treatment has stayed uppermost in my mind throughout the writing of this herbal, and at its conclusion I am left feeling that I have not drawn sufficient attention to that supreme law of natural medical treatment. 'Fast and pray' Christ ordained to the sick, and achieved miracles: He is the greatest of the healers. Today, except for some Eastern sects and the small minority who adhere to natural medicine, only the animals obey the paramount rule of Nature in the cure of disease: the domestic animals are generally prevented by man's ignorance, but the wild ones obey. A sick animal retires into a secluded place and fasts until its body is restored to normal. During the fast it partakes only of water and the medicinal herbs which inherited intelligence teaches it instinctively to seek. I have watched them at their self-healing so often. The Greek physician, Hippocrates, titled the Father of Medicine, taught fasting in diseases as well as the use of simple medicinal herbs.

There is a reason behind Nature's law: a strong reason. In sickness the body has little use for food during the first vital stages. The powers of the body are fully occupied with the restoration to normal of the diseased tissues. The work of food digestion takes a great amount of the daily energy; such energy in diseases is best used for curative purposes. Food itself does not give immediate strength. It is the use which the body makes of food which gives strength. Indeed food consumed during high fever creates exhaustion and weakness. I myself have achieved many fasts, the longest being over twenty-one days, taking lemon juice in water and a little pure honey only. During that time I continued with my usual strenuous daily work: care of my animals, land-work, writing, and so on. People have fasted forty days. Animals trapped in old pits or in bombed buildings have been rescued alive after being one and two months without food or water, and have fully recovered from such a severe fast.

As a student I was impressed by an incident in a travel book entitled: *One thousand five hundred miles in an Open Boat*, which is a true record of the experience of a party of shipwrecked men. The ship's cook had suffered for years from a discharging hip-bone which had almost crippled him. When rescued, his hip was fully cured and remained cured. The enforced fasting from food for over one week had given his body the chance to restore to normal the diseased tissues. That is just one small example which built up my belief in the value of fasting. I could write a long book on the subject, but I

427

am a herbalist, not a writer. Fasting is difficult for the human race, constantly assailed by appetite-provoking foods even during illness. Such was appreciated by Christ – 'Fast and pray'. It is simple for the animals. However, before ending the subject, I must state that I am not a believer in long fasts for the herbivorous animals with their capacious internal digestive system. Too much stomach and intestinal gas is generated, especially when they have for a long time been getting a diet of unnatural concentrates. When high fever is present, then certainly the witholding of food is a natural essential of successful treatment. Otherwise only a short fast of two or three days is recommended, and then semi-fasting maintained by means of a body-cleansing laxative diet: all fully dealt with in my chapters on animal diseases. The carnivorous dog can fast without discomfort for a week or more, provided it is not allowed to see or get the scent of food. And, indeed, wild dogs often endure weeks without food when prey is scarce and show no discomfort nor weakness at such times.

Nor is my attitude to orthodox medicine one of hostility, as readers of my herbal books sometimes think. My writings are mild in comparison to those of the famed Nicholas Culpeper when attacking human non-herbal medicine! I think that modern veterinary diagnosis and surgery is magnificent, and I owe much to it myself. I am only opposed to the Pasteur-inspired Germ Theory of Disease, on which modern veterinary medicine is based, with its attendant usage of chemical and inoculative therapy, and its acceptance of the amoral practice of animal vivisection. Louis Pasteur, who himself had inferior health and lost many members of his own family from disease, gave to the world his Germ Theory of Disease only so short a time ago as 1886, which theory ever since has been strongly backed by the vested interests of the big drug manufacturing companies with all of their enormous powers of finance, and the advertising and press space which finance can buy. Of Pasteur's germ theory, Mr J. E. R. McDonagh, FRCS, wrote in his prophetic book, *The Nature of Disease*: 'The theory has put back the clock of progress many years, and has led to abysses into which medicine has fallen and from which it will be difficult to extricate it.'

I was therefore pleased to read in the *Daily Telegraph* as long ago as December 1951, that in the ultramodern country of the United States of America, many of America's leading schools have banned all questions about the germ theory of disease from biology examinations. A law concerning this has been passed by the State Board of Regents: yet a further example, that doubt as to the true value of the Pasteur teachings, is growing in the minds of thinking men and women everywhere. Many doctors and veterinary surgeons are among the dissenters from the germ theory of disease. In theory the teachings are impressive; in practice they are killing to man and the animals under his care.

I am pleased that in my time I have witnessed the banning of DDT, the pioneer and the foremost of the dangerous chemical insecticides. World wide, leading agricultural countries have forbidden the use of DDT and all its derivatives. This terrible modern idea of killing weeds by herbicides is also now being condemned. In a book with the apt title *Chemical Scythe*, by an agricultural expert, the subject is examined. Diocine, a principal ingredient of most herbicides, is proved as a cancer danger.

I am further pleased that I began my veterinary herbal education and work in England. I have much admiration for English farming and livestock. My work with the sheep farmers of Swaledale remains unforgettable. And what a glorious achievement are the many species of English pedigree livestock, respected the world over. Consider too the speed of the English and Irish thoroughbred racehorse. I only regret the present-day scientification of farming and animal husbandry is destroying the great work of the past generations, who farmed and raised animals with such forethought and care. The modern chemical madness is fraught with dangers for the earth and all animals. Herbal medicine wants to play its part in stemming the development of all that is opposed to the age-old wisdom of Nature. I appreciate that in general the modern farmers of the world cannot afford to be idealists, for they are practical men rearing cattle and sheep for food. The attainment of the perfect health in animals which I stress throughout this book, is of only secondary importance for them. Food production and financial reward come first for the survival of their farms in the face of modern competitive methods and prices, and they have to remember that the present-day world respects quantity above quality. *But* the prevalent outbreaks of foot-and-mouth disease, fowl pest, and other animal plagues, with the great financial losses inflicted upon the farmer, must give the agricultural world reason for serious and intelligent thought. It pays to keep animals healthy. Natural diet and herbal treatments, which are never destructive to the body tissues, are the simplest method of keeping disease from all livestock and curing those which are diseased, as so many farmers have proved or are proving now, and in many countries today, especially in America, there are vets using herbs very successfully in their work.

Since the first edition of this book was published, over thirty years ago, herbal medicine has changed from being classified as 'eccentric' to being regarded as 'useful'. As yet this applies more to human herbal medicine than to veterinary; however, in such orthodox radio programmes as *Farmer's Weekly* one now often hears praise of herbs and recommendation of the organic method of farming.

I was agreeably surprised and pleased when the oldest

established and most austere canine group and rulers in the world, the Kennel Club of Britain, asked me to write for them and article on natural rearing and the use of herbs. I accepted, and my article was published in the November 1982 issue of the *Kennel Gazette*, the journal of the Kennel Club.

Then a group of German veterinary students in Frankfurt wrote to tell me that they were determined to utilize all branches of healing in their veterinary work, including herbs, and asked me for help. A Canadian vet also requested my help, as, having proved the value of herbs in disease prevention, he was being criticized by certain drug companies.

That is the great danger to herbal medicine today: the drug companies, fearing the challenge of herbs to their former almost total power over medicine, they are turning to herbs themselves, but in a destructive, not a constructive, way. One example is comfrey. Comfrey is one of the greatest of all the medicinal herbs. It is certainly a great favourite of mine and one which I use extensively.

A scientist working with rats claimed not long ago that comfrey was cancer-causing and that neither it not borage, a herb of the same Boraginaceae family, should be used further. His claim was given much publicity in the daily papers. The official advice was that neither herb should be prescribed for man or animal. (Further tests were undertaken – and, of course, unnatural ones on laboratory animals – to provide yet more evidence of the harmfulness of these two herbs.)

This is absurd. The foothills of North Africa and of the Spanish Pyrenees are literally covered with borage of several varieties, as I have seen on my travels there. The herds have grazed these foothills for centuries, yet the official advice is: do not use borage! I prefer the evidence of healthy herds that have flourished on those herbs to that of a thousand 'successful' laboratory tests.

431

Winter heliotrope is another member of the borage family, and that one is a baneful herb and should be avoided, but one cannot condemn a whole plant family because one of its members is poisonous. (Take the Solanaceae family, to which the potato belongs: the deadly nightshade, a known poisoner, is also a member.)

The other danger to herbs caused by modern interest in them is the desire to commercialize them so as to make large financial profits. Thus herbs are analysed and their active principle extracted (or produced synthetically – cheaper), and the now unbalanced herb gets a bad name. Foxglove leaves are mild and beneficial, but the digitalin extracted from them can prove dangerous. The same applies to the bark of the cinchona tree, from which quinine is derived. The former is safe; the extract can be dangerous. The poppy is a wonderful healing plant, but extracted heroin can be lethal.

Herbs need protection from the scientists. Let them keep to their chemical drugs for the making of fortunes in medicine. Herbs are not for large-scale commercialization.

There is an international farming commune at Massafra, Taranto, Italy, whose members call themselves the Gandhi Commune, and I like the way they describe their farming policy: 'We have taken ourselves away from the *frenzy* of modern farming, and cultivate our land in the old, careful ways, and likewise we care for our animals.' These people are making an Italian translation of my *Herbal Handbook for Farm and Stable* because, as they state: 'Your farm herbal could be really useful in Italy, in a cheap edition so that every farmer could read it.' In their letter they tell me further of good cures of various farm animals' ailments achieved by following my book.

Ann Petty, the pioneer Natural Rearing farmer, formerly of Quebec, Canada, whose impressive goats' testimonial I have already quoted (p. 241), wrote me, on the eve of publication of this book, another equally impressive letter:

> I am writing to tell you of a great breakthrough in herbal medicine, here in Quebec, involving a Canadian vet. I have long thought it impossible to teach herbal lore here and that all my words were falling on unheeding ears. But, lo and behold! Last Sunday a small miracle happened. A French graduate, whom I've known for eight years, Jacques Laberge, has opened at his own expense a small laboratory to make garlic powder, plus sage and thyme, plus vitamin A (his own formula) to market as a hog growth formula and herbal inoculant, and he is selling this in competition with the drug companies specifically.
>
> His former employer was a vet who, soon after graduating and working with pigs for two years, realized that he had to face squarely the issue of massive disease in the hog industry, resistant bacteria, huge mortality up to sixty per cent, etc.
>
> A year ago he came here in despair to talk with me, knowing my healthy goats. He declared, 'You were right. Now what do I do?' So I gave him everything I had, specifically your books, and my natural vitamin research.
>
> Now, after a year, this vet is back and with the marvellous news that he has had proper controlled tests on pigs who have had natural treatment, tests assessing growth gain, resistance to disease, quality of carcass, etc. *But* the problem is that orthodoxy is out to destroy him, so we want to know of people, preferably vets, whom he could contact for moral support.

I have thankfully witnessed the well-merited overthrow of DDT and its derivatives, as I have already mentioned, but I am also witnessing events which are very worrisome and ominous for the future of world herbal medicine. Discredited orthodox medicine is now taking an interest in herbal remedies, not from any wish to use them instead of their synthetic chemical pharmaceuticals (on which they make huge profits only comparable to the manufacturers of armaments), but in order to subject herbs to unnatural intensive tests in order to teach that they are dangerous! Medical scientists now have many of the most ancient and most trustworthy of the herbs on their condemned list, among them some of my most used and favourite herbs such as sage, wormwood, comfrey, borage. In time I expect that half the herbs in my Materia Medica chapter will have been blacklisted. And yet all my listed herbs have been well proved by medical scientists to be beneficial over the past forty years.

Mostly they now declare that the herbs are tumour-provoking. And on what have those scientists based their findings? Simply on unnatural and hasty experiments mostly on laboratory rats. Herbs have been with man since the creation of the world and are God's promise for medicine for man and animal. Their merits have been assessed during thousands of years of constant use. What can experiments on rats (disease-prone creatures anyway), experiments usually of a year's duration or less, prove? Rats are very tumour-prone and if force-fed anything in unusually large amounts, herbs included, they will very likely develop tumours. Also remember that all laboratory animals are in a condition of inferior health because they are deprived of a normal life: they suffer the mental stress of the caged, they lack sufficient exercise and their diet is unnatural, usually the totally denatured foods which most modern animals get from tins and packets; air is foul with an almost total absence of sunlight and moonlight.

Why should distorted findings be given official recognition whereas the age-long, careful and natural findings of herbalists are dismissed as 'unproved'. Unproved by what?

Because herbalists have not involved their medicines in cruel tests on imprisoned laboratory animals?

I have always refused any association of my work with laboratory tests on animals. Indeed, my total dislike of such testing and my deep pity for the millions (and sadly it *is* millions) of animals imprisoned in medical research places, have been among the principal reasons behind my veterinary herbal work. Very often have I planned to end such work – so time consuming, so isolating – but for the thought always with me of the helpless, frightened, hopeless animals under experiment, all of them crying out to someone to save them. *That* has kept me at my work, work to prove the benefits from the use of herbs, of a pure medicine, free from laboratory tests, and which has made its own tests through the centuries.

Now 'authority' has gained power over the herbalists. For example, I, as a long-time herbalist, can no longer improve my veterinary herbal formulae as I learn of more herbs on my travels. All formulae in Great Britain have to be registered with Food and Drugs Control. That is fair enough, but what is not fair is the ruling that no alterations to any of the registered formulae can be made *without* scientific tests on animals, tests of several years' duration, even though the herbs chosen may be in daily use. And, as I refuse such tests, my formulae cannot be improved. They are good enough as they are, but they could be far better – if I were 'allowed' to make them better!

In time, 'authority' may ban this book, my *Herbal Handbook for Farm and Stable*, because I would never delete from its pages the various herbs now on the ill-proved list of undesirable herbs.

In 1955, my *Canine Herbal* was almost banned because I would not mention within that book some herbal products which I had proved unreliable. The case against my book went to the High Court in London to be tried by the famed Mr. Justice Dankwaerts. The would-be banners of my book had a leading barrister to fight their case. I defended myself. I took along with me to the court a bunch of favourite herbs to give me inspiration. My book was not banned! But the future may not prove so fortunate.

I cannot complete this book without mention of modern 'factory' farming, although I cannot give much space to this in the interests of brevity and others have already written many leaflets, articles and books concerning and against this atrocious system.

The prophet/writer, Shelley, over a century ago declared that man's dominance over the unfortunate animals which he had domesticated was one of disease and pain; I can now add to disease and pain, *horror*. When I wrote the first edition of this farm and stable herbal more than thirty years ago, intensive farming was little known and it was certainly unknown to me, apart from the battery system of poultry keeping. I have kept hens as pets and companions, as one would dogs, and the hen is intelligent, a loving mother to her chicks and affectionate to her owners. But I have seen them confined in cages in which they could move only a few inches and that with difficulty. For added cruelty (and man's greed for money) those hens were subjected to unnatural hours of electric light to prevent them from sleeping at dusk in the manner of poultry, thus keeping them laying for longer hours. Their food was lifeless and totally without the green leafy stuff and the insects needed for normal health.

Factory farming of the larger animals – cattle, sheep, pigs and goats – is an abomination, not only for the cruelty inflicted on God's animals throughout their brief years on earth (made brief by man's commercial arranging), but also because it is a fraud upon the humans who buy eggs, milk and meat so produced. How can such fare be healthy eating? Not possible, because the animals from which it is obtained are living sorrowful, unnatural lives and deprived of all natural food, also proper exercise. Animals by nature are chaste and loving; yet widely they are subjected to artificial insemination, and often deprived of contact with their offspring.

This type of farming is a shameful, secretive thing, conducted behind closed doors and with a computer in control. Those who engage in it claim the animals do not suffer the hardships of inclement weather. But animals like such weather! Winds and storms and snow make them hardy and the weather is of daily interest to them. They enjoy and need to bathe in sunlight and moonlight and be cleansed by rain. The guilty ones declare also that their prisoners, poor concentration-camp animals, fatten well. Of course they fatten; fed on unnatural concentrates and deprived of all exercise. But fatness is *dis*-ease, not health; wild animals are always supple and lean.

Finally I want to state that in the writing of this herbal book I have had to curtail expression of my great admiration for the gypsy people. The farmer and the gypsy are rarely friends. A pity, because the Romanies with their quick hands and brains and strong bodies are tireless field-workers. The farmer misunderstands the gypsy and sees him only as a vagabond and thief. Horse owners see him as a great trickster. I, in my years spent with them, have found them people of great honesty, philosophers and skilled herbalists, and the most loyal of friends. I owe them much. But in view of the universal hostility to this strange and wonderful race of people, I will end my praise of them on those few words. Further praise is in several of my books about the gypsies, published by Faber and Faber.

I offer this herbal book to farmers and horse owners with the promise that it has been written from my long experience with animals and out of my love for them and for their good.

CONCLUSION

Since childhood, animals have been the central interest of my life, and I have raised many, and of all kinds. A large percentage of them distinguished themselves in health tests, in the show-ring and racing. I know that animals will always be dominant in my life, especially the wild ones, living examples of Nature's skill in the preservation of the rhythm of excellent health.

11

The Herbs in this Book

This appendix is for those who wish to gather their own herbs. Because most of the plants advised in the treatments are so common, no botanical descriptions are given, only the popular and botanical names, enabling readers to look them up in any book on wild flowers, where full descriptions will be given; botanical names are international and are the same in all countries and in all books of wild flowers, only popular names differ. As alternatives are given for many of the herbs in the treatments, those who cannot get one plant will usually be able to find another. My herbal for human use, *The Illustrated Herbal Handbook*, has nearly one hundred skilled drawings of essential medicinal herbs by a great botanical artist, Heather Wood.

Here are three lists: the first are all common weeds, trees, or shrubs growing wild; the second consists of garden plants and herbs; and the third, a few herbs that must mostly be purchased from herbal shops. Nothing is said about the part to be used as that is given in the treatments throughout the book. Many health foods stores in England and the United States and elsewhere stock supplies of dried, plain herbs, suitable for veterinary use.

439

COMMON WILD PLANTS

BILBERRY, WHORTLEBERRY (*Vaccinium myrtillus*. Vacciniaceae) Found on boggy heaths and on mountainsides. Its edible berries are well known.

BLACKBERRY, BRAMBLE (*Rubus fructicosus*. Rosaceae) A common thorny hedgerow and wasteland herb, known for its juicy and edible fruits.

BORAGE (*Borago officinalis*. Boraginaceae) Field and woodland, distinguished by rough leaves, intense blue flowers.

BROOM (*Cytisus scoparius*. Leguminosae) Found on dry heaths and sandy soils. Possesses yellow, pea-form flowers.

CATMINT, CATNIP (*Nepeta cataria*. Labiatae) Found in gardens, and wild in hedges and woodlands. Foliage greyish and pungent scented. Flowers pale blue, hooded, also strong scented with a mintlike odour.

CHAMOMILE (*Anthemis nobilis*. Compositae) Waste places and damp places. Fragrant, small, daisy-like flowers; very scented, feathery leaves.

CHICKWEED (*Stellaria media*. Caryophyllaceae) A tiny pasture herb with white, starry flowers.

CLOVER (Red) (*Trifolium pratense*. Leguminosae) A plant of pastures, with trefoil leaves and globes of red flowers.

COMFREY (*Symphytum officinale*. Boraginaceae) Inhabits ditchsides, though will also grow in dry places. Now often cultivated as a fodder crop especially in Russia. Large, rough leaves; pinkish or creamy bell-like flowers.

DANDELION (*Taraxacum officinale*. Compositae) Common weed found on waste ground, on banks, and in gardens.

DOCK (*Rumex sanguineus*. Polygonaceae) Common broad-leaf weed, spikes of loose, rusty-coloured, reedlike flowers.

ELDER, ELDERBERRY (*Sambucus nigra*. Caprifoliaceae) A small tree or shrub, with rich-scented, flat heads of creamy flowers, producing edible black berries.

ELDER, DWARF or GROUND (*Sambucus ebulus*. Caprifoliaceae) Grows in waste places, is also a persistent garden weed. Resembles small elder, but leaves darker, flowers scentless.

GOOSE-GRASS, CLEAVERS (*Galium aparine*. Rubiaceae) A trailing weed with round fruits and square stems, both of clinging nature.

GREATER CELANDINE (*Chelidonium majus*. Papaveraceae) Found by old walls and on rubble, also outskirts of woods. Grey leaves and small, frail, yellow flowers which shed their petals very easily.

HOLLY (*Ilex aquifolium*. Aquifoliaceae) A well-known red-berried bush or tree with prickly leaves.

HOREHOUND (*Marrubium vulgare*. Labiatae) Common in woodland and in hedgerows. Greyish, slightly woolly leaves; spikes of colourless flowers.

IVY (*Hedera helix*. Araliaceae) A well-known evergreen climbing plant with colourless, sweet-scented blossoms. Found on trees, banks, old walls, etc.

MALE FERN (*Aspidium filix-mas*. Filices) Likes woods and shady banks. Distinguished by its tall fern foliage which have numerous scales on their under surface of leaves, and bean spores.

MARSH-MALLOW (*Althea officinalis*. Malvaceae) Of way-sides, pink flowers, very round, dark foliage.

MEADOWSWEET (*Filipendula ulmaria*. Rosaceae) Grows in wet meadows. Has rose-form leaves, plumes of creamy, sweet-scented flowers.

NETTLE, STINGING NETTLE (*Urtica dioicia*. Urticaceae) A tall perennial, known by its leaves which sting sharply.

OAK (*Quercus robus*. Loganiaceae) A tree of woodlands. Has notable oval fruits in green cups, called acorns.

PLANTAIN (*Plantago major*. Plantaginaceae) Of pastureland and waste places. Distinguished by its flat-growing, oval-shaped and ribbed leaves, and unusual flowering spike, resembling a small bulrush, of greenish-brown hue.

RASPBERRY (*Rubus idaeus*. Rosaceae) A bramble-like woodland shrub, known for its juicy red berries.

THYME (*Thymus serpyllum*. Labiatae) Of moorland and sunny banks. Tiny leaves, the tufts of white-pink flowers of very sweet and aromatic scent.

TOAD-FLAX (*Linaria vulgaris*. Scrophulariaceae)   Of pastures and waste places, distinguished by its yellow and cream 'snapdragon' shaped flowers.

VIOLET (Sweet) (*Viola odorata*. Violaceae)   Of shady banks and woodlands. Well known by its fragrant purple flowers. The garden species is also used.

WATERCRESS (*Nasturtium officinale*. Cruciferae)   Well-known wild salad plant, growing in running streams, especially spring-water streams. If shop-bought, take care that it does not come from still, copper-sulphate water.

WILD ROSE, SWEET BRIAR (*Rosa* species. Rosaceae)   A well-known shrub of hedgerow and woodland. Distinguished by its sweet-scented pink flowers and hard, red, shiny, edible fruits – 'hips'.

WOOD SAGE (*Teucrium scorodonia*. Labiatae)   Of shady places and woodlands. Rough, dark leaves, spiky, greenish-yellow, hooded flowers.

YARROW (*Achillea millefolium*. Compositae)   A weed of lawns and pastures. Feathery leaves, flat heads of composite, tiny rose or cream-coloured flowers.

GARDEN PLANTS AND HERBS

ASPARAGUS (*Asparagus officinalis*. Liliaceae)   Known for its edible shoots. Also found wild.

BALM (*Melissa officinalis*. Labiatae)   Hairy leaves, whorls of creamy, hooded flowers: much sought by bees.

CRESS, GARDEN CRESS (*Lepidium sativum*. Cruciferae) The common salad herb with 'hot' leaves.

GARLIC (*Allium* species. Liliaceae) Easily grown in gardens or bought from greengrocers. The wild variety grows in damp woodland and pastures.

HOLLYHOCK (*Althea rosea*. Malvaceae) Well known for its tallness and large flowers of various colours with squarish petals.

HYSSOP (*Hyssopus officinalis*. Labiatae) An attractive, very aromatic border plant. Much celebrated in the Bible.

LAVENDER (*Lavandula vera*. Labiatae) Well known, very fragrant when dry or fresh, has small greyish leaves and spikes of blue flowers.

LILY OF THE VALLEY (*Convallaria majalis*. Liliaceae) Well known for its sweet-scented, white flowers; much planted in gardens.

MARIGOLD (*Calendula officinalis*. Compositae) The well-known hardy annual of bright, orange-hued, daisy form or double daisy flowers.

MARJORAM (*Origanum vulgare* or *onites*. Labiatae) Very aromatic, of mountain origin, and resembles a tall, wild thyme.

MINT (*Mentha viridis*. Labiatae) The common garden salad plant with mint scent.

MUSTARD (Black) (*Brassica nigra*. Cruciferae) A common garden weed, with bright yellow flowers and strong-tasting cress-like leaves.

PARSLEY (*Petroselinum crispum*. Umbelliferae)   Common garden salad herb, with flat or tightly curled leaves of intense green.

PEONY (*Paeonia officinalis*. Ranunculaceae)   It has distinct solitary red or pink, large, many petalled flowers, and large, fringed leaves.

POPPY (OPIUM) and WILD, RED (*Papaver somniferum* and *Papaver rhoeas*. Papaveraceae)   The former is a tall plant with grey-blue foliage and big, white-cream flowers; the latter, small, hairy stemmed, with small, brilliant red flowers.

RASPBERRY (see Wild Herbs, p. 442)

ROSEMARY (*Rosmarinus officinalis*. Labiatae)   A very aromatic plant of grey-green foliage and small, hooded light blue flowers.

RUE (*Ruta graveolens*. Rutaceae)   Distinguished by its much-divided flat, greyish leaves, and small yellow flowers of bitter scent.

SAGE (*Salvia officinalis*. Labiatae)   Popular garden culinary herb, also grows in abundance wild, on hills and plains. Grey, strongly scented foliage; spikes of blue flowers.

HERBS TO BE PURCHASED FROM SELLERS

Most of the herbs in this short list will have to be obtained from herbalists. Those readers who live in countries where they are native can, however, collect them for themselves from the countryside if regulations permit.

ELM (SLIPPERY) or RED ELM (*Ulmus rubra*. Ulmaceae) The pink-hued, very aromatic bark is famous for its medicinal properties.

EUCALYPTUS (*Eucalyptus globulus*. Myrtaceae) The extracted oil most used in veterinary medicine, has to be purchased. Leaves and bark can be gathered from the tree.

FENUGREEK (SEED) (*Trigonella foenum-graecum*. Leguminosae) The seed, except in Egypt and Tunisia, has to be purchased.

LIQUORICE (*Glycyrrhiza glabra*. Leguminosae) The root can be bought from herbalists or the black solid juice, usually called Spanish liquorice and sold in sticks.

QUASSIA CHIPS A very bitter wood from a shrub. Purchased finely flaked, and used as an insecticide, especially for lice. Can be ordered from herbal suppliers.

SENNA (*Cassia acutifolia*. Leguminosae) The foliage and flat seed-pods are sold by most herbalists and drug stores. The flat seeds are the part used mostly as a powerful laxative.

SKULLCAP (*Scutellaria galericulata*. Labiatae) The plant grows wild in Europe and North America, but is not widely distributed. In some parts it is rare. The dried herb is procurable from most herbalists.

WITCH HAZEL (*Hamamelis virginiana*. Hamamelidaceae) The bark is sold by herbalists, also its extract in alcohol. Most drug stores sell this famed astringent and antiseptic extract.

NATURAL REARING PRODUCTS (N.R.) As many farmers have not the time to gather and prepare their own herbs, and to satisfy wide demand, I have had a small range of proprietary herbal products made to my formulae. These products have been selling world wide for over fifty years. That they have existed so long and are still in big demand and have gained testimonials from the famous in agriculture and the canine world, shows that they were needed and that the formulae are good.

N.R. Herbal Compound Tablets A concentration of five highly antiseptic herbs, including wild garlic, the basic ingredient, eucalyptus, rue, sage, etc., in very careful proportions. In my opinion an improvement on plain garlic, as the companion herbs contribute new and powerful antiseptic and healing powers not possessed by garlic. They are certainly a more powerful vermifuge than plain garlic as many tests have shown for medicinal use and for herbal inoculation.

N.R. Herbal Gruel A blend of nutritious and healing tree barks, cereals, roots and herbs. A proved excellent weaning food for all young animals from poultry chicks to camel colts. Has saved the lives of many motherless animals. Also a powerful internal healer and invaluable in cases of dysentery and scour. Includes slippery elm bark (the basic ingredient), arrowroot, dill, barley flour, marsh-mallow, etc.

N.R. Seaweed Minerals Food The minerals-rich properties of seaweed are increased with the addition of the most chlorophyll and iron-rich nettle and comfrey herbs. An important food for giving powerful bone, good teeth and body hair, good dark pigment, and for fertility and milk and egg production.

N.R. All Herbal Insecticide Powder Five powerful insect repellent and aromatic herbs in powder form. Closely allied to the Herbal Compound tablets in formula. Will help free the body hair of parasitical vermin. When made into a liquid lotion is a

447

proved remedy for mange and ear canker, and for sores, wounds, etc.

A booklet giving details and prices of veterinary herbal products, many of them my formulae, is obtainable from Larkhall Natural Health plc, Forest Road, Charlbury, Oxford OX7 3HH. (They are not licensed for America.) Larkhall are long established in alternative medicine. They do *not* use animals in experiments. As herbs are long-time proved safe remedies, there is no need for herbal experiments and the cruel laboratory imprisonment of animals.

SOME HERB SUPPLIERS

Long established and with extensive supplies of herbs for mixing at home and on the farm:

ENGLAND Potters Herbal Supplies Ltd, Douglas Works, Leyland Mill Lane, Wigan, Lancashire, WN1 2SB; Fiddes Payne, The Spice Warehouse, Pepper Alley, Banbury, Oxfordshire

CANADA Wide World of Herbs Ltd, 11 St Catherine Street East, Montreal, Quebec H2X 1K3

UNITED STATES OF AMERICA Indiana Botanic Gardens, P.O. Box 5, Hammond IN 46325; Nature's Herb Company, 281 Ellis Street, San Francisco, CA 94102; Penn Herb Company, 602 North Second Street, Philadelphia, PA 19123

Postscript

I sincerely regret that it is no longer possible to answer readers' veterinary problems sent to me in the post. Because I travel so much, months often go by without mail reaching me and very many letters are lost as a result of my being out of reach of mail.

I have again, for this new edition of the *Complete Herbal Handbook for Farm and Stable*, studied carefully all the treatments given to make sure that all can be followed with ease and without needing any help from myself.

Of course there will be many ailments not dealt with in this book, which gives only the more general ones. To include all known ailments would make my book such a lengthy one that it would no more be a useful handbook, but would become a heavy tome too highly priced for most smallholders and farmers to care to buy and use.

Furthermore, this book is in many foreign translations, in addition to the British and American editions, and if all those countless thousands who now have a copy of it were to write to me for personal advice, my every day and most of every night would be fully taken in writing letters. Impossible! Nor can I, in fairness, answer a few chosen persons and not answer all. Unjust. Again impossible!

I have had a deep love for animals from early childhood to my present age, which has now reached the official one of retirement from work. I know that I can best serve animals by practical study of their needs in the field, during my continuing travels, and not monotonously, and *unwillingly*, confined to a room with a typewriter. Therefore, please do not write to me. I thank you for reading this book, all the thousands of you – 40,000 in America, for happy example – and I know that it will help your animals, as it has helped mine.

As I reach the end of another edition of my *Herbal Handbook for Farm and Stable* (the sixth edition), new things have been learnt and need to be included.

For instance, addresses of people mentioned have changed and some have given up their animals.

One of the best farmers lost to Natural Rearing is Ann Petty of Canada. She wanted to be free of the pain of sending her animals, cattle and goats, to be slaughtered when their numbers became too many for her to keep.

There are in this postcript bad things to report about land and animals, but there are also very good.

It is better to end with the good.

On the bad side are the words of a boastful chemist, heard over the radio from an international gathering of chemists. He was claiming to speak on their behalf and declared that chemists had saved the world, especially from starvation: 'We chemists have saved the world. We have made available in large quantities, chemical medicines, fertilizers, insecticides, herbicides'.

My opinion is totally contrary to that of the boastful chemist, and modern protectors of the environment likewise have no use for chemical spraying of the world. Remember the lesson learnt from the Union Carbide disaster in India, where thousands of humans and animals were killed or maimed for life by an explosion of chemicals for agriculture into their environment. But yet that lesson is not learnt. The poison-sprayers are at work even on this small and primitive island where I write this postscript: birds, wild animals, bees, butterflies, are all killed indiscriminately, and our underground water supplies are permanently polluted as is the near-by sea.

Take, for example, insecticides: insects are the natural, and main, food for birds and a bird will eat almost its body weight of insects daily. Poison that bird by use of chemical insecticides and herbicides and insects will increase. Indeed, it is now widely accepted that most insects speedily develop immunity to chemical sprays, whereas insects cannot be immune from the quick, trusting beaks of birds. So much for insecticides!

As for the herbicides of the chemist, they are yet worse as they are utilized over vast areas, especially when sprayed by planes or helicopters. Herbicides likewise kill the creatures of the world, winged and four-footed and those of the sea, into which poisonous chemicals are washed by rains.

The chemists teach people to destroy these so-called weeds, which encourages lazy farming. Before the days of chemists, farmers and gardeners ploughed and hoed into their land these weeds, valuing them as a natural fertilizer.

Nowadays, ploughing and hoeing of weeds has ceased in the main, poison sprays are in wide use, so the world's wells, streams, rivers and oceans are being poisoned. *The Silent Spring* of Rachel Carson's famous book is speedily approaching, when no birds sing.

In such a chemicals-dominated environment the health of all creatures, including human, is declining. Further harm is being done by the foods fed to farm animals. Chemicals make the preservation of all sorts of unclean substances possible to be turned into cheap foods. As a result, vegetarian cattle are getting part of their diet in the form of offal from slaughterhouses, with devastating results (see p. viii).

Almost gone are those days so well described in Thomas

451

Hardy's beautiful novel, *Tess of the D'Urbervilles*, when the great herds moved udder-deep through vast green pastures, waded in clean rivers, and rested under great trees. What excellence of creamy milk and butter were produced in those days! God, in his great love for all his creatures, strictly commanded Noah to provide the special foods which every animal in the Ark needed. Was dried blood, or was fish-meal ever the chosen food of the cow?

In consequence of unnatural, chemically-processed foods, the health of farmstock world wide, including England, is declining. In England, dangerous diseases are causing other countries to ban eggs and meat exported from British farms. Once the farms of England and their produce were the envy of the world.

That is some of the bad that has come along since the fifth edition of this book was published.

Now for the good! World wide there is now a reaching out to 'The Green'. Green stands for sane and safe organic farming, which means natural farming, such as the methods described in this book. Everywhere there are ever-increasing numbers of people determined to save the world from the poisoners. Their results in the improved health of the land and the animals (and people, of course) are impressive.

Long ago, and really continuing into today, the green was worshipped. There is 'El Hadr' of the Arabs 'the Green One', he who protects the animals, leading back to safety the lost ones, and comforting those bereaved by slaughter. He is also the rainbringer and patron of the nomads.

In Greece, there is St Menas, likewise 'the Green One' and protector of the herds, also of olive groves. His herbs are those known to us herbalists as being especially beneficial in medicine – southernwood, lavender, rosemary.

The special time of both these 'Green Ones' is mid November, which also happens to be the time of my birthday!

I need to add as my final lines for this edition that I have not included any of the 'new' ailments now found in farm-stock. Because they are caused by unnatural rearing, natural remedies are not likely to be successful.

Indexes

General Index

Herbal Treatments

Materia Medica Botanica

Achillea millefolium, 168–9, 443
Acorus calamus, 151–2
adder's tongue, 26
Adiantum capillus veneris, 102–3
Aesculus hippocastanum,, 48–9
Agrimonia eupatoria, 27–8
agrimony, 27–8
Agropyron repens, 57–8
Ajuga chamaepitys, 80–81
Alchemilla vulgaris, 95
alder, 28
alfalfa, 28
Allium ampeloprasum, 116–17
Allium schoenoprasum, 51
Allium species, 76–8, 444
almond, 28–9
Alnus glutinosa, 28
Aloe communis, 29–30
aloes, 29–30
Althea officinalis, 103–4, 442
Althea rosea, 86, 444
Anagallis arvensis, 122
anemone, 30
Anemone nemorosa, 30
Anethum graveolens, 62–3
angelica, 30–31
Angelica archangelica, 30–31
anise, 31
Anthemis nobilis, 47, 440
Anthriscus cerefolium, 48
apple, crab, 58–9

Arachis hypogea, 119
Arctium lappa, 43–4
Aristolochia clematitis, 38
Armoracia rusticana, 88–9
arnica, 31–2
Arnica montana, 31–2
Artemesia species, 146–7
Artemesia absinthium, 167–8
artichoke, 32
Arundo domax, 132
Arundo phragmites, 132
ash, 32–3
asparagus, 33, 443
Asparagus officinalis, 33, 443
Aspidium filix mas., 72–3, 442
Avena sativa, 115–16
avens, 34

balm, 34, 443
barley, 35
bed-straw, 35–6
beech, 36
Bellis perennis, 61–2
Betonica officinalis, 165
Betula pendula, 37–8
bilberry, 36–7, 440
bindweed, 37
birch, 37–8
bird cherry, 48
birthwort, 38
biting stonecrop, 149–50

465

467